teaching
health in
elementary schools

teaching
health in
elementary schools

MARYHELEN VANNIER, Ed.D.

Professor and Director, Women's Division
Department of Health and Physical Education,
Southern Methodist University,
Dallas, Texas

SECOND EDITION

Lea & Febiger 1974　　Philadelphia

Health Education,
Physical Education, and
Recreation Series

Ruth Abernathy, Ph.D., Editorial Adviser,
Professor Emeritus, School of Physical and Health Education,
University of Washington, Seattle, Washington 98105

Library of Congress Cataloging in Publication Data

Vannier, Maryhelen, 1915–
   Teaching health in elementary schools.
   (Health education, physical education, and recreation series)
   Bibliography: p.
   1.   Health education (Elementary)   I. Title.
[DNLM: 1. Health education. QT200 V268t 1974]
LB3405.V3   1974   372.3'7   73–18006
ISBN 0–8121–0351–3

Published in Great Britain by Henry Kimpton Publishers, London

Printed in the United States of America

This book is dedicated to my sisters:

Margaret Chambers

Mildred Busenhart

Maxine Harding

in remembrance of our wonder-filled childhood that we shared with Mother and Dad

preface

This book contains recommended methods and suggested activities for teaching health to elementary school pupils successfully through many new kinds of enriched educational experiences. It has been written mainly for four groups: (1) the college student who is preparing to be an elementary school teacher; (2) those studying to become health education specialists; (3) the beginning and experienced teacher searching for more productive ways to teach health to children; and (4) administrators and school health service personnel seeking new suggestions for helping teachers and parents so that they, in turn, can assist children to develop better health standards and improved health habits.

I am aware that there are many ways of teaching any subject area in the school curriculum, and that superior teachers will find their own successful methods by the slow process of carefully blending the ingredients of what is known about learning, the techniques used by former admired instructors, and their own trial-and-error attempts. It is hoped that they can profit from the many suggested activities and teaching methods presented in this book and tailor them to fit their own and their pupils' needs and their unique teaching situation.

Part I contains materials showing the pressing need for a greatly improved program in elementary school health education. Part II discusses the total school health program and points out many ways for teaching health more effectively through health appraisal activities as well as through the school environment. In Part III many new and creative teaching methods are discussed which can help teachers make health education become an exciting educational adventure for children. Part IV contains many specific suggestions and course outlines for teaching children in grades K-6 nutrition, dental health, body growth, structure and function, safety, mental health, communicable diseases, drugs, alcohol, tobacco, family life and sex education, and consumer education. The Appendix contains a list of sources of free and inexpensive teaching aids, recommended health textbooks for children, and a list of helpful teaching materials and guides to special media.

It is imperative that teachers join with parents to develop healthy, happy, vigorous children with initiative, resourcefulness, imagination, and courage. Like Diogenes, I contend that the foundation and real wealth of every nation lies in the education of its youth.

It has been said, in truth, that the final appraisal of any life must be based upon what causes have used it, what powers have surged through it, and what ideas have mastered it. May this book help teachers to discover, strengthen, and increase a dedicated desire to lead all children to the discovery of the beauty, joy, and miracle of life.

Dallas, Texas   MARYHELEN VANNIER

acknowledgments

I am indebted to many persons who have made this book possible. Appreciation is due my family, professional colleagues, and students for their encouragement and assistance during its creation.

Gratitude is expressed to all who gave permission to reproduce photographs, record forms, or other materials which appear in the book, especially to Mrs. Ora Wakefield, Health Coordinator and Director of Safety for the Nashville Public Schools; Blanche Bobbitt, Supervisor of Health Education and Health Services for the Los Angeles Public Schools; Vivian Weedom, Curriculum Consultant for the National Safety Council; Frances Mayes, Health Specialist in the Virginia State Department of Education; Robert Yoho of the Indiana Bureau of Public Health Education; Walter Graves, Assistant Editor of the *Journal of the National Education Association;* George Wheatley, Vice-President of the Metropolitan Life Insurance Company; Ella Wright and Nancy Kane Rosenberg of the AAHPER; Mary Ellis and Helena Hunt of the American Institute of Baking; Mildred Srnensky of the Wheat Flour Institute; and M. M. McDonald and H. D. Carmichael of the Dallas Health and Science Museum.

I thank the various publishers of Health Textbook Series who sent sample copies of various health readers along with a Teacher's Edition for each book.

The cover design was adapted from drawings by my young friend, Beth Floyd, seven years old, of Dallas.

The manuscript was typed by Mrs. Dorothy Jane Good.

contents

PART IV

THE PROGRAM—WHAT TO TEACH CHILDREN
IN SPECIFIC AREAS OF HEALTH

PART V

EVALUATING THE RESULTS

PART ONE

background

THE EDUCATED PERSON

—*understands the basic facts concerning health and disease.*

—*protects his own health and that of his dependents.*

—*works to improve the health of the community.*

Purposes of Education
in American Democracy

CHAPTER 1

the challenge

The real wealth of our nation is found in our children. Our future, as well as theirs, depends upon both the quality and quantity of their education and their resulting actions of doing what they believe is wisest and best for the benefit of all. Although yesterday, today, and tomorrow are linked and are dependent upon each other, our hopes and dreams as educators, parents, or other adults are focused upon that tomorrow when they all might come true. Our present children, with our adult help, can bring about this better tomorrow for the benefit of all in our society.

There are those who truly believe that education can change the world and each person in it. There are also those who contend that this can only become a reality if education itself changes to become better and more meaningful to every individual, regardless of age, who partakes of it. In spite of us, and in some cases because of us as teachers, rapid change is taking place in every phase of American life, for children, youth, and adults. Because of teachers, change can come about in education that will lead to real and greatly needed improvement.

One of the subjects in the total school curriculum that greatly needs a "new look," a new up-to-date body of knowledge, and a new kind of enthusiastic desire for teaching this important subject well, is health education. Of all of the subjects taught in our schools, this one too often is the most poorly taught of all, and far too many programs are a waste of educational time and the taxpayer's money. Yet students of all ages are keenly eager to learn how to get the most out of life, how to be successful, and how to keep well. The classroom teacher, aided by the health education specialist, can and must make a more significant contribution to the role an effective health education program will play in the lives of all students. Only when teachers, school administrators, parents, and the general public truly believe that helping children to learn how to live healthfully and abundantly is as important as teaching them to read, write, or learn anything else in school that school health education can become a vitally alive and productive program. Meanwhile, we are, as one sage has said, "reaping pigmy results from our pigmy efforts in a time of giant opportunities." If it is indeed true that "it is better to light one candle than to curse the darkness," we then need not only to look around to see what our feeble efforts have produced so far but to determine that we will do something of real value to make this program better.

Health education is required to be in the school curriculum by law in every state of America. Some significant accomplishments have been made since health education programs were added to the school curriculum: people are living longer, many diseases have been eradicated, more children and mothers survive from childbirth, and many more. These are real gains. They are due mostly, however, to many in the medical profession, and to some few teachers who have had good health education programs.

The need for a vastly improved school health education program is revealed in the following startling facts:[1]

There are 17 million mentally or emotionally disturbed Americans in need of psychiatric treatment.

Suicide has become one of the leading causes of death among young adults.

Accidents are among the major causes of death and disability to the school-age population.

Almost 1 million Americans cannot read newsprint even with the aid of glasses.

Probably about 3 million Americans have major hearing defects.

Cigarette smoking is the most important cause of chronic bronchitis, emphysema, and lung cancer.

Alcoholism among employees costs American industry and business approximately $2 billion a year. Even though the exact number of alcoholics is not known, the number is increasing.

Some authorities believe that 24 million Americans have used marijuana at least once in their lives.

At least half of the supply of amphetamines available in this country enters illegal channels in a year.

There are 10 million overweight teenagers. Adequate amounts of vitamins D, A, and C; iron; and iodine are lacking in the diets of many Americans.

Americans have an estimated 800 million dental cavities in need of treatment.

More than 2 million persons under 25 years of age are infected with the tubercle bacilli.

At least 1500 young adults become infected with venereal diseases each day.

About 17 million Americans have high blood pressure or hypertension.

The public water supplies of over 19 thousand communities, serving 58 million people, do not meet U.S. Public Health Service standards of quality.

Communities in the United States produce over 3.5 billion tons of solid wastes each day.

At least 150 million tons of pollutants are discharged into America's air every year.

More than 2 million people in the United States have food, meat, and milk-borne diseases each year.

At least $2 billion a year are spent on medical quackery, including more than $100 million spent on ineffective drugs and devices for weight reduction.

THE SCHOOL HEALTH EDUCATION STUDY

In 1961, under the direction of Dr. Elena Sliepcevich, the School Health Education Study, funded by the Bronfman Foundation, surveyed 1101 elementary schools with

---

[1] School Health Education Study: *Health Education—A Conceptual Approach to Curriculum Design.* Washington, D. C.: The Study, 1967, p. 11.

529,656 students and 359 secondary schools with 311,176 students to discover the effectiveness of school health education. The results were shocking, for they showed[2]

> a marked deficiency in the quantity and quality of health education in both the elementary and secondary schools. The problems confronting school personnel included: failure of parents to encourage health habits learned at school; ineffectiveness of instruction methods; parental and community resistance to discussions of sex, venereal disease and other controversial topics; insufficient time in the school day for health instruction; inadequate professional preparation of the staff; indifference toward and lack of support for health education on the part of some teachers, parents, administrators, health officers and other members of the community; inadequate facilities and instructional materials; student indifference to health education; lack of specialized supervisory and consultative services.

The study also disclosed that the health behavior of the students was appalling. Sixth graders could only answer half of 40 test questions correctly; only 1 in 5 brushed his teeth after meals; 3 out of 4 ninth-grade boys said that their parents or counselor would be the last person to talk with about sex. The misconceptions about health of 70% of the students were that fluoridation purifies drinking water; legislation guarantees the reliability of all advertised medicines; popular toothpastes kill germs in the mouth and prevent cavities; chronic diseases are contagious; pedestrians are safe under all circumstances in marked crosswalks; venereal diseases can be inherited; venereal diseases have never been a social problem; public funds support the voluntary health agencies; the best man to see for a persistent cough is a pharmacist.

The Minnesota Mining and Manufacturing Company (3M) has developed a suggested health education curriculum based upon the recommendations of the SHES Committee made up of health education experts. These 10 curriculum concepts were:[3]

1. Growth and development influence and are influenced by the structure and functioning of the individual.
2. Growing and developing follow a predictable sequence yet are unique for each individual.
3. Protection and promotion of health are an individual, community, and international responsibility.
4. The potential for hazards and accidents exists, whatever the environment.
5. There are reciprocal relationships involving man, disease, and environment.
6. The family serves to perpetuate man and to fulfill certain health needs.
7. Personal health practices are affected by a complexity of forces, often conflicting.
8. Utilization of health information, products, and services is guided by values and perceptions.
9. Use of substances that modify mood and behavior arises from a variety of motivations.
10. Eating selection and eating patterns are determined by physical, social, mental, economic, and cultural factors.

---

[2] Fulton, Gere, and Fassbender, William: *Health Education in the Elementary School.* Pacific Palisades, Calif.: Goodyear Publishing Company, 1972, p. 20.
[3] School Health Education Study: *Health Education: A Conceptual Approach to Curriculum Design.* St. Paul, Minn.: 3M Education Press, 1967, p. 20.

Behavioral objectives (progressions and sequence) for each of these 10 concepts were utilized to set up a suggested school health curriculum with four levels of progression to replace the traditional grade-level approach still being used in most schools. Obtainable from the 3M Company, this curriculum is complete with overhead project instructional materials and a guide for its use for teachers.

If health education in elementary schools will continue to be taught by classroom teachers, much improvement is needed in their academic preparation in order for them to enter the teaching profession. As Donald Read has pointed out:[4]

> Ultimately, all elementary teachers may be expected to have a minimum preparation of 6–8 credit hours of biology, 3 credit hours of college health, 3 credit hours of methods and materials in health education (perhaps including school health), and 3 credit hours of evaluation in health education.
>
> Since the health curriculum lends itself very well to team teaching, it is probable that a number of the larger elementary schools will move toward employing a health specialist to correlate and integrate all formal and informal health-related instruction. Such a curriculum specialist should be able to serve several schools.

Discussion Questions

1. Which facts presented in this chapter concerning the great need for an improved health education program were the most startling to you?
2. What were some of the astonishing results of the 1961 School Health Education Study regarding the health behavior of children?
3. Discuss the meaning and significance of each of the 10 concepts given in this chapter for the 3M Conceptual Approach to Curriculum Design in Health Education.
4. What academic courses related to health does Donald Read recommend be included in the professional preparation of elementary teachers?
5. In your own words define health, health education, classroom teacher, and health specialist.

Things To Do

1. In chart form, in column 1 make a summarized list of the behavioral objectives of each of the 10 concepts found in the 3M Conceptual Approach to Curriculum Design in Health Education. In column 2 show the recommended teaching progression for each of these concepts.
2. Role play a conference between the school health specialist and the classroom teacher in which the former tries to convince the teacher of the need for a better health program for her class.
3. Give an oral report of how you would go about getting the citizens in your community to become more interested in promoting a greatly improved school health education program.
4. Make a list of the changes which have occurred in America which have a direct relationship on the health behavior of adults as children.
5. As a panel member discuss the characteristics of an educated person.
6. Recently 50% of American adults taking the CBC National Health Test failed to pass it. Devise 10 true or false health fact questions (such as "Diabetes is caused by eating too much sugar," which is false). Give this test orally to any 10 adults in your community other than educators or fellow students. Share your findings with your classmates as well as give your own conclusions of what you have learned from this experience.

---

[4] Read, Donald: *New Directions in Health Education.* New York: The Macmillan Company, 1971, pp. 10–11.

7. Give an oral test to any 10 elementary children made of 10 true or false health fact questions suitable for this age group. Compare your findings and conclusions gained from this experience with your classmates.

Suggested Readings

Anderson, C. L.: *School Health Practice.* 5th ed. St. Louis: The C. V. Mosby Co., 1972.

Harrelson, Orvis: "Today's Children—Today's Health Education." *The National Elementary School Principal* 68:6–10, November 1968.

Mendelson, Harold: "What Shall It Be: Mass Education or Mass Persuasion For Health?" *American Journal of Public Health* 52:131–137, January 1968.

Oberteuffer, D., Harrelson, O., and Pollack, M.: *School Health Education.* 5th ed. New York: Harper & Row, 1972.

Read, Donald, and Greene, Walter: *Creative Teaching in Health.* New York: The Macmillan Company, 1971.

Shane, Harold: "Children's Interests." *NEA Journal,* April 1957.

Smith, Ralph: *The Health Hucksters.* New York: Thomas Y. Crowell, 1960.

PART TWO

health—a vital part of the modern school's curriculum

"Health and fitness as we understand them are must *needs for all persons. Enjoyed by the lowliest among us, they contribute to happy living and national morale. Missing in our leaders, their absence helps to precipitate world unrest."*

—Arthur Steinhaus

CHAPTER 2

the total school health program

Health education is a relative newcomer to the American school, in spite of the fact that man's chief concern since he first stepped upon this earth has been self-preservation. Although the problem of survival once pitted our primitive ancestors against ferocious beasts, man today faces his greatest foe among other human beings. To keep alive in our highly competitive society is increasingly becoming a major struggle. To survive in our polluted environment, highly competitive and rapidly changing society, one needs all the strength, courage, and total fitness he can develop.

Increasingly school administrators, teachers, and the public are giving more than lip service to the concept that the "whole child" goes to school and that the real task of education is to develop each student to his highest potential physically, emotionally, socially, *as well as* intellectually. Increasingly too, laymen and professionally trained educators are becoming more keenly aware that the main goal of education is to lead all students to a happier, healthier, and more productive life for the present and future, for all students while they are *in* as well as *out* of school.

Before 1900, the first concerns for school health centered around protective programs of controlling communicable diseases, medical inspection, classroom ventilation, and room temperature control. Although by 1880 most states had passed laws requiring that schools teach the evils of narcotics, tobacco, and alcohol, it was not until after World War I that health instruction gained a secure enough foothold to stay in the rapidly changing school curriculum. In 1918 the Cardinal Principles of Education stated the development and protection of health should be the primary objective of American education. It was also during this period that school physical education programs developed rapidly, due largely to the alarming statistical findings which disclosed that far too many youth were unfit physically for military service. Although school health services also expanded during this period, there was little cooperative action between teachers and parents, the school or the community. Health classes became large dumping grounds arranged to meet at any available free period in the pupil's daily class schedule or on a rainy day when physical education classes could not play outside. Frequently unprepared and uninterested teachers were saddled with the responsibility of teaching health or else it was conducted by a local physician or nurse who stressed the control, symptoms, and the prevention of communicable diseases, human physiology, or anatomy. Physical education and health education often became one in the eyes of school administrators and general public. Frequently the physical educator, who was assigned to conduct physical activity classes and coach winning athletic teams, as well as teach health classes, usually neglected the latter.

When it was disclosed by draft rejection figures of World War II, the Korean War and the Vietnam War that the physical, mental, and emotional health of youth of military age had not improved over the years regardless of an exposure to school health education and physical education programs, public criticism at these two fields became extensive. Experts in both areas, however, have by now convinced most of the general public that the vast majority of American schools did not have even the barest minimum program requirements in either area, and that all too often many existing makeshift programs were directed by teachers unprepared in either field or that the physical education program consisted mostly of an athletic sports program for the few highly skilled players. Then, too, people are becoming increasingly aware that many of the draft rejections were due to faulty vision, hearing, illiteracy, poor nutritional status, and other factors more directly connected with the school health service program than with either physical or health education.

Americans are fast awakening to the fact that we are far from being as physically strong or as healthy as we must be if we are to survive as the leading nation in a rapidly changing world. Consequently, it is now the educator's task, whether he be the school administrator, or the classroom or specialized teacher, on all educational levels to lead the way by providing adequate and greatly improved health education and physical education programs in *all* schools throughout this vast land, as well as to convince the people that *every* student has the right to go to school in a safe, hygienic environment, receive periodic physical checkups, and partake in richly rewarding educational experiences which will enable him to learn to live abundantly and productively throughout his *entire* life. Although most parents want the best for their children, they often are unaware and confused as to what *is* the best or *how* to obtain it. Americans have always bought what they really wanted and supported the causes in which they really believed. To sell them now of the need for and the values of a superior total school health program conducted in a safe, hygienic school environment by professionally well-prepared teachers is the duty of every educator, regardless of whether he is teaching children or older youth, for the development of a "sound mind in a sound body" of each and every school student *is* a major goal of American education.

THE MEANING OF HEALTH

Children with health problems are found in every classroom of every school in every state of America. Yet medical authorities are agreed that no one, regardless of age, can live effectively or efficiently unless he has a well-functioning body and is able to meet successfully the many problems and crises which arise throughout his life.

Good health means far more than the absence of disease or infirmity, for it is a state of complete physical, mental, and social well-being.[1] Health results from fitness—to have it enables one to live a full, fruitful, and joyous life. To become healthy is no easy task, for it takes self-discipline and applied "know how." To stay healthy, man also needs the desire to do so, good medical care, and something to live for and to live by. Possessing total fitness enables one to "live most and serve best,"[2] for the healthy individual can do his daily work without undue fatigue, face his daily problems, is happy, has an energy reserve for emergency situations which may arise, and is concerned about maintaining his own health status as well as improving that of others. Such a healthy child or adult radiates and shines; the sickly one droops and is dull. Those with abundant buoyant health work, play, and live with zest! They have a sense of well-being, personal worth, and can adjust to ever-changing life situations.

Good health is far from accidental. It results from heredity, environment, and following carefully planned, routinized habits. Adequate rest and sleep, a balanced diet, normal waste elimination, freedom from infection, strain, and worry, coupled with the right amount of exercise are the ingredients necessary for obtaining and maintaining it. Parents, however, cannot give their offspring the wonderful gift of lifelong health, for each child must learn to assume ever-increasing responsibilities for his own health and his own behavior throughout life. A good parent, like a good teacher, becomes progressively unnecessary.

When the child enters the new, exciting, and ever-expanding world of the school, the administrators, teachers, school doctor, nurse, and other health specialists should become as concerned about his health status and well-being as his parents, family doctor, and dentist should continue to be. The school and community health agencies must work together as a team in order to provide:

1. Meaningful educational experiences for learning how to live healthfully in the home, school, and community.
2. Better methods for detecting children needing medical attention through improved techniques for screening, diagnosing, and treating those who deviate from normal.
3. Diagnoses and treatment of youth with impaired hearing; defective vision; epilepsy; dental, emotional, and other health problems.
4. Safe drinking water and sanitary toilets in schools.
5. Nutritional school lunches which meet recommended sanitary standards.
6. A safe total school environment.
7. Educational programs for children with physical and mental handicaps.

THE SCOPE OF THE HEALTH PROGRAM

The total school health program consists of three closely related and interdependent facets: (1) healthful school environment, (2) health and safety instruction, and (3) health services. It should be a program of instruction, guidance and counseling, and services which protect and improve the health status of each individual. Such a total program must be informative, shape positive health attitudes and values, and develop meaningful health habits.

---

[1] From the Preamble of The World Health Organization, 1946.
[2] This definition of health was coined by Jesse Fiering Williams, former Chairman of the Department of Health, Physical Education and Recreation, Columbia University.

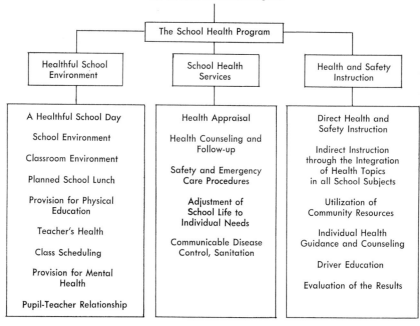

Figure 2-1. The total school health program.

Healthful School Environment includes the provision of a wholesome, safe environment, a healthful school day, sound teacher-pupil relationships, and all other environmental factors necessary for the best development for pupils and all school-employed personnel.

Health Instruction is the teaching of health facts, values, and concepts in such meaningful ways that individual and community health patterns improve. The end product of such instruction should be the motivated action of each pupil to use the basic health information he has acquired by applying what he *knows* to what he *does* in his daily life. The mere memorization of facts is of little, if any, value unless the child applies what he has learned, for the real and only true test of any educational experience is what a person *does*. Although one may know the many facts concerning tooth decay and oral hygiene, unless he brushes and cares for his teeth, the information he can give back to the teacher in a parrot-like or squeezed-sponge fashion when questioned is of little value. Education is for use. Its goal is self-directed behavior which will develop and improve both the individual and the community. Health education classes must become more student oriented in terms of their problems, interests, and needs. It must prepare students to be receptive to new scientific facts and time-tested, improved ways to solve daily life problems.

Health Services include determining the health status of each pupil, enlisting his cooperation in maintaining and protecting his own health, informing parents of defects, preventing diseases, and correcting remedial defects.

RESPONSIBILITIES FOR THE SCHOOL HEALTH PROGRAM

No other person can make a greater contribution to the school health program on the elementary level than the classroom teacher. Her first responsibility is to plan and conduct learning experiences for children. In order to do this effectively, she must make a careful study of the pupils in her class as well as of all those in the school, the school environment, and analyze the school program in its relationship to promoting health. She should also make a daily health inspection of each pupil, plan and teach health units, assist with screening tests, health records, work closely with parents and others in the community, as well as cooperate with the entire school staff in making the health program an inseparable, invaluable part of the total school program. Although she should be primarily responsible for health instruction, the total health program should be the responsibility of the school board, school administrator, school physician and/or nurse, and all teachers. The specific obligations of each toward this program are as follows:

The School Board
1. Provides adequate funds for qualified health personnel, instructional materials, teachers, and for the proper maintenance of buildings and grounds.

The School Administrator
1. Directs and coordinates all phases of the school health program.
2. Secures the services of school-employed medical personnel.
3. Provides and maintains a safe and healthful school environment.
4. Provides for an in-service health training program of all school personnel.
5. Appraises continuously the total school health program in terms of improved health status, improved group and individual health behavior, and adequacy of the school plant.
6. Establishes good home and community relationships by assisting the medical and nursing staff in interpreting the health needs of children, acquainting the home and community with the school health program, and organizing programs for parent participation and education in that program.
7. Enforces existing laws regarding school health and works toward obtaining new and better ones.
8. Acquaints school personnel with community facilities and resources obtainable for meeting the health needs of children.
9. Provides for an adequate program of health examinations and remedial follow-up.
10. Provides changes or adaptations in the school program for those with special needs.
11. Ensures an adequate health record-keeping system.
12. Conducts periodic surveys for evaluating the total school health program, the adequacy of the school plant, the efficiency of the teachers, and custodial services.
13. Develops plans for emergencies such as fires, tornadoes, and atomic nuclear fallout.
14. Assigns only qualified teachers to teach health.
15. Enforces a well-organized program of school safety and emergency care.

The School Physician
1. Conducts health examinations for all school children, keeps adequate records, establishes remedial programs, and secures medical and dental care for children needing them.
2. Conducts an in-service health educational program for teachers in the techniques of daily health observation, in detecting negative behavior

symptoms, screening tests and measurements of growth and development, and for keeping needed health inventory records.

3. Develops policies and procedures for the control of communicable diseases and accidents.

4. Assists the school administrator and public health officials in evaluating the school plant and gives skilled leadership in helping to provide a safe and hygienic school environment.

5. Works with parents in helping them maintain, protect, and build good health in their children.

6. Assists the administrator and teachers in evaluating the total school health program.

The School Nurse

1. Assists in conducting health examinations.

2. Administers and instructs teachers in giving needed screening tests for vision, hearing, and in other areas.

3. Works with the physician, school personnel, parents, and others in the community to carry through with adequate follow-up measures recommended as the result of health examinations.

4. Keeps adequate cumulative health records.

5. Assists in the special control of communicable disease.

6. Assists in providing a safe, healthful school environment.

7. Contributes to the health education program in as many ways as possible.

8. Helps coordinate community and school health efforts and resources.

9. Helps plan the overall total school program.

10. Works with parents for improving the health of their children.

11. Cares for the injured and sick in the school in accordance with the school policy.

The Teacher

1. Gives health instruction through carefully planned class sessions and at teachable moments throughout each school day.

2. Assists the nurse by giving screening tests, keeping records, and helping to provide a safe, healthful environment.

3. Guides and counsels students in personal health matters.

4. Works as a vital team member with all school-employed personnel in developing fully the three interdependent facets of the total school program.

5. Prepares children for physical and dental examinations and screening tests for vision, hearing, and posture.

6. Observes the health practices of children.

7. Weighs and measures each child at least twice yearly.

8. Isolates those coming down with communicable diseases.

9. Integrates and correlates health education with as many other subjects as possible.

10. Assists in evaluating the total school health program.

The Physical Educator

1. Assists in developing a good total school health program and a school health council.

2. Assists in giving screening tests for vision, hearing, posture, and in physical examinations.

3. Assists in weighing and measuring pupils periodically and in keeping health records.

4. Conducts classes in first aid and in other areas of health instruction.

5. Assists in emergency care, giving first aid and accident prevention programs.

6. Conducts remedial and adapted physical education programs for those with handicaps.

Other Participants

The Custodian

1. Maintains a clean, sanitary, and safe school building.
2. Regulates the heating, lighting, and ventilation of the school plant according to school and public health standards.
3. Assists all school personnel in all matters pertaining to health and especially in the teaching of children, through example, the importance of good health and safety practices in daily life.

The Nutritionist

1. Conducts and supervises the lunch and cafeteria services.
2. Participates in an in-service training program for teachers in nutrition.

The Dentist

1. Makes his program an educational one.
2. Provides services aimed primarily at teaching children intelligent self-direction and secondarily at providing dental treatment.

The School Health Coordinator

1. Helps teachers make wise selection of supplementary educational materials to the textbook and course of study.
2. Works toward planning for greater emphasis of certain health education areas at certain grade levels in order to avoid duplication.
3. Assists in developing close working relationships between teachers and those personnel working in the area of school health service and closer school-home and school-community relationship.
4. Conducts in-service health education programs for all who are concerned with pupils while at school.

RELATIONSHIP TO PHYSICAL EDUCATION

Although the specific goals of physical education, like those of all other subjects in the school curriculum, are to develop students physically, socially, mentally, and morally so that they will become well-rounded, healthy, responsible, happy citizens in our democracy, nevertheless each subject area in the curriculum makes a definite and unique contribution to the attainment of this end. The major contribution of physical education is in the area of physical and skill development. Objectives of the physical education program are to develop: (1) organic vigor; (2) physical motor skills; (3) increased knowledge concerning sports and games, one's body, and of life itself; (4) greater appreciation of one's self, the values of physical activity, and of others. The outcomes of such a program should result in better, more productive use of leisure time through taking part in recreational activities, and improved health.

On the other hand, the objectives of the school health program are to (1) teach basic facts concerning health; (2) shape positive attitudes toward health; (3) develop daily routinized habits for the maintenance, protection, and improvement of one's own health; and (4) learn to develop and protect one's own health throughout life.

In every physical education class numerous moments for instruction in health education arise. The very nature of this activity requires adequate safeguards, for the well-being and safety of those taking part in the program. Frequently the physical educator is the most popular, admired, and respected teacher in the entire school and has a closer relationship with more students than most teachers. It is imperative that this leader be worthy of emulation, for youth copies those admired.

The example that this leader sets provides vast opportunities to make a major contribution to the health of all participants in the physical education and school program.

THE RELATIONSHIP TO GENERAL EDUCATION

Every member of the entire school staff must understand and contribute team effort to the health program. Likewise, healthful practices should be woven into every part of the child's living. The school should provide a learning atmosphere that is relaxed, cheerful, and attractive wherein students are both "seen and heard." Any program of education, including health, conducted in such an environment is unsatisfactory and meager if it revolves around facts alone, or merely studying a textbook. Education can and should be an exciting adventure!

The school has three major responsibilities in the area of health. These are to (1) develop an improved health status of each student; (2) provide a safe, hygienic, and stimulating environment wherein learning experiences take place; and (3) aid in correcting remediable defects by informing and encouraging parents to secure medical services for their children with defects, as well as to provide a special, modified educational program for children who need it.

Although each school should develop its own objectives for the total school health program, the following may serve as a guide for the formulation of these objectives:

The program should strive to:
1. Inspire the child to be well and happy.
2. Convey to the child a public and personal health ideal, designed to ensure for him the continuation throughout life of wholesome and effective living, physical and mental.
3. Educate the child, according to a definite plan, in the cultivation of those habits of living which will promote his present and future health.
4. Impart health knowledge and attitudes to the child so that he will make intelligent health decisions.
5. Develop in the child a scientific attitude toward health matters, and an understanding of the scientific approach to health problems.
6. Maintain adequate sanitation in the school, the home, and the community.
7. Protect the child against communicable and preventable diseases and avoidable physical defects by providing effective public health control measures, both individual and social, throughout the school and the community.
8. Bring each child up to his own optimal level of health.
9. Extend the school health program into the home by obtaining family and community support for the program.
10. Discover early any physical defects the child may have, secure their correction to the extent that they are remediable, and assist the child to adapt himself to any residual handicap.
11. Provide healthful school living for the child.
12. Relate the school health program to the health program in the community so that it may deal with real, current, and practical problems.
13. Organize effectively not only the program of direct health instruction but the equally important indirect learning experiences of the child in the field of health.[3]

---

[3] Illinois Joint Committee on School Health: *Health Education and the School Health Program.* Springfield, Ill.: Illinois Department of Public Health, 1972.

Cooperation of the school, home, and community is essential if any effective health program is to be developed. Likewise, the health education program in the elementary school must be a primary responsibility of all teachers and staff members. All must work as members of a united team, bent upon helping each child assume greater and more intelligent responsibility for the development and maintenance of his own health in a safe and healthful environment.

THE NEED FOR INCREASED HEALTH EDUCATION IN ELEMENTARY SCHOOLS

Although medical authorities consider American children to be among the healthiest in the world, there is an abundance of evidence that far too many of them are not living at a peak health level or as totally functioning human beings. Many are not benefiting from disease-prevention measures now available at low cost or provided free of charge. It has been estimated that only around 20% of all children have received the Salk polio vaccine. Many youths tend to be physically soft from sedentary living of riding instead of walking to school, and sitting indoors watching television instead of playing rugged games out of doors. Likewise, too many American adults tend to be discontent, avid pill-gulpers, victims of stress, and frenzied consumers of quick-cure remedies advertised through the media of second-rate television or radio programs and inferior reading materials. If it is true that the "wealth of any nation is found largely in the health of its citizenry," and that "as a twig is bent, so grows the tree," it is equally true the education of all children in areas of healthful, wholesome living is of paramount importance. The very foundation and the continuation of our way of life depend largely upon the quality and quantity of the education of our children. The following health problems are prevalent in our American elementary schools:

Physical and Mental Defects

Suffering from these defects include those with postural defects, the orthopedically crippled (post-polio, cerebral palsied, post-encephalic, muscular dystrophied, or subject to convulsive seizures), the blind and the partially sighted, the deaf and the hard of hearing, those with speech deviations (articulation, voice, language, rhythm),

TABLE 2-1.   NUMBER OF HANDICAPPED CHILDREN, 1960-1970

Handicap	1960	1970
Epilepsy	360,000	450,000
Cerebral palsy (under 21)	370,000	465,000
Mentally retarded (under 21)	2,180,000	2,720,000
Eye conditions needing specialist care including refraction errors (5–17)	10,200,000	12,500,000
Hearing loss (under 21)	360,000–725,000	450,000–900,000
Speech (5–20)	2,580,000	3,270,000
Cleft palate–cleft lip	95,000	120,000
Orthopedic (under 21)	1,925,000	2,425,000
Congenital heart disease	About 25,000 born each year, of whom 7,000 die in the first year.	
Emotionally disturbed (5–17)	4,000,000	5,400,000

Arnheim, Daniel, Auxter, David, and Crowe, David: *Principles and Methods of Adapted Physical Education.* St. Louis: The C. V. Mosby Co., 1969, p. 11.

those with respiratory diseases, cardiac patients, those with nutritional deficiencies, those with rheumatic fever, and those with arrested tuberculosis.

It is estimated that between 5 to 10% of all school children should be in some program of special education. The following table shows the handicapping conditions under which these children are classified:[4]

Low physical fitness	20 to 25%
Poor body mechanics	50 to 60%
Nutritional disturbances	1 to 2%
Visual handicaps	1 to 2%
Auditory handicaps	1 to 2%
Cerebral palsy	Less than 1%
Cardiac conditions	1%
Arrested tuberculosis	Less than 1%
Diabetes	Less than 1%
Anemia	Less than 1%
Asthma and hay fever	2 to 4%
Hernia	Less than 1%
Mental retardation	1%
Other	1%

Mental retardation affects nearly 6 million Americans. In the chart above, therefore, even those conditions which apply to only 1% of all school-age children are found in large numbers (Table 2-1). The vastness of this and other handicaps requires that these children be given much more educational attention than ever before.

The most common handicaps found among school-age children and youth are the results of congenital defects, cardiac conditions, cerebral palsy, polio, accidents, epilepsy, cancer, osteomyelitis, tuberculosis, and diabetes.

Nonwhite children and youth in low-income groups are often the most permanently damaged. Those living with migratory parents or in ghettos within our crowded major cities are unlikely to have defects corrected. Many are labeled as mentally retarded when actually they have faulty vision or cultural deafness (a technique of tuning out the noise of many persons living in close quarters in slum conditions). Overcrowding, the population explosion, inadequate medical care, and lack of income are now being recognized as the serious national economic, health and cultural problems that they are. It is estimated that 20 to 40% of all school children in our nation suffer from one or more chronic health conditions. As one authority has pointed out, about 30% of these handicapping conditions could be prevented or corrected through good medical care during the first five years of life and that, if care could be continued to the age 18, as much as 60% of all found defects could be corrected.[5]

Accidents

The chief cause of death among school children is accidents—most of them preventable. It would be foolish to restrict the activities of children because they

---

[4] Joseph, Douglass: "Is Man Free To Make Choices for Health?" *The School Health Review*, September 1969, p. 6.

[5] Fait, Hollis: *Special Education, Adapted, Corrective, and Developmental*, 3rd ed., Philadelphia: W. B. Saunders Co., 1972, p. 40.

might get hurt or to remove all hazardous equipment so that they would never learn how to cope with danger. They might then be afraid to take chances or might develop dangerous emotional quirks and behavior patterns which ultimately might bring about their own destruction. The school, however, does have a great responsibility to teach children to take chances wisely, as well as to teach them to live and play safely in a hazardous environment. Safety appeals to the aged, danger attracts youth. This does not mean that just growing old (if one survives) will enable a person to be safety wise, nor does it mean that we shove children into the paths of fast-approaching cars in order for them to gain experience in how to survive in dangerous situations. It does mean that the school must play a greater role in teaching children both the necessity and "know how" for avoiding unnecessary and foolish risks. Studies show that:

about 43 percent of all school age accidental deaths occur either at school or going and coming to school. Of these accidents 20 percent happen in the school building, 17 percent on the school grounds, and about 6 percent going to and from school. In school buildings, the gymnasium is the location of the most frequent accidents, making up about one third of the fatal accidents within the building. Another 2 percent of the fatal indoor accidents occur in halls and stairs. Shops and laboratories account for about 18 percent and other classrooms add another 14 percent. On the school grounds, 41 percent of fatal accidents occur in unorganized activities, 20 percent in football, 12 percent in baseball, 9 percent on playground apparatus and 18 percent in other organized activities. The 6 percent of school age fatal accidents which occur while the pupil is going to and from school are mostly pedestrian-motor vehicle and bicycle-motor vehicle accidents.[6]

The following table shows the severity of the accident problem among children and youth in our society:

TABLE 2–2. ACCIDENTAL DEATHS OF SCHOOL AGE CHILDREN 5–14 YEARS PER 100,000 POPULATION (1968)

	Deaths	Rate
Total	8,400	20.3
Motor vehicle	4,200	10.2
Pedestrian	1,900	4.6
Home	1,400	3.4
Public nonmotor vehicle	2,600	6.3
Work	200	0.5

National Safety Council: "Accident Facts." 1969.

The number of deaths by poisoning among young children are astonishing. As one authority points out:

Childhood curiosity, like childhood enthusiasm, needs guiding. Every 24 hour period more than 750 children in the United States are poisoned by their own curiosity, which impels them to gulp aspirin and sleeping pills, sip floor polish and kerosene, swallow kitchen detergents, rubber cement and cos-

---

[6] Anderson, C. L.: *School Health Practice*. 4th ed. St. Louis: The C. V. Mosby Co., 1968, p. 228.

metics, and gnaw peeling paint from furniture and walls. Children, it has been said, will eat just about anything—and there are some 15,000 substances which are, to some extent, poisonous.[7]

Considering that 10,000 school children lose their lives yearly through careless preventable acts, these percentages are staggering!

Deviations from Normal Growth

Although every child has his own growth pattern, teachers can quickly spot the child who is markedly taller or shorter, skinnier or fatter than others. Normal growth deviates (and there are many of them in our public schools) often are victims of an uncontrollable appetite, malnutrition, malfunctioning glands, or deep-seated emotional problems. Many of these defects can best be remedied or controlled by both early discovery and treatment, for most of these problems are both physiological and psychological. Contrary to the belief of many parents that their child will "outgrow his trouble," most children usually do not and greatly need expert medical help. The teachers and school personnel should do their utmost to convince parents of the necessity of obtaining medical assistance as quickly as possible. The obese child will become the fat adult and needs help.

Cardiovascular Disorders

It has been claimed that every year more than half of the teachers of the nation have at least one child with a serious heart disorder in their classrooms. Rheumatic fever and congenital heart defects account for the major portion of these disorders. It is estimated that around 500,000 children have or have had rheumatic fever and that it accounts for two-thirds of all heart conditions found in children. There is a tendency for the disease to recur. Consequently, it is vital that every precaution be taken to withstand or prevent a second attack. Many cardiac cases can participate in regular school activities, but some should not. Although this is a decision for the medical specialist to make, it is imperative that the child live as normal a life as possible and that he learn to capitalize upon his capabilities and work around his limitations. Rheumatic fever is far more serious and common among school children than has been formerly believed. Since heart disease is the chief cause of death in America, it is evidently true that rheumatic fever does, indeed, "lick the joints and bite the heart of children." It is imperative that teachers know about the major kinds of cardiovascular deviations and how to plan and conduct educational programs for children suffering from defects.

Dental Disorders

Dental disorders constitute the major health problems among public school pupils, for it is estimated that 9 out of every 10 school children suffer from dental disease. According to the American Dental Association, the first grader usually has 3 or more cavities, and by the time this child has reached the age of sixteen he will have 7 decayed, missing, or filled teeth involving 14 tooth surfaces. Thousands of children have serious dental difficulties ranging all the way from carious or missing teeth, abscessed gums, pyorrhea, and gingivitis, to malocclusion with a

---

[7] Willgoose, Carl: *Health Education In The Elementary School.* 4th ed. Philadelphia: W. B. Saunders Co., 1974, p. 17.

marked overbite or underbite. A conscientious teacher will do her utmost to help the child receive the dental care he must have and to teach him ways he can protect both his teeth and general health throughout life.

Neurological Disorders

Epilepsy and chorea (St. Vitus's dance), with the former being more common, are serious neurological disorders with which the teacher usually will come into contact sometime during her professional career. Epilepsy is due to a disturbance in the electrochemical activity in the brain. Seizures may last only a few seconds (petit mal or "little sickness") to twitching and convulsions in which the persons become unconscious (grand mal or "big sickness"). Afflicted persons are educable, many are extremely intelligent, but a few are feeble minded and noneducable or nontrainable. It is estimated that one-quarter to one-half of a million Americans are victims of this disorder and that 80% of all those afflicted are below twenty years of age. It is estimated that one in every 30 to 40 children has this malady. Epilepsy occurs as frequently as diabetes and tuberculosis and four times more than infantile paralysis. Consequently, since this condition is more common than once supposed and since epileptic pupils who have mild attacks are often placed in school with normal children (while those with more serious difficulties are in special classes, schools, or hospitals), teachers must know what to do should an attack occur in the classroom. They should also be aware that epileptics are greatly in need of special attention and security, for the majority of them are fearful, ashamed, shy, and awkward socially. Those who are engaged in satisfying activities are less apt to have a seizure than those who fearfully and passively anticipate them. Rapid, successful advances are being made in treatment for epileptics. These include anticonvulsive medication, diet, education, psychotherapy, improved environmental conditions, and surgery. Here again, the classroom teacher is morally and professionally obligated to see that somehow the parents of the afflicted youngster in her group are made aware of these newly opened avenues of hope for their child, as well as to see that the pupil himself is working and playing in an educational environment which will prove most beneficial both for himself and the class.

Visual and Auditory Handicaps

One out of every 20 children has some kind of a hearing impairment or is deaf. Although most youngsters who have some hearing loss acquire it gradually, this difficulty can be detected early and treated before the afflicted child develops feelings of inferiority and becomes shy and withdrawn or defiant and rebellious. Many cases of defective hearing among elementary children may be due to psychological rather than physiological reasons such as mental retardation, cultural deafness, or retarded development of normal speech. Almost every school teacher has children in her classes who turn their heads to one side, cup the ear, wear worried puzzled expressions, are inattentive, fail or do poorly with their school work, have faulty posture with the head and torso held forward, show poor word pronunciation, or have faulty speech habits. The majority of these children have hearing difficulties.

Partially sighted pupils exist in greater numbers than most adults realize, for almost every school has children enrolled in it whose vision is faulty. Studies have shown that approximately 20% of elementary school children have visual problems requiring professional care. These problems include problems of refraction (nearsightedness, farsightedness, astigmatism, or eye imbalance), strabismus, cross-eye, or other eye deviations. Since 85% of our learning comes through the eyes, the fact that one out of every four school children has a visual defect presents a major problem teachers must both recognize and help solve. Normal vision is 20/20. Those with partial sight can be enrolled in most public schools if their vision is between 20/70 or 20/200 or there is no prognosis of vision deterioration, if they have an intelligence quotient of 70 or more, can take care of their own toilet needs, can communicate, have no behavior disorders, can hear, and are ambulatory. Simple screening tests can quickly detect those children who have more serious vision defects, whereas teacher observation can easily spot those whose poor posture, squinting, inattention, and poor school progress may be due to their inability to see.

Mental Health Deviations

The rapid increase in mental illness is the most serious health problem in this country today. Over 52% of those persons ill enough to be hospitalized are mentally and emotionally sick. Mental illness and emotional disturbance among children are increasing. It is estimated that 10 to 12% of all children have maladjustment and emotional problems requiring psychiatric help, and 3% more children have serious psychotic or pre-psychotic problems. Further, experts claim that in a class of 32 pupils, 3 to 4 will have emotional problems and one will need psychiatric assistance.[8] It is estimated that one out of every ten Americans is emotionally unbalanced enough to need psychiatric care. It is also known that one does not suddenly "go off the deep end" and become a raving maniac or completely withdraw from reality; the mentally ill adult usually showed abnormal behavior as a child. His case history is filled with experiences, terrifying to him, particularly during his early years at home and in elementary school. According to psychiatrists, those who show early, but markedly significant, behavior patterns of withdrawal or aggressiveness can and must be singled out and helped earlier, during their formative years. Certainly the building of bigger and better mental institutions is not a preventive answer to the problem of the increase in mental illness.

The role the classroom teacher can play in the prevention of disease and human tragedy is tremendous. Every elementary school teacher is already engaged in the field of health education—whether it be half-heartedly because of ignorance and "I don't care" attitude or actively because of knowledge and a desire to see that *all* children have a "square deal" at school. In every classroom throughout the nation health problems do exist, regardless of whether we ignore them or want to do something about them.

Never before have there been so many children enrolled in our public schools. Never have the opportunities of the real educator been greater!

Discussion Questions

1. Why should health be taught in school?
2. What are the health effects of poverty or being a member of a minority group?
3. When do most school-connected accidents occur? How can these be prevented?

---

[8] Cornacchia, Harold, Staton, Wesley, and Irwin, Leslie: *Health in Elementary Schools*. 3rd ed., St. Louis: C. V. Mosby Co., 1970, p. 316.

4. What are the three divisions of the total school health program? Which one do you think is the most important?
5. How serious is the problem of dental disorders in our society? How can this problem be solved?
6. What should a teacher do if one of her class members has an epileptic seizure in her classroom?
7. Defective hearing among children may be due to psychological rather than physiological reasons. What are these reasons?
8. Discuss the seriousness to a student of having faulty vision. What should the teacher do to help that child?
9. Why do you think that mental illness and serious emotional problems are increasing among children? How can these be prevented?
10. What are the duties of the classroom teacher in the various areas of health?

Things To Do

1. Visit an elementary school health class. Report your findings to your classmates.
2. Find out the health education laws in your state. Do you think that these laws are being upheld? Support your answer.
3. Interview an elementary school classroom teacher in order to learn what she is doing in health education. Report your findings to the class.
4. Bring to class and read aloud any newspaper article which relates to a health problem among children.
5. Read and report on any article in *School Health Review* or *The Journal of School Health* or the first chapter from any book in the suggested readings found below.
6. In groups of four present a panel discussion on any aspect of school health given in this chapter.
7. Bring for the class bulletin board any cartoon or comic strip which shows the need for health education among adults as well as children.
8. Divide into buzz sessions to discuss areas in which health instruction needs improvement.
9. Make a survey of safety hazards at your campus. Report your findings to the class. Discuss how such a survey, if made by children at their school, could become a rich educational experience for them.
10. Give an oral report of any health lesson you remember at school or home when you were a child. Why did this experience remain in your memory?

Suggested Readings

Anderson, C. L.: *School Health Practice*. 4th ed. St. Louis: C. V. Mosby Co., 1968.
Cornacchia, Harold, Staton, Wesley, and Irwin, Leslie: *Health in Elementary Schools*. 3rd ed., St. Louis: C. V. Mosby Co., 1970.
Grout, Ruth: *Health Teaching in Schools*. 5th ed., Philadelphia: W. B. Saunders Co., 1968.
Haag, Jesse: *School Health Program*. 3rd ed., Philadelphia, Lea & Febiger, 1972.
NEA–AMA: *Health Education*. Washington, D.C., National Education Association, 1961.
Nemir, Alma: *The School Health Program*. 3rd ed., Philadelphia: W. B. Saunders Co., 1970.
Oberteuffer, Delbert, and Beyer, Mary K.: *School Health Education*. 4th ed., New York: Harper & Row, 1966.
Willgoose, Carl: *Health Education In The Elementary School*. 4th ed., Philadelphia: W. B. Saunders Co., 1974.

CHAPTER 3

teaching through health appraisal activities

Every single child in a group of five children is as different and unique as each of the five fingers of a person's hand. It is imperative that the teacher recognize these differences, for each pupil will react to both adults and his peer group according to his own growth patterns, his developmental stage, his special needs, interests, and abilities. Fortunately, teachers can glean greatly needed health information about each student from a variety of sources. These include (1) daily observation and evaluation of how each child looks and acts, (2) the pupil's health history, (3) screening tests, (4) medical and dental examinations, and (5) psychological tests.

School health appraisal activities abound in numerous opportunities for real health education, such as when the child asks why he should have his teeth examined by a dentist at school or how much he should weigh in comparison to what he does weigh or the weight of his classmates. All health appraisal activities should be utilized fully by the examining school doctor, nurse, and the teacher at every opportunity throughout the school year. Since we only learn when we want to, the role of the teacher is to capitalize upon as well as to arouse each pupil's curiosity to find out about himself. Children are eager to find out "why we are doing it this way" about things done to them. Health appraisal activities offer ripe educational opportunities which can yield a harvest of rich learning. During such procedures the child should be seen *and heard*. The basis for health education course materials can be laid preceding and during these activities. Each testing and measuring experience produces many opportunities for on-the-spot teaching, which can make a lasting impression on the child and provide a more valuable educational experience for that pupil than a health lesson given to the whole class.

TEACHER'S OBSERVATIONS

Teachers play a vital role in the development of a child's physical and emotional health. She must learn how to detect deviations from the normal appearance and behavior in her entire class as well as of each child in that class. Unlike the parents, the educator can see the unique individual differences of each pupil against the background of those of his many peers of approximately the same age and school grade. The teacher learns from the child himself what to expect from him as an individual, as well as a group member, and often her expectations are more objective than those of the parents. Although the teacher, when a normally bright-eyed appearing youngster comes to school looking droopy-eyed and dull, or a usually cooperative pupil suddenly becomes inattentive and defiant, cannot and should not attempt to diagnose what is wrong, it *is* her obligation to see to it that this change is called to the attention of the school health authorities. Then, too, she often can become aware of any change in general health and inform the school medical personnel or parents of the situation. Likewise, she should see to it that parents realize the seriousness of their child's poor posture, crossed eyes, or protruding teeth, which they have taken for granted or ignored, for sometimes parents are unaware that these deviations are of real importance and often can do serious emotional damage to a youngster. Such defects are largely correctable when the child is young, growing, and pliable. As it is pointed out in the splendid pamphlet "What Teachers See":[1]

> The school physician all too often has time only to see that a child has a physical condition which is interfering with the normal functioning of his body. The nurse is concerned chiefly with the ways and means of getting the condition corrected. The teacher is more likely to see the child held back from what she knows he can be and do by something which is interfering with his expected progress.
>
> School physicians, nurses, and parents are coming to recognize the important place held by the teacher as an observer who may be depended upon to find children in need of medical or dental care. To make the best use of her strategic position as an observer, the teacher herself should be aware of the service she is peculiarly equipped to give, and she should be taken into the confidence of the physician and nurse as a working partner.

The teacher can learn how to observe the daily health status of each person in the class by first being able to pick out deviations in the appearance of one child and then in each of the groups of children encountered daily. She should practice observation for the specific purpose of detecting departure from good health, realizing that she can act for the school nurse as the mother of the child does for the family physician. It is imperative that she knows how the child normally looks, whether he usually has a pale or ruddy look, or if he ordinarily comes to school a happy, smiling youngster or a shy, withdrawn, timid one. Also, the teacher, if she wishes to be a successful health observer, must want to assume the responsibility for the health of her class group, be able to recognize abnormalities, as well as know the constructive things to do when deviations occur.

The daily health inspection may be done informally by the teacher as she greets each pupil as he enters the room. She should carefully note at the same time the

---

[1] *"What Teachers See."* New York: Metropolitan Life Insurance Company.

Directions: 1. Put an X after the item when there *seems to be* deviation from normal or a defect.
2. Circle the X (X) when the defect has been corrected and/or the pupil is under medical care.

YEAR IN SCHOOL	1	2	3	4	5	6	7	8	9	10	11	12	13	14

General
Does not look well (physically)
Very fat
Very thin
Tires easily
Posture seems poor in general
Lacks appetite
Frequent headache
Other

Behavior
Very withdrawing—seems afraid or shy
Cries easily
Usually gives in (submissive)
Fails to play most of the time
Often very restless
Daydreams excessively
Very inattentive
Very hostile and/or destructive
Excessive bragging
Irritable—most of the time
Excessive use of the toilet
Bites nails or chews objects
Usually does not get along with others
Has many accidents
Stutters or other speech defect
Other

Eyes
Styes or crusted lids
Crossed
Squints or frowns
Holds book very close—or very far
Other

Ears
Discharge
Earache
Turns head to side
Other

Mouth Teeth
Obvious cavities
Obviously irregular
Need cleaning
Inflamed gums
Other

Nose Throat
Persistent mouth breathing
Frequent sore throat
Frequent colds
Persistent cough
Constant clearing the throat
Other

Skin Scalp
Rashes or sores
Extremely rough and dry
Other

Orthopedic
Chronic limp
Toes pointed in or pointed out
Stiff or swollen joints
One shoulder higher than the other
Holds head to side habitually
Other

Number of days absent due to illness
(record at end of year)

* (Courtesy, North Carolina State Department of Education.)

Figure 3-1. Teacher observation health form.

hair and face of each child, whether he seems happy or sad, tired or rested, and whether the eyes are clear and bright instead of red and inflamed. Throughout each day she should be frequently observant of each child's posture, the contents of his lunch-box if he brings one, as well as note if the pupil usually takes time to eat or bolts his food, whether he is usually a quarrelsome social outcast or a person the other children like and readily accept as a group member.

In a self-contained classroom, the teacher has a golden opportunity to observe children as she directs them in periods of physical education. Educators discovered long ago that if you want to find out what a child is really like, you should *watch* him play, but if you are concerned as to what he will become, you should *direct* his play. Children are their true selves when they are so engrossed in the game that they forget to be the "goody-goody" their mother and teacher expect them to be. Since what a child *does* is far more important than what he says, all classroom teachers should observe as well as direct children at play.

The teacher should be aware of the following disorders in various parts of the body, as well as of behavior symptoms and emotional problems, as she observes each child daily in her class:

EYES

Sties or crusted lids
Inflamed eyes
Crossed eyes
Repeated headaches
Squinting, frowning, or scowling
Protruding eyes
Watery eyes
Rubbing of eyes
Twitching of the lids
Holding head to one side

NOSE AND THROAT

Persistent mouth breathing
Frequent sore throat
Recurrent colds
Frequent nose bleeding
Chronic nasal discharge
Nasal speech
Frequent tonsilitis

TEETH AND MOUTH

State of cleanliness
Gross visible caries
Stained teeth
Gum boils
Offensive breath
Mouth habits such as thumb sucking

GENERAL CONDITION AND APPEARANCE

Underweight—very thin
Overweight—very obese
Does not appear well

Tires easily
Chronic fatigue
Nausea or vomiting
Faintness or dizziness

GROWTH

Failure to gain regularly over
    3-month period
Unexplained loss in weight
Unexplained rapid gain in weight

GLANDS

Enlarged gland at side of neck
Enlarged thyroid

EARS

Discharge from ears
Earache
Failure to hear questions
Picking at the ears
Turning the head to hear
Talking in a monotone
Inattention
Anxious expression
Excessive noisiness of child

SKIN AND SCALP

Nits on the hair
Unusual pallor of face
Eruptions or rashes
Habitual scratching of scalp or skin
State of cleanliness
Excessive redness of skin

HEART

Excessive breathlessness
Unexplained fatigue
Any history of "growing pains"
Bluish lips
Excessive pallor

POSTURE AND MUSCULATURE

Asymmetry of shoulders and hips
Peculiarity of gait
Obvious deformities of any type
Abnormalities of muscular development

BEHAVIOR

Overstudious, docile, and withdrawing

Bullying, overaggressive, and domineering
Overexcitable, uncontrollable emotions
Unhappy and depressed
Stuttering or other forms of speech difficulty
Lack of confidence, self-denial, and self-censure
Poor accomplishment in comparison with ability
Lying (imaginative or defensive)
Lack of appreciation of property rights (stealing)
Abnormal sex behavior
Antagonistic, negativistic, continually quarreling

It is not enough, however, for the teacher to spot the child who is coming down with an illness, for although she can do much to prevent the spread of communicable diseases, she should teach the children how to protect themselves from germs, that they should say in bed when they have a cold, that they should cover their mouth when they cough, that they should get plenty of rest and sleep, and so forth. Every aspect of the health observation program abounds with opportunities for individual health counseling and teaching. Group instruction can become developed from any part of such a program. If increasingly more pupils are having colds, it is a good time to stress cold prevention techniques. Epidemics, accidents, and other types of disasters can also be put to positive educational use.

Teachers should be aware of the range of pupil differences before they recognize these specific differences. The more each teacher knows about the needs and interests of each pupil, the better she can guide him to rich learning experiences which can help him find a solution to his own problems, including those in health. This discovery of each pupil's health and safety needs is basic to any sound school health education program. These must be discovered by each teacher herself. She must also find out what the child already knows and does as well as how he feels about himself, life in general, other people, what he wants to be when he grows up, what he fears, and as much other kinds of information as possible. The more she talks, the less she will learn about each child; the more each child talks about himself, the more she will learn about him. The resulting instructional program should be chiefly concerned with everyday health and safety practices as they will affect all the children in the class.

SCREENING TESTS

Although in large school systems the nurse is usually responsible for giving screening tests with the classroom teacher working as her assistant, the teacher in a small or rural school often must assume this responsibility. It is important that those conducting such tests be aware of all teachable moments as they arise, as well as knowing what and how to answer the questions children ask, for it is then that they *want* to learn. It is at this time, too, that fears can be assuaged. Educators call this "having a need for learning" and have discovered that "wanting to know" is basic to "getting to know."

Vision Tests

Children having vision difficulties often display this through the appearance of the eyes (crusted lashes, red or swollen eyelids, sties) or by their behavior (fre-

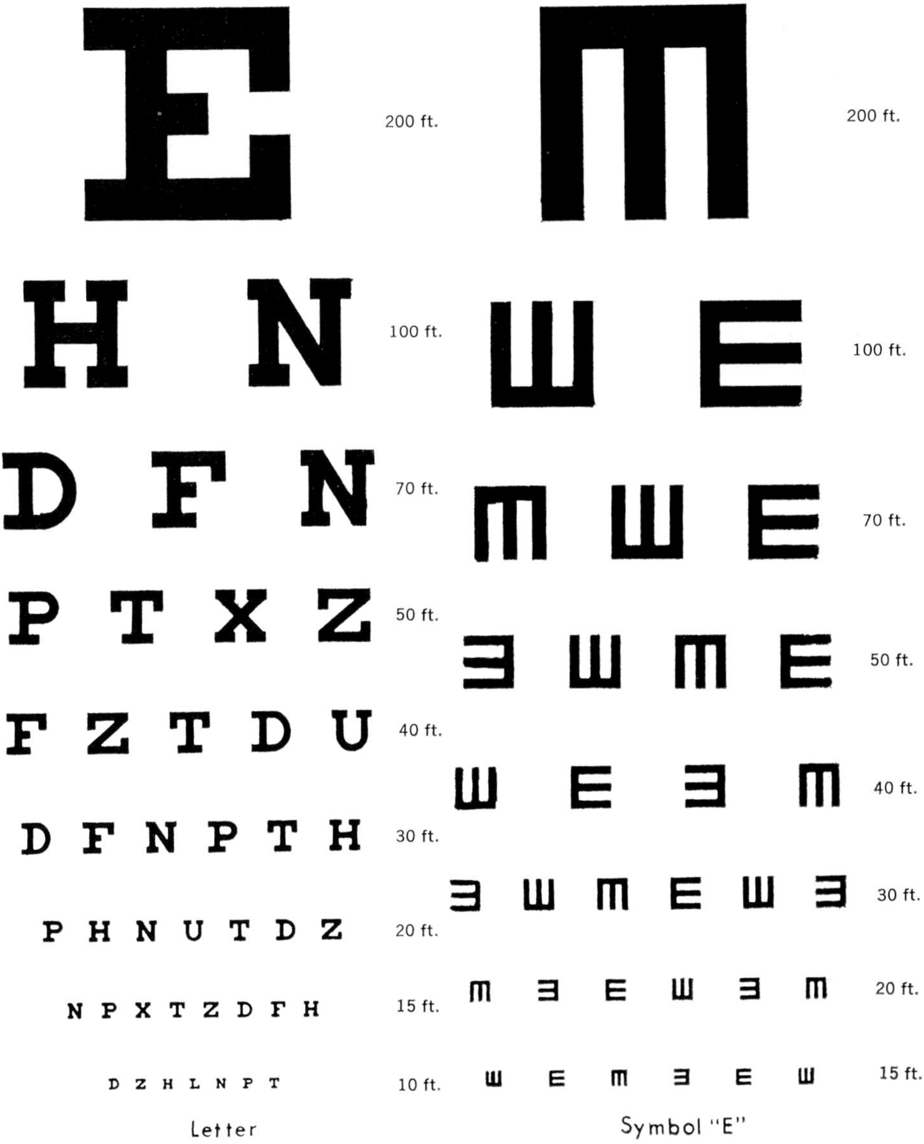

Letter   Symbol "E"

Figure 3-2. Snellen charts. (Courtesy of the National Society for the Prevention of Blindness)

quently rubbing of the eyes, signs of inability to see well or do close work, irritability, inattentiveness, holding of a book too close or too far away, shutting or covering one eye, cross-eyes, and many other signs).

A number of vision tests are available. The Snellen test is recommended for elementary schools, for it is easily given and inexpensive, and it enables the teacher to pick out quickly the child who is having vision difficulties and should be referred to an eye specialist. The chart is available in letter or in the "E symbol" form. The latter is for children who cannot read letters but who can point the direction the "legs" of the letter *E* are turned.

Each child should be tested standing 20 feet from the chart.* He covers one eye with a card and looks out of the other one and attempts to read several letters before the opposite eye is tested. The teacher must be sure that the child understands what he is to do, has not memorized any part of the chart, and is not afraid to take the test. If he can read the letters in the 20-foot line on the chart, his vision is normal and is recorded as 20/20. If he can only read the letters in the 100-foot line, his vision is 20/100. This means that the pupil is greatly in need of seeing an eye specialist.

Although the Snellen test does not test color blindness, depth perception, or other vision difficulties, it does enable the tester to pick out those who cannot see from a distance of 20 feet, or those who have eye muscle imbalance causing one eye to be used more than the other.

Other recommended screening tests for vision are the telebinocular test (which measures the extent to which the eyes work together), the Massachusetts vision test, and the Holmgren wool test for color blindness.

Numerous educational opportunities arise each time a child has his eyes tested in school. The teacher should prepare each group for this experience. In younger children, interest in eyes and how we see can be aroused by showing pictures of eyes of different kinds of animals and birds, having each child then look at his own eyes in the mirror, and discussing how our eyes function and can be protected. Older children can become interested in learning about the importance of good lighting and vision by using a light meter and finding the candlepower present in various rooms or parts of them in the school building. Regardless of the type of teaching methods used to teach how our eyes work and should be protected, each pupil should gain from this experience a new appreciation for his own eyes and use this new knowledge of how to care for them properly in his daily life.

Hearing Tests

Pupils who have hearing difficulties often turn their heads to one side or cup the ear, seem dull, have a worried facial expression, or speak in an unusual-sounding voice. Hearing tests include audiometer (by far the most accurate), the watch tick, and the whisper test. The most satisfactory testing instrument is the discrete frequency audiometer, which can be used to test groups as well as individuals. Such instruments can be borrowed or rented from hearing specialists, the local or state health department, or often from a local college or university.

---

* Complete directions for administering the test are available with the chart. It can be obtained from a number of sources including state departments of health, local eye specialists, local or county health departments.

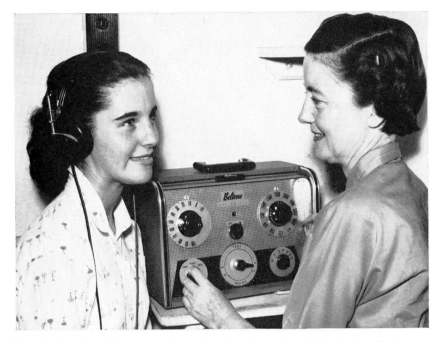

Figure 3-3. An audiometer test is an educational experience in itself. Its effectiveness can be increased if the teacher capitalizes upon teachable moments during the test. (Courtesy of Los Angeles Public Schools)

Other tests include:

Massachusetts group pure-tone test

This is an audiometer group test for hearing deficiencies. It can quickly point out those pupils who have normal hearing acuity. Those who fail the test should subsequently be given an individual pure-tone sweep-check test as a means of double checking the results.

Pure-tone sweep-check test

This test, using a pure-tone audiometer, establishes the ability of the pupil to hear several different tones or pitches at a given intensity. Should he fail to hear certain pitch levels, the pure-tone threshold acuity test should be made. Pupils who can hear all test tones at the prescribed intensity have satisfactory hearing acuity and need no referral.

Pure-tone threshold acuity test

This test, given by machine, determines what intensity or loudness is required before it is possible for the child to hear the test tones of varied pitch. Failure to hear certain test tones indicates that the pupil does not have normal hearing and should receive attention by a medical specialist.

Speech test

This test measures the most important function of the ear. Under ordinary conditions, however, it is unsatisfactory, for often poor acoustics and unavoidable noise may make it impossible to secure meaningful results. It is especially important to have a quiet room with as little outside noise as possible. The whisper should be about one-third as loud as the voice used in ordinary conversation.

Coin-click test

In this test, three coins are clicked together behind the head of the examinee several times, and the pupil is asked to count each click. Reports should be kept of those who fail to hear all three clicks and these students referred to a specialist. A quiet room is necessary for this test.

Audiometer tests

In recent years the audiometer has replaced all other methods of testing hearing because it is more accurate, constant, and reliable than any other hearing examination. The tests are made by setting the dial of the audiometer at one intensity point and changing the pitch or frequency. At each change, the child presses the signal button when he hears the sound.

It is not enough, however, merely to give each child a hearing test, for each class should be prepared for this experience. Lessons or units on the human ear and how it functions should be planned by the class through teacher-pupil planning and carried out by individual or small committee assignments. This educational experience should enable each pupil to understand better how the ears work and how hearing can be tested and protected.

Height and Weight Charts

Children should be weighed and measured each month and an accurate record be kept for each pupil. A scale with an accurate height-measuring device may be used, or a permanent wall marking may also be used. Although charts of weight norms are available from insurance companies, the teacher should use these only to compare the height and weight records of *each* pupil in relationship to those of many students of the same age and grade in school. Whether a child has a small, large, or medium skeletal frame should also be considered, as should recent or lingering illnesses or deep-seated emotional strains—all of which may influence growth patterns.

The Wetzel grid is often used in elementary schools for recording a child's growth over several years. It is a card on which horizontal channels are drawn to represent body types: (a) stocky, (b) average, and (c) frail, and vertical lines are drawn on which height and weight results are recorded. Such a chart is kept for each pupil, and his growth patterns are plotted. It is an excellent way to record and observe the normal growth and deviations from the norm. Pupils who skip from one channel to another, or who fail to grow over a period of time, should be referred to a physician. Although the school nurse usually records and keeps a Wetzel grid for each child, in some schools this is the duty of the class or homeroom teacher. Numerous teachable moments occur each time a child is weighed and measured. The wise teacher takes time to capitalize upon them.

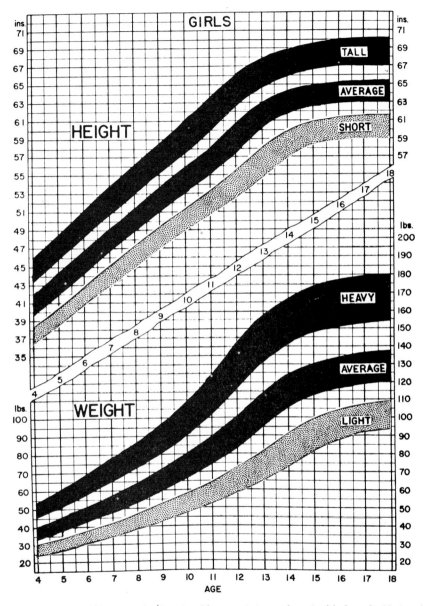

Figure 3-4.   The Wetzel grid. (Reprinted by permission and attainable from the National Education Association Service, Inc., 1200 West Third Street, Cleveland, Ohio.)

It is not enough to weigh and measure a child. Weighing and measuring experiences can be educational as through each experience health education can become both personalized and more meaningful. Children are extremely interested in growth, and most of them are eager to accelerate the process as much as they can. Checking the height and weight of each pupil and of the entire class provides opportunities to build health units into which nutrition, the value of exercise, sleep, and rest, and other aspects of health can be incorporated.

Although most children are interested in growing up, many are unaware of how this process takes place or what happens to them as they do grow. Individual and class interest in this process can be evoked in a number of ways, such as having each pupil bring his baby picture to class, asking such questions as "How much did you weigh when you were born? How much do you weigh now? What caused you to weigh more now?" or by having the class become interested in performing plant and animal experiments to show the relationship of proper food, sunshine, and other factors to growth. Cattle breeders, farmers, or even rural children can share much valuable information with a city group concerning the types of food given to fatten cows, pigs, or other animals. Visits to farms, dairies, or other types of food plants can make lasting impressions upon children, especially when they hear other adults at these places stress the same good health habits as does their teacher.

HELPING CHILDREN UNDERSTAND THE IMPORTANCE OF GROWTH

School camping is especially valuable as a means of providing youngsters with meaningful educational experiences. The program in such camps might well include caring for animals, for such an adventure can give children an opportunity to see for themselves the role that good food and care plus other factors play in growth. Those who can be given opportunities to gather and candle eggs, milk a cow, or feed baby turkeys have rich learning experiences which remain meaningful, valued, and bright in memory throughout life. Learning to plan menus, shopping, and cooking their own food (whether it be over an open fire or on a kitchen stove) makes education become alive and far more significant in the lives of boys and girls than the teacher telling or reading aloud about these things to a class; those methods of teaching have value too, but only when used at the right time, just often enough, and in small amounts.

Children need to learn that they grow in many other ways, other than just physically. Units on growing up socially, emotionally, and intellectually can help the class learn that growth is more than just an increase in size, nor is it confined only to the body.

Posture Tests

Good posture means comfortable efficient body alignment when one is both stationary and moving, standing as well as walking. Causes of poor posture are faulty nutrition, poor environmental conditions, fatigue, mental or emotional strain, faulty vision or hearing, or orthopedic defects.

The most common types of posture defects are:

Scoliosis or curvature of the spine
Lordosis or hollow back
Kyphosis or round shoulders
Kypholordosis or round upper back and hollow back

Faulty arches which are too low or high
Flat feet
Pronated or supinated ankles
Carrying the head too far forward, back, or to the side
A hollow or deformed chest
Winged shoulders
Protruding stomach which throws off body alignment

Although there are many good screening tests for posture, the posture test included in the New York State physical fitness test is recommended* In this test the teacher compares the various standing postures of each pupil with drawings on a card and rates him accordingly. Since few teachers have been trained to pick out postural defects and cannot readily detect deviations, the use of the drawings which clearly show any abnormalities is most helpful. The test determines if the child's head is held correctly, shoulders are level, the spine straight, hips level, feet pointed straight ahead, arches normal, neck erect, chest elevated, shoulders correctly centered, trunk erect, abdomen flat, and lower back curved normally.

The plumb-line posture test can also be used. The pupil stands by a weighted line while his posture is checked from lateral, anterior, and posterior views. From the lateral view, the line should fall about one-half inch away from the center of the hip, shoulder, and through the lobe of the ear. From the anterior view, the line should fall an equal distance between the knees and in the center of the chin, nose, and head. From the posterior view, the line should fall in the center of the back, ankles, knees, buttocks, cleft, head.

Posture education for many children is dull and uninteresting, for it too often consists of warnings of impending doom if one does not stand up straight. Actually it can become an exciting area of study, especially when related to what one wants to be or become. At every grade pupils have a fairly good idea of what they do want to be when they grow up, even though many fields are "sampled" along the way. Helping the child see the role his posture can play in his success of what he does tomorrow can be an effective way to help him improve his own posture.

There are many effective ways to help pupils become posture conscious. It is the teacher's duty to provide the right conditions in which healthy growth can take place and wherein the child can make correct or desired responses. Educators call this "getting the act performed with satisfaction" and stress the importance of having children do things which bring not only personal satisfaction but also praise by the teacher. Since good posture is an important health factor closely related to mental and physical efficiency and well-being, there should be an emphasis upon this aspect of health in each grade. Good posture results when the mind works well with the body. There are many postures each person assumes besides the static ramrod once considered to be ideal. It means proper body alignment in standing, sitting, and lying positions—all done with a minimum of fatigue, with ease, grace, and efficiency. The body should be properly balanced, the head erect, the hips tucked under rather than thrust out, and the shoulders held straight. The key words to stress when talking about good posture are *balance*, *rhythm*, and *grace*.

---

* Available at small cost from C. F. Williams and Son Printing Company, Albany,
   N. Y.

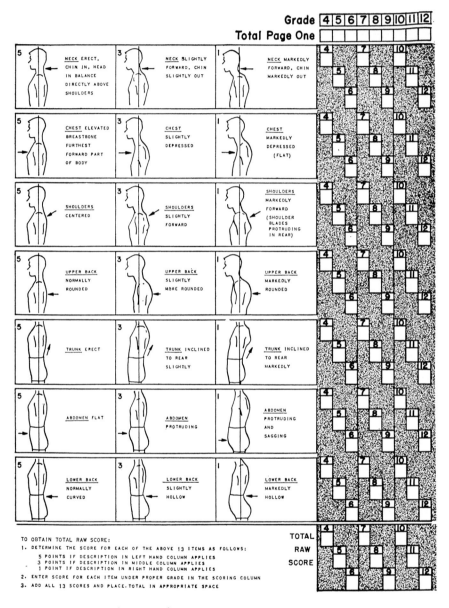

Grade 4 5 6 7 8 9 10 11 12

Total Page One

5 NECK ERECT, CHIN IN, HEAD IN BALANCE DIRECTLY ABOVE SHOULDERS **3** NECK SLIGHTLY FORWARD, CHIN SLIGHTLY OUT **1** NECK MARKEDLY FORWARD, CHIN MARKEDLY OUT

5 CHEST ELEVATED BREASTBONE FURTHEST FORWARD PART OF BODY **3** CHEST SLIGHTLY DEPRESSED **1** CHEST MARKEDLY DEPRESSED (FLAT)

5 SHOULDERS CENTERED **3** SHOULDERS SLIGHTLY FORWARD **1** SHOULDERS MARKEDLY FORWARD (SHOULDER BLADES PROTRUDING IN REAR)

5 UPPER BACK NORMALLY ROUNDED **3** UPPER BACK SLIGHTLY MORE ROUNDED **1** UPPER BACK MARKEDLY ROUNDED

5 TRUNK ERECT **3** TRUNK INCLINED TO REAR SLIGHTLY **1** TRUNK INCLINED TO REAR MARKEDLY

5 ABDOMEN FLAT **3** ABDOMEN PROTRUDING **1** ABDOMEN PROTRUDING AND SAGGING

5 LOWER BACK NORMALLY CURVED **3** LOWER BACK SLIGHTLY HOLLOW **1** LOWER BACK MARKEDLY HOLLOW

TO OBTAIN TOTAL RAW SCORE:

1. DETERMINE THE SCORE FOR EACH OF THE ABOVE 13 ITEMS AS FOLLOWS:

    5 POINTS IF DESCRIPTION IN LEFT HAND COLUMN APPLIES
    3 POINTS IF DESCRIPTION IN MIDDLE COLUMN APPLIES
    1 POINT IF DESCRIPTION IN RIGHT HAND COLUMN APPLIES

2. ENTER SCORE FOR EACH ITEM UNDER PROPER GRADE IN THE SCORING COLUMN

3. ADD ALL 13 SCORES AND PLACE. TOTAL IN APPROPRIATE SPACE

TOTAL
RAW
SCORE

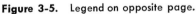

Figure 3-5. Legend on opposite page.

POSTURE RATING CHART

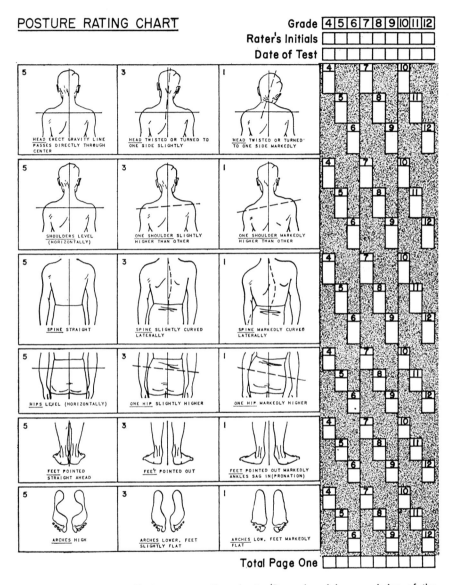

Figure 3-5. The New York posture-rating chart. (Reproduced by permission of the Albany, New York, State Education Department.)

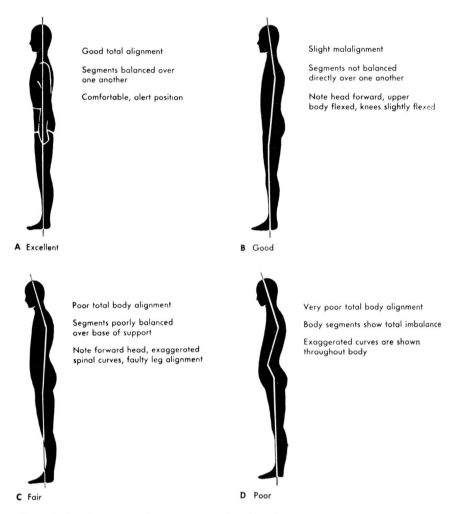

Figure 3-6. Four types of posture as seen by plumb-line test.

There are as many as seven causes of poor posture—all of which cannot be corrected upon command, for the student with bad posture can only develop good posture by developing muscular strength, energy, and self-confidence which will lead to good carriage and body mechanics. Causes of poor posture are: (1) an *improperly balanced diet* which causes the muscles of the body to lack the necessary supportive power to hold the person up; (2) *environmental conditions*, including poor lighting, a sagging bed mattress, or the use of a large pillow; (3) *rapid growth*, which is especially apparent in adolescence; (4) *fatigue* due to strain, faulty health habits including lack of sleep and rest, eating irregularly, and lack of exercise by riding and sitting too much; (5) *mental and emotional tensions*, for worry, insecurity, inferiority, and fear all tell on the body; (6) *poor vision and/or hearing*, which may cause the child to carry his head to one side or crane his neck; and (7) *structural and orthopedic defects*, which may be congenital or may be due to accidents or disease after birth. Poor posture can best be eradicated when the child is young, for his body is more pliable and flexible than it will be as he becomes older.

Since good posture is an indicator of health, teachers should be aware of how each pupil stands, walks, moves, and sits. Lighting, seating, work and play habits, and the pace of all school activities should be geared toward providing a favorable environment in which each pupil can use his body and grow healthfully. Since young children are restless and tire easily, opportunities should be given to them frequently throughout the school day to move about the room and do simple relaxation exercises. Their recess periods must be closely supervised by the teacher, who should also teach the children many kinds of vigorous activities, including relays and team games. The physical education instruction period should consist of rugged play activities, and the children should be taught conditioning exercises, rhythmical and self-testing activities, swimming, and outdoor camping techniques.[1] It is unreasonable to expect a program of health education in posture or corrective exercises to cure postural defects brought on by fatigue, malnutrition, or emotional difficulties, for these must first be eliminated before the child's posture can ever be improved.

There are many ways to arouse the child's interest in posture education. Slogans, bulletin board pictures taken from magazines or, better still, actual photographs of the children themselves taken at work and play, all can help do this. Individual learning activities might well include:

1. Making posters.
2. Learning exercises in school to be done at home; telling the class about teaching these exercises to neighborhood friends or to the family.
3. Practicing good posture before a full-length mirror.
4. Keeping personal improvement charts.
5. Drawing cartoons showing pictures of *poor* posture.

Suggested group activities include:

1. Composing and dramatizing poems and short plays.
2. Judging of posture by the children of their own group.
3. Demonstrating sitting posture showing the correct and exaggerating the incorrect way.
4. Using blocks to show the relationship of balance to the "straight man" and to the "crooked man."
5. Forming a password club and have the class decide on a secret word to be whispered to anyone who is seen slumping.
6. Playing a variety of games to develop strength, balance, and coordination such as the duck-walk relay, prancing horses, and the inch-worm race.
7. Doing a wide variety of relaxation mimetic activities such as rag doll, floating on your back, swinging the elephant's trunk.
8. Keeping unsigned reports on each child's own weekly sleep records. Having groups act out the correct and incorrect ways to get ready for bed.

---

[1] See Vannier, Maryhelen, Foster, Mildred, and Gallahue, David: *Teaching Physical Education in Elementary Schools*. 5th ed. Philadelphia: W. B. Saunders Co., 1973, for suggested materials and methods of teaching physical activities for this age group.

    9. Demonstrating body "uneven-ness" and "one-sidedness."
10. Making a cardboard skeleton using heavy paper and string to show the bones of the body; discuss how muscles move bones, what makes muscles grow.
11. Setting up a posture obstacle course in the classroom which has ropes at varying heights to jump over or crawl under, areas in which to walk with a book on the head, areas to jump over, etc. Discuss the relationship to body alignment of physical movement.
12. Use a doorway bar for hanging by the hands or by the knees.
13. Teaching rope climbing and chinning activities.

HEALTH EXAMINATIONS

Although some school authorities believe in giving annual physical examinations, others contend that each child should have a minimum of four periodic examinations. These should be given when the child enters the first grade, during the middle elementary experience, at the beginning of adolescence during junior high school years, and before leaving the senior high school. However, throughout a child's experience at school he should be referred to either the school physician or a specialist if a teacher's observation or the results of a screening test show some health problem. Each school district should determine how often, by whom, when, and where the physical examinations should be given.

The kind of medical examination given will, of course, vary from school to school. In general, the examination should include the following:

Nutritional status	Muscle tone
Eyes and eyelids	Posture
Ears and eardrums	Bones and joints
Skin and hair	Abdomen
Heart	Nose, throat, and tonsils
Lungs	Thyroid gland
Nervous system	Lymph nodes
Pulse rate when resting and after exercise	Teeth and gums

Teachers can and should make a great contribution to this phase of the school health program. Their chief contribution can be in helping each child understand (1) *why* he needs to be examined, (2) *what* the doctor will do (look into your ears, listen to your heart beat, etc.), and (3) by *talking with each pupil after the examination has been given* so that he gains an understanding of what the doctor told him. Although less such preparation is needed with older children who have previously been examined, it is still an important function of the elementary teacher. Some children magnify previous negative experiences among their peers, and thus a whole cluster of children can become upset over having an examination. However, the neglect of the teacher to capitalize upon teachable moments which evolve from the physical examination can cause many other similar types of disturbances and emotional upsets to arise. Ideally the parents should accompany their child when the examination is made. Since this is impossible for some parents, the teacher should do so, especially with primary youngsters. Unfortunately, the examining physician too often does not discuss the examination with the child or does not spend as much time with each person as he should. Consequently, the teacher can be of valuable assistance in making the examination an educational and personalized experience of major significance.

Form 3J.6—6-59—20M

LOS ANGELES CITY SCHOOL DISTRICTS
Auxiliary Services Division — Health Education and Health Services Branch

PHYSICIAN'S REPORT*

School_____   Date_____

GENERAL DATA   Totals

1. Routine physical examinations (complete)... _____
2. Physical examinations of children specially referred by school personnel................... _____
   Total Physical Examinations... _____
3. Health inspections for contagion, cafeteria work, readmissions, etc.................... _____
4. Routine athletic inspections.. _____
   Total Inspections... _____
5. Consultations with school personnel... _____
6. Consultations with parents **at school or by telephone**................................... _____
7. Consultations with private physicians, dentists, or others............................... _____
   Total Consultations.. _____
8. Home notices sent... _____
9. First aid given... _____
10. Sanitary inspections of school plant... _____
11. Lectures to faculty.. _____
    to parent-teacher associations.. _____
    to pupils... _____
    Total lectures.. _____

CONDITIONS FOUND	Needing Correction †	Under School Physician's Observation ††	Under Care *	Irremediable **
		CHECK ONLY ONE COLUMN		
1. Malnutrition				
2. Obesity				
3. Defective vision				
4. Diseases of the eyes				
5. Defective hearing				
6. Diseases of the ears				
7. Diseases of the nose and throat				
8. Tonsils (greatly enlarged or diseased)				
9. Dental defect (a) caries				
(b) malocclusion				
10. Heart defects (organic)				
11. Heart defects (functional or questionable)				
12. Chest diseases				
13. Chest deformities				
14. Orthopedic defects (a) posture				
(b) foot				
(c) miscellaneous				
15. Neurological diseases				
16. Nervous and emotional disorders				
17. Speech defects				
18. Skin diseases (communicable)				
19. Skin diseases (non communicable)				
20. Endocrine disorders				
21. Miscellaneous				
TOTALS				

†Definite recommendation is being made to parents
††For recheck or health counseling at school only
*Under care of private physician or clinic. No recommendation to be made at this time
**A congenital or acquired defect where medical or surgical treatment is not indicated.

Remarks_____

_____

_____M.D.
Examining Physician

Figure 3-7. Sample of physician's report. (Courtesy of Los Angeles Public Schools)

Health appraisal should be a continuing process which ranges from the health examination to the observations by the classroom teacher and to the last health evaluation in the final year of high school. Yet this appraisal is not an end to itself, but rather a means to helping each pupil gain better health.

The purpose of the school health examination should be to ascertain the state of each pupil's health, to discover defects, to provide the pupil with information concerning any existing deviation, to discover if the child can participate fully in

Form 33.364 (6-55)

LOS ANGELES CITY SCHOOL DISTRICTS ✱
Auxiliary Services Division — Health Education and Health Services Branch

Dear Parent: Your answers to the following questions will help the school to meet your child's needs in planning his school program and provide valuable information for our school records. Please fill out the answers and bring them with you or send them with your child.

HEALTH HISTORY FORM *

Date_____

School_____ Room_____

Name_____ Address_____ Phone_____

Birth Place_____ Birth Date_____ Grade_____

Family Doctor_____ Address_____
                                                    Date of last visit

Family Dentist_____ Address_____
                                                    Date of last visit

Please check any of the following conditions that your child has had:

Asthma		Chickenpox		Tires Easily	
Hayfever		Measles		Fainting	
Eczema		German Measles		When?	
Diabetis		Whooping Cough		Recent Bed Wetting	
Heart Disorder		Mumps		Nose Bleeds	
Poliomyelitis		Hernia		Growing Pains	
Pneumonia		Frequent Colds		Operations — what?	
Rheumatic Fever		Frequent Sore Throats			
Scarlet Fever		Frequent Coughs		Accidents	
Tuberculosis: Child		Frequent Headaches		Other Serious Illness	
Tuberculosis: Family		Wears Glasses		What?	

Has the child been immunized against the following: No   Yes   If Yes, give date or dates

Smallpox		
Diphtheria		
Whooping Cough		
Tetanus (Lockjaw)		
Poliomyelitis		
Others		

Family History:

Who lives in the home?	Yes?	No?	Health Condition
Father			
Mother			
Brothers — Ages			
Sisters — Ages			
Others			

Health Habits

Appetite _____ How much milk daily?_____
Any food allergies?_____ What?_____
What does child eat for breakfast?_____
What time does child go to bed?_____
What time does child get up?_____
Give any other health or behavior information you feel we should have:_____

_____
Signature of Parent

Figure 3-8. Sample health history form. (Courtesy of Los Angeles Public Schools)

SCHOOL:

Child's name:	Birth date:
Address:	Location:
Father's name:	Occupation: Business phone:
Mother's name:	Occupation: Home phone:

Emergency Care Plan

Physician's name:	Phone:
Address:	
Dentist's name:	Phone:
Address:	
Hospital:	Phone:

Health History			Immunization History				
	Kind	Date		Date	Date	Date	Comment
Measles			Diphtheria				
Poliomyelitis			Booster diph-				
Rheumatic			theria				
Fever			Whooping cough				
Tonsilitis			Tetanus				
Tuberculosis			D.P.T.				
Contact			Booster D.P.T.				
Operations			Poliomyelitis				
Accidents							
Other				Date	Result	Date	Result
			Smallpox				
			Tuberculin test				

Dental Health

Grade									
Date									
Needs attention									
Care received									
Decayed perm. teeth									
Missing perm. teeth									
Filled perm. teeth									

Health Appraisal by Physician   Code: O—satisfactory   X—needs attention

Grade					
Date					
Height (inches)					
Weight (pounds)					
Nutrition					
Skin and hair					
Eyes					
Vision					
Ears					
Hearing					
Nose and throat					
Teeth and gums					
Thyroid gland					
Lymph nodes					
Heart					
Lungs					
Abdomen					
Genitalia					
Nervous system					
Bones and joints					
Muscle tone					
Posture					
Any restrictions on physical activity					
Parent present					
Examining physician					

Figure 3-9. Sample cumulative school health record. (Courtesy of Bureau of Public Health Education, Indiana State Board of Health)

the school program, and to recommend modifications if he cannot, and most important of all, to provide a valuable positive health education experience for the child potent enough to develop within each youngster an appreciation of the importance of similar examinations throughout life. Unless parents, school authorities, and other adults are informed of the physical examination findings, few changes or real benefits can accrue from this experience.

Throughout the examination it is the physician who is the educator, with either positive or negative results, of the child being examined. Although ideally as much time as possible should be spent with each child, the large number of pupils to be examined usually prevent this ideal from becoming a reality. The examination itself should take a minimum of ten minutes per pupil, with a comparable amount of time given for counsel and health instruction.

Although health information and findings should be recorded by the school nurse as directed by the examining physicians, in smaller schools this duty is performed by a teacher. All examination records should be available to qualified school personnel. It is important that, since the health status of each child can greatly affect his success in school, each teacher closely examine the record of every child in her group each year. This not only will enable her to better understand the behavior of each individual in her class but also will assist her to know more about what to expect from each one; such records can also aid her in quickly spotting deviations from what is normal in the appearance and behavior of each child.

PREVENTION AND CONTROL OF COMMUNICABLE DISEASES

All schools should have written policies concerning the exclusion and readmission of students who have communicable diseases, the kinds of immunizations required for school admission, and procedures to be followed in the event of an epidemic. Teachers, the school administrator, the public health department, local physician, and parents should work closely together in formulating such policies and help enforce these policies once they have been adopted.

The classroom teacher is the key person in the prevention of the spread of communicable diseases in the school. It is her duty to teach children the reasons *why* they should cover their mouths when sneezing or coughing, wash their hands after going to the bathroom, keep disease-transmitting objects such as pencils, pens, and crayons out of their mouths, not drink from another's cup or use another's personal toilet articles, or avoid getting too overheated, chilled, or too tired. Furthermore, they should supervise their pupils as much as possible, to see that these desirable health habits are carried out, for what a child does with what he learns is the key to a successful health education program.

This is real health education and is far more important than following a daily health lesson plan and/or ignoring health education opportunities which have arisen in the meantime. Children must be reminded over and over again to do things before habits are formed. The building of positive daily health habits should be the chief objective of the health education program on the primary level.

The daily health observation program is invaluable for the early detection of those coming down with a contagious disease. If the school nurse is unavailable (some schools share one nurse with several buildings) and the teacher knows that both parents of the child work and would not be home, she should see to it that the child is isolated at school and, if ill enough, put to bed. Here again the child should be taught why he is being isolated and why he must go to bed. School health policies should contain written directives concerning procedures for removing an ill child from school and what to do with him if he cannot be taken home, as well as what to do in other types of emergencies. Such policies should be drawn up by a committee of teachers and the principal. Those who have had courses in health education should take a leading role in the formulation of these and other similar policies regarding health and its protection in the school. It is during such experiences that they can teach and guide their colleagues. The skilled educator can, should, and does work with people of many ages and educational backgrounds in many kinds of environments both in and away from the school building.

Signs of the early stages of most communicable diseases include:

Flushed or pale face, "glassy eyes," runny nose
Excessive sneezing and coughing
Light blue or pale lips and fingernails
Rash or other unusual skin conditions
Swollen glands
Body temperature above 99 ° F
Listlessness or unusual overactivity

Both the teacher and her pupils must not only be able to recognize these signs but also know exactly what to do when they appear. Several class lessons about communicable diseases can be built, and emphasis should be placed in each of these units upon preventive measures.

HEALTH RECORDS

Carefully kept health records provide the teacher with valuable information regarding each pupil. They should also serve as a means of making a careful study of the health needs of each class group as well as of each child in each grade. This information should guide the teacher's selection of materials to teach to her class and be the basis upon which the health education program is built. These records should be kept by school physicians, nurses, dentists, secretaries, and teachers. They also enable the instructor to better adjust the school program to the limitations of those needing such an arrangement. The records should be cumulative from the time the child enters until he leaves school, and they should follow him from one school to another. Most states have adopted such records, which are relatively standardized in schools within each state. The cumulative records should contain:

The name, age, and correct address of each pupil
The name and address of the parents
The name of the family physician, dentist, and the preferred hospital in case of an emergency
How and where the parents or guardian of the child can be reached in case of an emergency
Where the father works and type of work he does; if the mother works, where, and type of work she does
A health history of all communicable diseases, operations, and other pertinent information
Immunization record
Allergies or other conditions which affect health
Height and weight records; body (Wetzel grid)
Remediable defects, recommended corrections, and a follow-up record

Date_____

Dear Parent:

    In planning a school health program which meets the individual needs of your child, it is necessary for the school to secure from you certain information about your child. Please fill in and return to the school the information requested on this sheet.

_____School

General Information

Name of Pupil_____ Date of Birth: Year____ Month____ Day____
School_____ Race_____ Sex_____
Name of Parent — Guardian_____
Residence Address_____ Phone_____
Business Address_____ Phone_____
Family Physician_____ Dentist_____

In case of accident phone $\left\{ \begin{array}{l} \text{Father} \\ \text{Mother} \end{array} \right\}$ at_____

                          Family Physician at_____

In case the child requires emergency care while at school, phone_____ or take to Dr._____

Diseases that child has had: (If year unknown, write **yes**).

Disease	Year	Disease	Year	Disease	Year
Measles		Infantile Paralysis		Running Ear	
German Measles		Sore Throat (Frequent)		Worms (Type)	
Mumps		Rheumatic Fever		Rupture	
Chickenpox		Heart Disease		Typhoid Fever	
Whooping Cough		Headache (Frequent)		Convulsions	
Diphtheria		Asthma and Hay Fever			

Other Diseases, Injuries, or Operations (Explain):

_____

Inoculations child has had: (If year unknown, write **yes**).

Basic Series	**Booster**
Diphtheria_____	_____
Whooping Cough_____	_____
Tetanus_____	_____
Smallpox_____	_____
Typhoid Fever_____	_____

Request for Health Services

_____School, through its approved facilities, is given authority and hereby requested to serve my child when clinics are held for any of the following:

(**Note to School Personnel:** List here all the health services rendered through your school such as smallpox vaccination, typhoid inoculations, etc.)

Signed_____
                           (Parent or guardian)

Figure 3-10. Sample health history form for parents to fill out. (Courtesy of Los Angeles Public Schools)

Recommendations concerning nonremediable conditions (birth injuries, etc.) and suggestions concerning a modified school program, and a record of such program

Teachers' daily observations of permanent and/or significant deviations which will lead to better understanding of the child

Dental examination results

Physical examination results

Physical fitness test results

Results of social tests in which children reveal how they feel about themselves and others

Record of emotional problems

Attendance reports

Individual cumulative health records should be filed in a central office and be easily accessible to all teachers and other authorized personnel for professional use.

HEALTH GUIDANCE

The health history, physical examination results, and other valuable information contained in each pupil's cumulative health record are the basis upon which an adequate group as well as an individual health guidance program should be built.

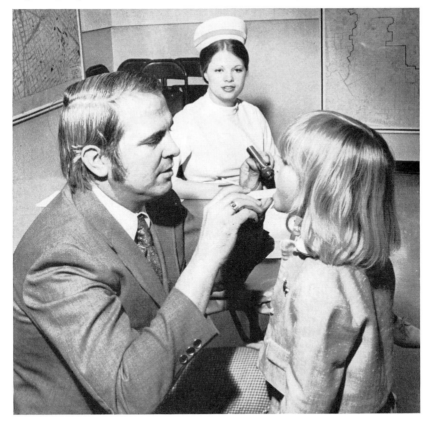

Figure 3-11. All children should have their teeth examined by a dentist at least once a year. (Courtesy of Dallas *Morning News*)

In cases requiring the school program to be adjusted to meet the needs of any pupil, it is the duty of both the school nurse and teacher to see that such changes are made. There are many possibilities for the development of a splendid program in health guidance built around the teacher's daily health appraisal of each pupil through observation, tests, and physical examinations. Such a guidance program in the elementary school must also reach the parents. Clearly children do not know what to do, nor can they correct decayed teeth, faulty vision, or malnutrition, so that teachers must motivate parents to act in the best interests of their children's health. In some cases, formal written notes to parents sent by the school nurse or doctor will get results.* Personal interviews, at school or at home if necessary, make for a warmer, more productive atmosphere wherein the teacher can often gain the cooperation of the parents in seeing to it that their child's health deficiencies are corrected so that he will do well in school. A determined teacher will keep trying to reach parents who are almost impossible to motivate into desired action for the well-being of their own child.

Throughout the school day, the teacher has many opportunities for group or individual health guidance. A chat before or after school with the pupil who returns to class following a long illness, or with the girl who is obviously getting a cold, or a boy who needs glasses—all constitute guidance opportunities geared to help the child desire to reach to obtain better health. Class discussions during or following a health lesson or a film or at the many other teachable moments in every school day open up numerous guidance channels and opportunities. Guidance is more than giving advice or warning, preaching or praising in an attempt to motivate action, for it requires mature judgment, a deep understanding of human behavior, and a knowledge of ways in which the individual can be directed toward and helped to obtain professional assistance when needed.

As has been often pointed out, each child comes to school wrapped up in a package of his social and economic background, his cultural heritage, and the era into which he is born, and although each child appears to sit alone on his little red chair in the classroom, he is far from alone for:

> his family came with him. Their values are present, coloring his values, and therefore his behavior. What he possesses, acquired in a few years, is largely the values current in his household. It is through these meanings that he gives significance to the things that happen in the classroom. The skills learning which he brings in are home-made. The teacher who receives him, the society which requires his presence, the future which banks on him, must remember this in anything they do for him, or in anything they expect him to do for himself.[2]

Just as each child takes his family to school with him, the teacher must get to know and gain the cooperation of the parents if she is to teach each individual youngster successfully. Every teacher should not only know as much about each of her pupils as she can find out but also as much about his home environment as she can discover. Likewise, she and the parents of each child must be closely working partners, striving for the development of each youngster.

---

* See the Appendix for the suggested form letter to the parents.
[2] Ramsey, Marie: *Toward Maturity, How Children Think and Grow.* New York: Barnes & Noble, 1947, p. 4.

PARENT-TEACHER CONFERENCES

Conferences between parents and teachers can yield a rich harvest of understanding and help build a team approach for helping children with problems, as well as produce feelings of mutual respect and admiration. All such meetings must be carefully planned for desired results. Found below are suggestions for making such a conference become a rich learning experience for both parties concerned:

WHO: There may be times when the conference should be parent-teacher-pupil, but it is usually better if conferences can be parents-teacher conferences.

WHAT: Planned meeting between parent and teacher to report on the child's progress and/or discuss mutual problems.

WHY: "To develop a closer relationship between teacher and parent so that through mutual understanding and cooperation they may work for the child's benefit."—Highland Park PTA Book

WHEN: Preferably at some permanently scheduled time—that is at a time set aside by the teacher for conferences—after school, off-periods, etc., particularly at the beginning of the year and when occasion demands.

WHERE: If possible, in the home of the child, as well as at the school.

HOW: The PTA might give special notices to all the parents informing them of the parent-teacher conference plan. The teacher might call each parent or write a note, on the report card perhaps, giving the parent the teacher's schedule and issuing an invitation for a conference. The follow-up might be a phone call, or the parent may be invited to call the school office and make an appointment with the teacher.

DO

1. Do plan conferences with *all* parents.
2. Do tell the parents the aim of the conference.
3. Do expect and welcome both mother and father at parent conferences: they should be *parents-teacher* conferences.
4. Do be friendly, interested, relaxed, and to the point.
5. Do accept and respect the personalities of the parents.
6. Do listen to what parents have to say.
7. Do try to find out all you can about the child without trying to pry.
8. Do be completely honest in matters of fact.
9. Do begin and end in a positive manner.
10. Do have representative material of the child's work, a fair sampling containing examples of both good and bad work to show parents.
11. Do have physical test information in lay language to give to the parents.
12. Do have the child's cumulative record, or information contained therein, on hand for reference.
13. DO PLAN CONFERENCES IN ADVANCE.

DON'T

1. Don't try to confer with parent when either parent or teacher is emotionally upset.
2. Don't try to crowd a conference into too short a time.
3. Don't try to cover too much material.
4. Don't compare the child with other children or with brothers or sisters in his family.
5. Don't try to "out-talk" the parent.
6. Don't quote capacity or mental ability (I.Q.) test scores to parents.
7. Don't make conferences too formal.

8. Don't alarm parents with "norms," "means," or other statistics of a professional nature which they may not understand; i.e., avoid use of professional jargon.
9. Don't repeat any personal material.
10. Don't sit behind the desk if at all possible.
11. Don't say anything to the parent that you would mind the child knowing.

Discussion Questions

1. What are differences between a screening test and a physical examination in relationship to personnel, time, cost, activities, and recommendations?
2. What is the role of the classroom teacher in daily observation of the appearance of each member of the class?
3. What is the Snellen E-symbol chart used in a screening test for vision? For whom should it be used?
4. How is hearing tested by the use of a discrete frequency audiometer?
5. What is the Wetzel grid? How can it best be used?
6. Explain and illustrate by giving examples of the statement that "children need to grow in many ways other than just physically."
7. What are the most common posture defects? How can they be discovered?
8. Discuss the seven causes of poor posture given in this chapter.
9. Which of the suggested individual learning suggestions mentioned in this chapter seem to you to be best for arousing a child's desire to have good posture?
10. What information should the cumulative health record contain?

Things To Do

1. Using the plumb-line test, check the posture of five classmates.
2. Using the Snellen eye chart, discover if any of your classmates should be referred to an eye specialist.
3. Write a two-page report on any chapter in any book in the suggested readings for this chapter. Read your paper aloud in class.
4. Using the coin click or whisper test, screen test the hearing of your classmates.
5. Role play a parent-teacher conference showing first the wrong and then the right techniques the teacher should use in order to get the best results.
6. Refer to the Red Cross First Aid textbook. With a partner, demonstrate the first aid treatment for a broken bone and for arterial bleeding.
7. Weigh and measure your classmates in order to find which ones are below or above the norms for their ages.
8. Interview a school nurse about her duties, problems, and the role she plays in health education. Report your findings to your classmates.
9. Using the list of the areas to be covered in a daily observation of health status, observe any five persons other than your classmates twice in one week. Share your conclusions in class.
10. Bring to class magazine pictures for a bulletin board on "Teaching Health through Appraisal Activities."

Suggested Readings

Alonso, Lon: "What the Classroom Teacher Can Do for the Child with Impaired Vision." *NEA Journal* 56:42–43, 1967.
Bothwell, Hazel: "What the Classroom Teacher Can Do for the Child with Impaired Hearing." *NEA Journal,* 56:44–46, 1967.
Byrd, Oliver: *School Health Administration.* Philadelphia; W. B. Saunders Co., 1964.
Katzin, Herbert, and Wilson, Geraldine: *Strabismus in Childhood.* St. Louis: C. V. Mosby Co., 1968.

Lowman, Charles L. and Young, Carl H.: *Postural Fitness.* Philadelphia: Lea & Febiger, 1960.

Metropolitan Life Insurance Company: *Absent from School Today; What Teachers See; The School Administrator; Physician and Nurse in the School Health Program.* New York: The Company.

National Society for the Prevention of Blindness: *Screening, Eye Examinations, and Follow Up; An Eye Health Program for Schools; The Snellen Eye Chart.* New York: The Society.

Nemier, Alma: *The School Health Program.* 3rd ed. Philadelphia: W. B. Saunders Co., 1970.

Rogers, J. F.: *What Every Teacher Should Know about the Physical Condition of Her Pupils.* Pamphlet No. 68. Washington, D.C.: United States Office of Education, 1945.

Turner, C. E., Sellery, C. M., and Smith, Sara: *School Health and Health Education.* 6th ed. St. Louis: C. V. Mosby Co., 1970.

Wheatley, G. M., and Hallock, Grace: *Health Observation of School Children.* 3rd ed. New York: McGraw-Hill Book Co., 1971.

CHAPTER 4

teaching health through the school environment

There is no justification for forcing children by law to attend schools conducted in dirty, drab, unsanitary, or even dangerously unsafe buildings. Nor is there logic in teaching children the necessity of washing their hands after going to the bathroom if the school does not provide soap, warm water, and towels. Whether the school building is well kept or neglected, school housekeeping adhered to or ignored, the school lunch program properly or improperly conducted, play space assigned and facilities designed wisely or foolishly, precautions taken or avoided for safety protection from fire or other disasters, will, along with other facets of school environmental conditions, accelerate or deter the development of proper health attitudes, appreciation, and understanding. The total school environment and teachers must serve as models if children are to *want* to develop good health practices they can carry out at school and at home, or when they become adults. Emerson's statement, "What you *are* sounds so loudly in my ears that I cannot hear a word you are saying," is well worth remembering as is our old folk saying of "Actions speak louder than words." The school administrator, teachers, and all other school personnel must practice what they preach if children are to learn through indirect as well as direct health teaching methods. Educators know that the "whole child" who goes to school is greatly affected by the "whole school."

The members of a class of teachers in training were recently required to write a paper recalling their most potent learning experiences during their own elementary school years. The majority of these experiences resulted in fears and foolish concepts, although some remembered the use of the fun approach to learning by some ingenious educator. One girl believed for years that she would have a baby if she kissed a boy, for her little friends were convinced and, in turn, "taught" her that this was so. Another student believed that a pregnant woman was one punished by God for sucking her finger—a practice he was taught at home would cause the stomach to swell. Many of the class wrote that they could still "see" and even "smell" how certain classrooms looked, for either they were unpleasant, poorly ventilated, or made suddenly a place of magic by a color-appreciative teacher who, with a few cut-out red, yellow, or green figures, could capture the attention of a child and long keep in mind's memory *that* room, *that* teacher, and *that* time in life. Delia Sharp's splendid book *This I Remember, Teacher* is full of such lasting learning experiences, as is Leo Deuel's *Teachers Treasure Chest* or Alice Humphrey's *Heaven in My Hand*. Most of the memorable childhood experiences related by these authors took place not only in the classroom, but also on the playground, in the toilets, or while coming to or going from school.

Teachers must realize that there is learning wherever there is life, but that learning can be positive or negative, depending largely on leadership. Education is by no means confined to a school or classroom or can be gained only from reading a book, for children often learn more outside than inside schools and more from their playmates and parents than from their teachers. The school buildings, grounds, and other parts of the total school environment, like a bulletin board, can be silent but powerfully effective teachers. Educators do not have sole possession of education. Because of their professional preparation, skill in imparting knowledge and shaping attitudes, and sensitivity and belief in children, they can, however, become a potent and positive factor in the total development of the children with whom they work.

THE USE AND MAINTENANCE OF SCHOOL BUILDINGS

The one-room rural school of yesterday is rapidly disappearing in America. It is being replaced by consolidated community schools that are much larger, more attractive, and more functional. Increasingly, all environmental factors which influence health are being taken into consideration by architects and school-sponsored committees who plan new buildings or the reconstruction of old ones. Since all plans for new buildings and their sanitation must be approved by the state board of education and state board of health, children are now being taught in an improved environment.

Whether the building is old or new, it must be *more* than just a building, for it is a vital part of the environment in which children are educated. It is imperative that the school be a healthy, happy place which children will look forward to coming to throughout their entire education with as much eagerness and joy as they did as first graders. The sharp increase in school vandalism in the past decade is not only a national disgrace, but should be a warning signal to educators as well as parents that children need more than increased discipline. Children must somehow regain the almost reverent feelings the earliest Americans had not only for education but also for the schoolhouse itself, for this building was preceded only by the erection of the church in any newly established community settlement. In our time of distorted values, wherein the rights, privileges, and property of others never become the concern of the "me-first" individual striving to get ahead at any cost, children must be given opportunity to do things for themselves instead of being waited on and pampered by adult servants (teachers and parents included) who rob any child of rich learning experiences every time they tie his shoes or zip up his snowsuit. There is wisdom in Bernard Shaw's statement, "If you teach me, I shall never learn."

One reason the Tyler Public School Camp and other school camps throughout the nation rarely have walls defaced or ruined by children is that the youngsters at these camps are given increased responsibility for the care and maintenance of their own living environment. The program at many of these camps is built around (1) learning to live with others in the out-of-doors, (2) healthful personal and community living, (3) basic campcraft skills, (4) work experiences, and (5) conservation projects. According to many school camp directors, the favorite camp activities are taking care of animals (what a rich health education opportunity this is), cabin clean-up duties, making erosion check dams, meal planning and outdoor cooking, milking, and weather forecasting.

Although millions of children do not attend any kind of a camp, educators might well seriously consider why the educational experience found in camping is so appealing to children, or why research has disclosed that a child can learn more in an eight-week camp under good leadership than he can in a whole year in school. The reason could well be that children at camp are given *real* responsibility for their own well-being and that of others. Every teacher, whether she works as a camp counselor or classroom educator, must provide opportunities for children to form desirable health habits in their daily lives and instill in them a feeling of responsibility for controlling and improving their own working, playing, and living environment.

THE TEACHER'S EXAMPLE

Although an abundance of well-selected teaching aids coupled with an attractive, sanitary, and well-kept building are vastly important in teaching health and instilling positive health habits, without a good teacher these are of little value. A real teacher is one who not only sets a healthful example worthy of pupil emulation but also provides an exciting and stimulating classroom atmosphere. All children need teachers who enjoy being and working with children, who respect them as unique individuals, and who set firm but secure behavior boundaries. Such teachers are loved by children, who want to be like them.

Teaching requires good health, stamina, patience, a sense of humor, plus many other qualities which will enable an older person to work patiently and successfully with youngsters. It is important that educators have recreational outlets during their leisure hours every day, as well as legitimate outlets for feelings of hostility and rejection through sports, games, or other types of recreation. Those who balance work and play in their daily lives will be less apt to project feelings of aggression felt toward a superior down upon their smaller charges who cannot fight back. Interests in many outside school activities and periodic health checkups help teachers to maintain an even keel in the classroom, as well as help them become outstanding leaders for children. Such teachers are both fun and profitable to be with and are the ones most eagerly sought by children.

THE CLASSROOM AND OTHER FACILITIES

Children who go to school in a relaxed but controlled learning environment feel both secure and happy. In such an atmosphere of security they are being given freedom of movement, responsibility in planning what they are to learn (guided by the teacher), and greater responsibility in helping to make and keep the classroom their own—a place of friends, fun, adventure, and beauty. The modern schoolroom is full of enchanting equipment and movable furniture sized correctly for each pupil, and a happy, cheerful atmosphere permeates it. Here the curriculum is both carefully planned and flexible, and each child is made aware that what he learns today or this year will dovetail into tomorrow and the next grade and into what he wants to be and do when "grown up." Each child finds that planning what he will do in order to learn is an adventure in itself. Helping children plan for, select, and carry out what they will experience is masterful teaching and requires far more skill than telling children what to do and how to do it.

Students should be encouraged to move their seats around in the room in order to obtain the best light. Since so many health learning opportunities are inherent in the care of plants and animals, pupils should become responsible for the daily care of fish, birds, hamsters, rabbits, a garden, flowers, etc. Facilities should also be provided for the group so that each can hang up his own hat and coat and put his rubbers or boots in an assigned space. Each child should be encouraged to become increasingly independent from adults by receiving praise from his teacher for taking such good care of himself and his possessions.

The emotional climate of the classroom is of paramount importance. Learning can be greatly spurred on or reined back by teacher enthusiasm and encouragement or pupil frustration and fear. Jealousy, lying, cheating, tattling, and obvious signs of inferiority feelings are warning signs that pupil-teacher relationships are strained. All children should feel secure and adequate and believe that going to school is a great adventure. The slow learner must feel as secure as the rest of his classmates. Although the teacher should discuss with the children behavior standards that are to be maintained in order that the classroom and school be a place in which the best kind of learning can take place, the pupils should also help devise conduct rules which will provide a desirable educational and living environment. All adopted rules must be promptly, firmly, and consistently enforced and pupils made well aware that all such standards have been established primarily for their benefit. The teacher should treat each child alike. Studies show that children like teachers best who are firm, fair to all, and consistent in what they do. The most successful educators are those who can share magical things with children, can make them excited about what they are learning, and who expect success for each learner in each group. Children, as well as adults, respond to such an adventure and such challenge. It is imperative that each pupil feels that he is making progress, for nothing destroys learning desire and self-confidence more than repeated failure without hope of success or motivating words of encouragement to keep on trying. It is unwise to take away the recess periods from those who misbehave or fail to complete their work, for either is often a sign of pent-up tensions and rebellion which can best be relieved through increased physical activity.

Although the physical maintenance of the room is the responsibility of the school custodian, the teacher and children should make every effort to see to it that their classroom is as healthful and attractive as possible. Included below are suggestions of things pupils can do to make this phase of the total school health program functional and meaningful:

Lighting
1. Adjust the window blinds according to changing light conditions.
2. Move seats around so that the light can be used most advantageously.

3. Keep windows free from pasted-on pictures or curtains which interfere with proper lighting.
4. Do not pile boxes or books on window sills.

Ventilation

1. Assign to one student the honor of reading the room thermometer or regulating the thermostat properly under supervision. Rotate this privilege among different members of the class.
2. Adjust windows, if the building is not air conditioned, to changing weather conditions. Use air deflectors when necessary so that no child sits in a draft.
3. Open doors into halls and ventilate the room frequently.
4. Adjust seating according to temperature readings, if need be.
5. Help children become conscious of the weather and room temperature. Teach those in the upper elementary school how to forecast the weather. Have a daily or weekly forecaster.[1]

Drinking Facilities

1. Provide adequate facilities (one drinking fountain for every 75 pupils).
2. Teach children to use the fountains properly.
3. Devise a few but strongly enforced rules regarding pushing and shoving around the fountain or while someone is drinking.
4. Insist that no one drop gum or other objects into the basins.
5. Keep fountains clean and sanitary at all times.
6. Provide individual paper cups.

Hand-washing Facilities

1. Provide adequate facilities (one wash basin for every 50 pupils).
2. Demonstrate the correct way to wash one's hands; supervise each child as he does so the first day at school, and frequently thereafter.
3. Provide adequate warm water, soap, and paper towels.
4. Enforce the rule that those who soil the basin must wipe it clean again and all other rules devised by the class.
5. Provide mirrors near the basin and encourage children to keep themselves neat and clean at all times.

Toilet Facilities

1. Provide adequate toilet facilities (one commode for every 30 girls and one for every 60 boys, one urinal for every 30 boys).
2. Teach children the necessity of flushing the toilet every time it is used; build in them a feeling of civic pride for having a well-cared-for restroom.
3. Take all children on a complete tour of the school building and grounds the first day of school so that they know which is the boy's restroom and which one is for the girls. Explain carefully the reason each has a room for themselves, in contrast to the family bathroom.
4. Train and encourage children to report uncleanliness in use of facilities or writing of "dirty words" on the walls to the teacher, janitor, or principal.
5. Supervise frequently the use of toilet facilities by class groups. Be sure that each child knows how to use each facility properly.

THE SCHOOL LUNCH ROOM

Although the consolidation of small schools into larger districts has resulted in lunchroom service in many rural areas, there are still isolated one-room school-

---

[1] Fisher, Robert: *How About The Weather?* New York, Harper & Row; *Weather.* Boy Scout Handbook, No. 3816. New York: Boy Scouts of America; Girl Scout Weather Handbook, No. 19-503, New York: Girl Scouts of America.

houses to which children come on horseback or foot instead of by school bus or in the family car, and there are many areas where pupils bring their own lunches in a paper bag or lunchbox, instead of buying it at low cost from the school cafeteria. Regardless of where the children eat or who prepares the food, the lunch period should be a time for rich learning experiences, for this period in the child's school day abounds in many daily life-related educational opportunities. Although basic nutritional principles can be taught in the classroom, the lunchroom is the laboratory for those principles to be put into practice, and teachers can see for themselves how effectively the children have learned and are applying what was taught them about nutrition. The school lunch offers a wide variety of opportunities to integrate materials gleaned from all areas of the curriculum, but especially in social studies, arithmetic, health, and physical education. The whole program should be far more than merely a feeding one. Its success depends primarily upon the knowledge, desire, and interest of the classroom teacher, who should either eat with her group or supervise them as they eat, and her cooperation with all other school personnel who are connected with this phase of the school program.

Learning experiences which are inherent in the school lunch program include:

1. Developing proper hand-washing habits as actually carried out and supervised before each meal.
2. Creating an interest in choosing food wisely.
3. Selecting a nutritious lunch in the classroom as guided by the teacher from the menu written on the board before the actual lunch period begins.
4. The proper way to store lunches brought from home.
5. Enlisting the cooperation of parents in helping their children select or bring to school a nutritious lunch by sending them in advance the weekly lunch menu and encouraging them to guide their children into selecting the right foods.
6. Encouraging children to eat new kinds of food and making efforts to develop good food selection an intelligent habit; gauging serving size to fit child-size appetites.
7. Helping children learn the value of eating slowly, the necessity of chewing food thoroughly, and being relaxed and happy when eating.
8. Encouraging the practice of good eating habits:
   a) correct use of silverware and napkins
   b) not talking with food in the mouth
   c) contribution to the conversation and listening to what others say
   d) keeping one's voice low and avoiding unnecessary noise
   e) waiting until all are served before starting to eat
   f) saying "thank you," "please," or "excuse me" at the proper time

THE SCHOOL PLAYGROUND

Playground activities should do more than merely add fleeting pleasure, for they should enrich the leisure time of all children as well as develop physical fitness. By teaching obedience to rules, taking turns, accepting defeat as well as victory, children learn to get along with others as well as gain a working set of values. No child can live in a world by himself, even though some few may escape through daydreams to such a desired place. The school playground can be a place where the child learns the give and take of life, a lesson he must learn if he is ever to grow up.

For all recess and supervised free-play periods, pupils should be assigned a specific play space. Many activities can be dangerous if unsupervised. Although children are not as interested in safety as they are in being daring, adults must help them realize that they can have the most fun over a longer time period if they remain free from accidents or injury. Safety education means learning to take chances wisely. Accidents can often be the most teachable moment to impress upon others why they should be careful, for then children can see what actually happens when a person has not done the right thing.

The teacher and pupils must jointly assume responsibility for safety on the playground as well as in the gymnasium. The specific duties of each might well include the following:

The Teacher

1. Check and keep all equipment in good repair at all times.
2. Find all hazards with pupils and mark in bright yellow paint.
3. Direct all pupils in safety measures to be taken.
4. Teach all children how to use apparatus and equipment correctly.
5. Discuss with the class why they should not do certain things while on the playground which might interfere with the safety of anyone else.
6. Use activities which minimize accident possibilities.
7. Insist that all children wear suitable apparel for all activities.
8. Do not permit pupils to try new, more dangerous activities until they become skilled enough to do so.
9. Insist that all game rules be obeyed at all times.
10. Never leave an assigned group.

The Children

1. Stay in assigned play areas.
2. Assist the teacher in discovering and painting all hazards with bright yellow paint.
3. Take turns using swings and other equipment, and report to the teacher those who do not.
4. Report to the teacher any equipment which is broken or is faulty.
5. Come to the teacher when hurt in any way so that needed first-aid treatment can be given.
6. Serve as a member of a school playground safety-patrol club.
7. Tour the grounds accompanied by the teacher discussing and discovering safe and unsafe play places.
8. Dramatize going to the right person in case of an injury.
9. Dramatize safe and unsafe ways to play.

Since the vast majority of all accidents which occur at school happen on the playground during unsupervised play periods, it is imperative that children become especially safety-conscious during recess and play periods before and after school. The school administrator and teacher assigned to teach physical activities or supervise free-play periods are legally responsible should an accident occur, if it can be proven they were negligent, which can easily be done if they were not with the group they were assigned to supervise. Likewise, the school administrator and teacher must work closely together and plan recess activities wisely, provide safe play equipment, and assign playground space in the area for each class. Areas should be assigned so that there is opportunity for the greatest number to play safely at one time. At least five acres should be provided for elementary schools or a minimum of 100 square feet per pupil. The grounds should be fenced in, and the youngest grades assigned space closest to the building and widely separated from the older children. Regardless of whether the surface is cement, blacktop, grass turf, or sawdust combined with asphalt, it should be an area where the play will be safe and healthful. Backstop fences for softball and enclosed swing and apparatus areas are recommended. Space should be provided for sandbox play. All outdoor equipment should be chosen from the viewpoint of safety. Jungle gyms and horizontal hanging bars should hang 36 inches from the ground for primary children but may be up to 54 inches for older groups. Canvas-seat swings hung 10 to 12 inches from the ground, slides, monkey rings, parallel bars, merry-go-rounds, manila or hemp climbing ropes, horizontal ladders, low graded to high circular traveling rings, and a heavy rope giant stride are exciting facilities on which children love to play. They also enjoy playing with big boxes, climbing on old logs laid parallel to the ground, and jumping over things. One reason, of course, they are so attracted to these types of activities is that their use presents a challenge, contains elements of danger, and are fun to master.

SCHOOL SANITATION

One of the best ways to impress upon pupils that their school is a sanitary place and that they have an important part in keeping it that way, is to take them on a complete tour of the building. They should visit the furnace and air conditioning rooms in order to learn how temperature is regulated, see how the school disposes of its sewage, garbage, and rubbish, observe how school lunches are prepared, food stored, dishes washed, and the procedures used for proper food handling. A visit to the city water department and water filtering plant will help impress upon young minds the value of pure water, as well as inform them of the methods used to make and keep it safe.

Thus we see that children can and should be taught valued health practices through the school environment itself by (1) giving them direct purposeful responsibilities in the care and maintenance of their own assigned areas at school, and (2) having them actually visit and see for themselves, rather than reading or hearing about, the environment at school in which they learn, work, and play.

SCHOOL SAFETY

School safety is a must, for the chief cause of death among children is accidents. Accidental death is more prevalent than death caused by the total of the five leading diseases affecting children aged 1 to 14.

There must be a balance between safety protection and safety education. Overprotection can be damaging to youth. Gradually each child should be given more opportunities to assume responsibility for his own safety and to know what to do in case of an emergency.

The main goals of the school safety program should be to help all students to:

1. Prevent accidents.
2. Eradicate hazards.
3. Develop safety habits at home, school, and play.
4. Learn what to do and from whom to seek help in case of an emergency.
5. Realize the relationship of saftey to individual and group success and happiness.

Home Safety

Home accidents cause discomfort, harm, and even death to thousands of children yearly. Most injuries occur in the kitchen. Cuts, burns, and falls constitute the major portion of these accidents. In the bathroom it is falls, electric shock, and poisoning. Falls and injuries to hands, feet, and toes by power mowers are also common accidents which happen to people of all ages at home. Children should be taught at school as well as in the home to be careful while there as well as at school and especially so in certain areas of both places.

Safety Coming to and from School

Children in the primary grades are especially vulnerable to accidents and are most apt to be seriously injured by morning traffic coming to and from school. Many are bitten by dogs or injured by other animals or insects. All elementary school children are also in danger of being picked up and molested by sex perverts. Pushers are increasingly trying to "hook" children on drugs and will often entice them to become so by offering candy mildly sprinkled with narcotics to them.

Although there are many advantages found in having children walk to and from school, in large cities many parents now drive their children back and forth, even though this, too, is also taking a risk.

The School Safety Patrol

Safety-patrol uniform usually is a white San Browne 2-inch wide belt and a white or yellow helmet. Patrols composed of sixth-grade or older boys should be supervised by an on-duty policeman or woman or volunteer parents when children are crossing streets or highways going to or from school. Patrol boys should stay behind the curb and guide the pupils safely across the street. All children should remain on the curb until the signal is given for them to cross safely. Patrol rules should be taught and reviewed every school year and be strictly enforced at all times.

The School Bus

Although the major responsibility for the children's safety is that of the bus driver, children should be taught many safety practices when riding in the bus. Increasingly schools are using adult volunteers or older boys as school-bus patrol members. The duties of such persons include helping children on and off the bus, checking attendance, seeing that all passengers have stay-in assigned seats, seeing that all carried items are securely placed in racks, helping pupils to cross streets when leaving the bus upon the signal of the driver, and assisting the driver in all emergency situations.

Fire Drills

Fire and nuclear fallout drills are required to be held periodically by local as well as state laws. In areas where floods, cyclones, and tornadoes are frequent, safety drills are also a must. All children should know exactly where they are to go and what they should do when such a catastrophe occurs. Legally both the school and its teachers are responsible to (1) remove all school environmental hazards; (2) cooperate with local emergency agencies such as firemen or policemen; (3) teach emergency safety practices; and (4) inspect periodically all fire prevention devices and correct all deficiencies.

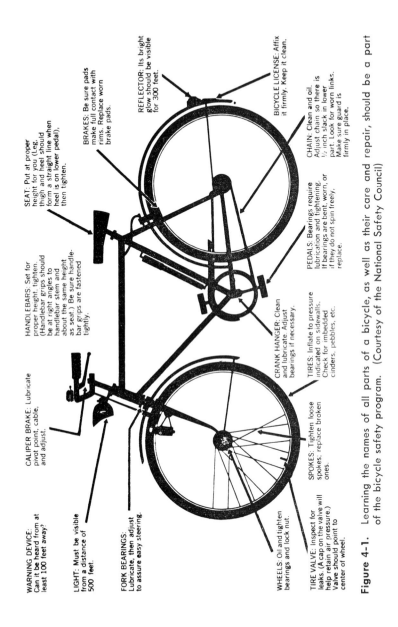

REFLECTOR: Its bright glow should be visible for 300 feet.

BICYCLE LICENSE: Affix it firmly. Keep it clean.

BRAKES: Be sure pads make full contact with rims. Replace worn brake pads.

SEAT: Put at proper height for you (Leg, thigh and heel should form a straight line when heel is on lower pedal), then tighten.

CHAIN: Clean and oil. Adjust chain so there is ½ inch slack in lower part. Look for worn links. Make sure guard is firmly in place.

HANDLEBARS: Set for proper height, tighten. (Handlebar grips should be at right angles to handlebar stem and about the same height as seat.) Be sure handlebar grips are fastened tightly.

PEDALS: Bearings require lubrication and tightening. If bearings are bent, worn, or if they do not spin freely, replace.

CRANK HANGER: Clean and lubricate. Adjust bearings if necessary.

TIRES: Inflate to pressure indicated on sidewalls. Check for imbedded cinders, pebbles, etc.

CALIPER BRAKE: Lubricate pivot point, cable, and adjust.

WARNING DEVICE: Can it be heard from at least 100 feet away?

LIGHT: Must be visible from a distance of 500 feet.

FORK BEARINGS: Lubricate, then adjust to assure easy steering.

WHEELS: Oil and tighten bearings and lock nut.

SPOKES: Tighten loose spokes; replace broken ones.

TIRE VALVE: Inspect for leaks. (A cap on the valve will help retain air pressure.) Valve should point to center of wheel.

Figure 4-1. Learning the names of all parts of a bicycle, as well as their care and repair, should be a part of the bicycle safety program. (Courtesy of the National Safety Council)

Bicycle Safety

Three out of four youngsters under age 15 ride bicycles. Every 19 minutes a rider is involved in a serious accident; every 21 hours a cyclist is killed by an automobile.[2] Although boys have far more accidents than girls, members of both sexes frequently ride bicycles to and from school and, for their protection, should be taught bicycle care and safety rules.

The term "bicycle driver" instead of "rider" is now commonly used, for the former term implies responsibility for the control and use of the bike. According to the National Safety Council, collisions between motor vehicles and bicycles occur as follows:

1. 50% occur at intersections.
2. 70% happen during daylight hours.
3. 80% of the bicyclists killed or injured in traffic accidents are violating traffic laws at the time of the accident.
4. 50% of the motor vehicle-bicycle accidents involve a violation on the part of the motor-vehicle operator.
5. 20% of the bicycles involved in accidents have some mechanical defect.

The most common traffic violations of cyclists are:
1. Riding in the middle of the street.
2. Failure to yield right-of-way. (In most cases, the cyclist didn't "see" the car; in some cases he intentionally infringed on the motorist's right-of-way.)
3. Riding too fast for conditions.
4. Disregard of traffic signs or signals.
5. Riding against the flow of traffic.
6. Improper turning.
   Other injuries are caused by falls on slippery surfaces, deep ruts, sand, gravel; collision with pedestrians or fixed objects; falls from defective or overloaded bicycles.

Every bicycle driver should know:
1. The laws governing bicycling in his community.
2. One should carry parcels in a basket or carrier and have both hands on the handlebar.
3. That learners especially should coast with pedals horizontal in readiness to stop and to avoid scraping the pedals on turns.
4. All signals for turning (left turn—hand and arm extended horizontally; right turn—hand and arm extended downward).
5. To walk the bike across busy streets.
6. Two on a bike greatly increases stopping distances and is unwise.
7. Never hold on to a moving vehicle nor attach the bike to it.
8. Always ride single file.
9. To be especially alert when passing parked cars.
10. To keep the bike locked in a rack or a kick stand.
11. Report all vehicle-bicycle accidents to the police.
12. To use a horn or bell for signaling; never use a siren.
13. To wear white or light-colored clothing when riding at night and have a headlight and red tail reflector in good working order.
14. To always give pedestrians the right-of-way.
15. That wise bike drivers don't "horse around."

---

[2] Willgoose, Carl: *Health Education in the Elementary School.* 4th ed. Philadelphia: W. B. Saunders Co., 1974, p. 225,

ACCIDENT REPORT FORM*

PART A. Information on All Accidents

1. Name: Home address:
2. School: Sex: M☐   F☐   Age: Grade or classification
3. Time accident occurred: Hour   A.M.;   P.M.   Date:
4. Place of accident: School building ☐   School grounds ☐   To or from school ☐   Home ☐
   Elsewhere ☐

5.

Nature of injury			Description of the accident
Abrasion	Fracture		How did accident happen? What was student doing? Where was student? List specifically unsafe acts and unsafe conditions existing. Specify any tool, machine or equipment involved.
Amputation	Laceration		
Asphyxiation	Poisoning		
Bite	Puncture		
Bruise	Scalds		
Burn	Scratches		
Concussion	Shock (el.)		
Cut	Sprain		
Dislocation			
Other (specify)			

Part of body injured	
Abdomen	Foot
Ankle	Hand
Arm	Head
Back	Knee
Chest	Leg
Ear	Mouth
Elbow	Nose
Eye	Scalp
Face	Tooth
Finger	Wrist
Other (specify)	

6. Degree of injury: Death☐   Permanent impairment☐   Temporary disability☐
   Nondisabling☐
7. Total number of days lost from school: (To be filled in when student returns to school)

PART B. Additional Information on School Jurisdiction Accidents

8. Teacher in charge when accident occurred (Enter name):
   Present at scene of accident: No: Yes:
9.

Immediate action taken	
First-aid treatment	By (Name):
Sent to school nurse	By (Name):
Sent home	By (Name):
Sent to physician	By (Name):
Sent to hospital	Physician's Name:
	By (Name):
	Name of hospital:

10. Was a parent or other individual notified? No: Yes: When: How:
    Name of individual notified:
    By whom? (Enter name):
11. Witnesses: 1. Name: Address:
               2. Name: Address:
12.

Location			
Specify activity	Specify activity		What recommendations do you have for preventing other accidents of this type?
Athletic field	Locker		
Auditorium	Pool		
Cafeteria	School grounds		
Classroom	Shop		
Corridor	Showers		
Dressing room	Stairs		
Gymnasium	Toilets and		
Home econ.	washrooms		
Laboratories	Other (specify)		

Teacher: Signed: Principal:

Figure 4-2. Sample accident report form. (Courtesy of the National Safety Council)

The school bicycle-safety program should include (1) knowledge of safety rules, (2) the testing of riding skills, (3) periodical inspection of the mechanical operation of all bicycles, and (4) the licensing and registering of all vehicles.

Bicycle-safety units should be taught at every grade level as part of the elementary school and community health program.

INJURIES AND EMERGENCIES

The school is responsible for the emergency handling of sudden illness and accidental injuries and should have written policies detailing the measures that are to be taken.

Every teacher and upper elementary pupil should be trained in first aid. Even first graders can be taught what to do in an emergency, how to give simple first-aid treatment for their skinned knees or minor cuts and bruises. All children injured at school should receive first-aid attention. Accidents, when they do occur, can often be the best time to instruct youngsters to be safety conscious. Units of study on playground safety, safety at home, safety measures to follow when coming to and from school, and other aspects of safety education should be included in health education program on every grade level in the elementary school. There should be a review of previously learned materials yearly. New aspects of any major safety topics should be introduced at every grade level. Individual attention and frequent talks should be given to each pupil as needed, and especially to the accident-prone youngster. Such personalized education is often the most effective way to teach certain pupils difficult to reach in a class. Accidents, the chief health hazard to children, can and must be prevented through effective educational programs.

Teachers should remember that they are not doctors and can neither diagnose nor treat injuries. A complete record must be kept of all injuries, filled out in duplicate or triplicate; the teacher should keep one copy of this report and send the other to the administrators. The report form might well include:

> The name of the injured and accident date
> The place of the accident and condition of the environment
> What first aid was given
> The names and addresses of two or more witnesses

First-aid Supplies

Every school should have first-aid supplies as well as written policies concerning their use because of the danger of legal liability suits. Ideally every school should also have a nurse on duty at all times to handle emergencies. The first-aid chest or kit should not contain medicine of any kind.

Suggested supplies include:

Absorbent cotton	Tourniquets
Adhesive tape	Tincture of green soap
Compresses and sterile gauze	Wooden applicators
Roller and triangular bandages	Elastic bandages 2 and 3 inches wide
Packaged sterile cotton swabs	Blankets
Scissors	Splints
Eye droppers	Pillows
Aromatic spirits of ammonia	Safety pins
Needles for removing splinters	Tweezers
Paper cups	Ice bag
	Instant cold chemical bags

First aid is the first temporary treatment given to an injured person in an emergency by one trained and certified by the American Red Cross. Additional aid should only be given by a physician. Any person other than medical personnel giving additional aid is legally liable because he is not licensed.

THE HEALTHFUL SCHOOL DAY

Every aspect of the school environment should contribute to the health and comfort of the pupils and all school personnel. The building should be attractive, clean, and colorful. Heating, lighting, and ventilation systems should be provided by competent specialists in these areas. The air temperature for classrooms should be 68° to 72°; for corridors 66° to 70°; for gymnasiums 60° to 70°. A room that is too warm is both a health and learning hazard. Since children have lower metabolic rates than adults, room temperatures should be set for their comfort, not primarily for those of teachers, as is the usual case.

The custodian is a vital member of the school health and safety team. Although teachers may stress the necessity of hand washing after toilet use, unless the janitor sees to it that soap and paper towels are available, the children will be cheated out of opportunities to put into practice what they have learned.

The Schedule of the School Day

The most difficult subject should be either scheduled early in the school day or on an alternate basis with less difficult ones. Recess periods should be included both in the morning and afternoon and be well supervised by the classroom teacher. When children have playground periods and physical education classes, the classroom teacher assigned for recess duty or teaching physical activities to them cannot do so by remote control. Some older teachers, as well as a few unprepared younger ones, believe the recess period is the time to stay in one's warm classroom or the teacher's lounge. They then peer out to watch the children playing on the cold playground and tap on the window if there are fights. Such persons are window tappers, not teachers, and are very vulnerable to being sued for negligence should an accident occur when they were not with a group they were assigned to supervise.

No child should ever be denied a recess period as a form of punishment. Every youngster needs opportunity to take part in vigorous physical play in order to maintain health and stimulate growth.

Care should be taken that no child take part in more than two after-school extracurricular activities, for childhood should be a time for free, unstructured hours to wander and to wonder.

The Classroom Experience

Some teachers gang up on children by telling their colleagues, "Wait until you get Johnny next year. He is really something!" Thus Johnny is "labeled" and his next teacher already is leery and prejudiced against him. Some educators also either knowingly or not single out one child as a scapegoat for wrath. Students sense this attitude and copy the teacher's behavior toward this individual. The victim usually is too weak or unintelligent to fight back and often is doomed to a school life of great misery. Fortunately, there are many teachers who do treat all children fairly and alike, one who loves them all and is exciting to be around.

Nonteaching personnel are in some schools the best educators there. Often it is the school janitor or the cook that children delight in being near. All school employees, regardless of where they work, should be selected for their concern for children.

Discussion Questions

1. Describe the classroom and school wherein you had your happiest and your poorest experiences. What made the difference, and how was this accomplished?
2. Recall a memorable childhood experience that happened not in a classroom but on the playground, in the toilets, or while coming to or going from school.
3. In what ways can a school building be a silent but powerfully effective teacher?
4. What is a school camp? What are some of the most popular activities at such camps?
5. What role does the teacher's example play in the area of health education?
6. What are the educational advantages of taking all first-grade children on a complete tour of a school building?
7. What other learning experiences other than nutrition are inherent in the school lunch program?
8. Why should teachers carefully supervise playgrounds and recess periods?
9. How can the teacher and pupils jointly assume responsibility for safety on the playground and gymnasium?

Things To Do

1. Interview an elementary school principal to learn of the accident procedures at his school. Report your findings in class.
2. In groups of four, make a safety survey of your school building and play areas. Compare your findings with others.
3. Make a survey of the toilet facilities at your school from the standpoint of cleanliness and good sanitation. Report your findings in class.
4. Observe any elementary school recess period. Give a brief report in class of your findings from the standpoint of school safety.
5. Devise an accident report form you would like your school personnel to use if you were principal.
6. Make a sketch of a safe playground for an elementary school.
7. Bring to class a school safety poster on any subject discussed in this chapter.
8. Discover what provisions are made at your school to handle a major catastrophe such as a fire, flood, or tornado.
9. Interview a school safety-patrol boy or a school bus driver to discover what his specific duties and major problems are. Report your findings in class.
10. As a class project, plan and conduct an after-school bicycle-safety clinic in a nearby elementary school. Write a report on what you have learned from this experience.

Suggested Readings

Florio, A. E., and Stafford, G. T.: *Safety Education.* 3rd ed. New York: McGraw-Hill Book Co., 1969.

Kilander, H. Frederick: *School Health Education.* New York: The Macmillan Company, 1968.

National Education Association: *School Safety Education Checklist.* Washington, D. C.: The Association, 1967.

National Safety Council: *Accident Facts* (Annual edition issued in July); *School Safety* (A monthly magazine for elementary school teachers); *School Safety Handbook; Using Standard Student Accident Reports*

Vannier, Maryhelen, Foster, Mildred, and Gallahue, David M.: *Teaching Physical Education in Elementary Schools.* 5th ed. Philadelphia: W. B. Saunders Co. 1973.

PART THREE

new and creative ways for teaching health

"*If you have ever seen the light of understanding shine in another's eyes where no light shone before, if you have ever guided the unsteady and unpracticed hand and watched it suddenly grow firm and purposeful, if you have ever watched a young mind begin to soar to new heights and have sensed that you are participating in this unfolding of the intellect, then you have felt within you the sense of being a humble instrument in the furtherance of mankind.*"

Samuel Gould, "*Definition Of A Teacher,*" *from* Why Teach?

CHAPTER 5

what children want and need to learn about health

Children are in love with life! Watch any child having his very first "finding-out-about" experiences—he inspects and smells a strange flower, holds a brand-new baby sister, first touches timidly and then finally ever so softly pets a cow, kitten, puppy, or any other animal, or tries to turn a somersault or roller skate. Such total absorption, delight, and sheer determination! Look closely at two of the most beautiful books ever written about children throughout the world at play, work, or school in *The World of Children* or *Teach Me*,* and note how totally absorbed these children are in what they are doing to learn about the wonderful world of which they are such a vital part.

The desire to learn trickles through the brain of all normal human beings, but in youth it is a strong flood. To learn means to discover—to find out that you could do things all the time but did not know you could. Learning also means changed behavior. If you do not change in what you do or believe, you have not learned. Children do not need to be driven to learn the things *they* want to learn. They sometimes must be prevented from learning about or experiencing harmful things too early or not at all in life. Our old folk saying that, "you can drive a horse to water but you cannot make him drink," is much truer than you think. The pupil, not the teacher, controls the learning situation. Children discover early in school how to tune the teacher out, or to give the impression of full attentiveness when far away in the golden land of their daydreams. They size the teacher up long before she labels them as smart, dumb, or lazy as poor teachers do.

---

* Hamilyn, George, et al.: *The World of Children*. London: Drury House Publishing Co., 1969.
  Purchell, Carl: *Teach Me: A Photographic Essay on the Joys and Challenges of Teaching and Learning*. Washington, D. C.: N.E.A., 1966.

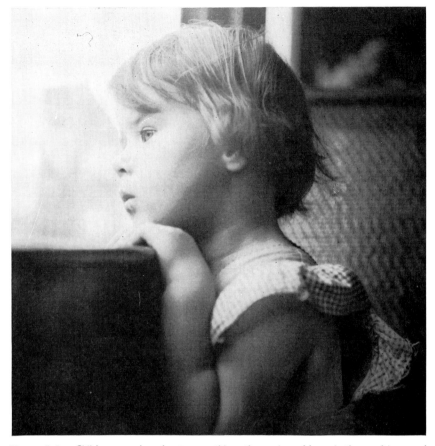

Figure 5-1.   Children wonder about many things they see and hear in the world around them. (Courtesy of the American Association of Heatlh, Physical Education and Recreation)

The desire to learn spurs the child on and often gets him into all kinds of trouble, for he usually acts first and thinks later in his attempts to satisfy his curiosity and find out. Every living child can learn something. Any child who fails to learn in school may be stymied by physical or emotional blocks, which must be removed before any real progress can be made. Sometimes these clogs are due to an inability to see or hear, fear of failure, or the dread of loss of parental love. The six-year-old boy who refused to take part with his class in any type of supervised play activities on the playground, finally, after many tears, confessed to his teacher that he was afraid to play for fear he would get dirty, knowing that if he did so, "Mamma wouldn't love me anymore; she hates dirty boys!" Regardless of present deterring factors, these must be removed before the child will give his whole attention to learning.

Learning involves the entire child; there is no physical Johnny, no mental or emotional Johnny. There is just one boy. One cannot draw a picture, catch a ball, read a book, or master any learning task by only using one's head or "learning it through one's body." The mind of man is a central clearinghouse, a transfer station, a switchboard which can only function when messages come to it, are received, sorted, clarified, or filed, and sent back out again. As William Kilpatrick, the famous educator from Columbia University, once said: "What we live, we learn. Where we live, with whom we live, toward what ends we live—these determine what we learn." The whole community educates, but the learner teaches himself. No one can really "teach" anyone else to do anything.* Each person teaches himself by some magical process which includes his own mistakes and fumbling attempts. Most of our learning comes from making errors first and then discovering how to avoid them. Without failure there can be no success. The role of the teacher is to (1) guide the pupil around learning pitfalls that are sure to stymie him and lead to failure, as well as to (2) "egg him on" to keep trying until he succeeds (riding the bicycle after falling so many times, or finally pronouncing and spelling a new word correctly), and (3) to lead him to new learning thrills and adventures he never dreamed existed. Learning can be speeded up when the learner sees the relationship between what he is trying to learn and his own chosen goals. Although children change their minds many times before actually selecting a life goal or a chosen profession, most know definitely what they want to be or do at every grade in school. The fourth-grader who wants to be a traffic policeman must see the necessity for developing good health habits, learning arithmetic, or doing anything else in relationship to that desire to be a policeman. What matters if he wants to be a truck driver or baseball player in the fifth grade? Nothing, if what he learns as a fifth-grader is in keeping with his long-range goal. Past experiences, goals, and drives are the foundation upon which new and often more lasting experiences are built. Each child, in order to succeed as a student, must clearly see where he is in relationship to where he wants to go, as well as have carefully selected and well-planned educational experiences which will enable him to arrive at his goal.

TYPES OF LEARNING

Most of what children learn comes through the senses of hearing, seeing, tasting, and touching. The more these senses can be used, the richer and more lasting the learning experiences will be. For example, the child being taught the new word "papaya" will more quickly gain an understanding of it if he sees it written (sight), hears it spelled and pronounced correctly (hearing), and actually eats the fruit (taste and touch). A child learns when he:

Understands words and their meanings.
Can communicate with others.
Develops and uses new skills.
Forms new habits.
Develops new attitudes.
Builds new interest.
Gains new understanding.
Makes generalizations and uses learned facts.
Develops social skills.

---

* For an eye opener regarding this truism, read the delightful book *Nobody Can Teach Anyone Anything* by W. R. Wees, published by Doubleday and Company, Garden City, New York, in 1971.

Becomes more concerned about his environment and other people around
him.
Develops favorable attitudes toward himself and others.
Shows concern for the rights of others and has good conduct.

Although experts differ as to the number of different kinds of learning there are,
most agree that the various types are not wholly dissimilar and that some of the same
factors operate in all of them. All stress that one only learns by doing, or from his
own experience. One learns when he responds correctly, such as when he jumps a
rope without missing, or recognizes the word "cat" when he sees the symbols
c - a - t written out. The most frequently found types of learning are (1) *conditioned
responses* (the result of forming a patterned reflex), (2) *autogenous responses* (the
result of self-initiated actions), (3) *sociogenous responses* (the result of social stimula-
tion), (4) *incidental learning* (the result of exposure to a set of stimuli or to a single
stimulus), and (5) *insightful learning* (the result of seeing relationships and meaning
in what is being learned, or suddenly catching on, such as how and when to swing
a bat to hit a ball).

The central task of the teacher is to help each pupil develop self-discipline. Although this cannot be imparted directly from one person to another, it can often be
instilled best by setting high standards and by example. A self-directed learner,
who is strongly motivated to attain goals he has clearly in mind, can and usually
does obtain them. It is the job of the teacher to provide the stimulus which sets off
this magical process of self-learning, studying, developing ideas and concepts, reading, thinking, and creating. Education, then, is a long, slow process that lasts a
lifetime. It should be shared by the school, the home, and the community. If in
these places there is a real respect for learning, education becomes easier and more
enjoyable and fruitful, for as Plato has said, "What a nation honors it will cultivate." Much of the child's attitude toward school and his own ability as a learner is
a reflection of those closest to him—his family, friends, and members of the school
and community.

There are four significant elements in the learning process: the *drive* (the stimulus
that triggers action), the *cue* (the stimulus that guides action), the *response* (the
action itself), and the *reward* (the result of action). If the child is to learn, he must
(1) *want something* (the drive), (2) *notice something* (pick up a cue and relate it to his
past knowledge of similar words or experiences), (3) *do something* (the response), and
(4) *get something* for his efforts (the reward). A skillful teacher uses positive motivation and is adept at providing children with cues which they can readily pick up and
use in their own learning attempts. Such an educator also provides the drill necessary for retention of what has been previously learned, and establishes a warm and
friendly classroom environment so that positive attitudes can be shaped and
healthy emotional responses can be established. Lucky, indeed, is the pupil who
knows as well as feels that his teacher likes him and is there to help him grow.
Parents who daily ask their children, "What did you learn in school today?" and
who are sincerely interested in the reply can do much to help teachers aid children
gain a great respect for both education and the pupil's progress as he strives to become educated. What the child learns in the primary grades is the most important
of all. It is here that children gain concepts of self, how to read, write, "figure,"
play with others, and a host of other magical fundamental things upon which his
future attitudes toward school, himself, and others are built. These are the magic

years. The spark of individuality each had when he came to school for the first time and first year will either catch flame or be smothered by someone. That person has the most valuable as well as the most dangerous job cf anyone in the total school system, from grade one on up to a university graduate school. That person is the teacher of very young children.

CONDITIONING

The simplest type of learning is conditioning, or establishing a patterned reflex response to a repeated stimulus. Pavlov, in his famous experiments, proved that dogs could be conditioned to salivate when a bell was rung and food was expected. We all show that we have been conditioned when we automatically pick up the phone when it rings, stop at the red light, turn over and sleepily shut the alarm off at our bedside when it awakens us, or do numerous other automatic acts to the same repeated stimuli. The pupil who can give back the right response when asked to spell the word "boy," or how much is $2 + 2$?, or what is the capital of Texas? has been trained to do so. However, education which stresses understanding far transcends such training, for it makes paramount the full development of each person in relationship to all communicative symbols. Educators are not trying to train robots or talking parrots, who can repeat a dictated and meaningless vocabulary. The role of the educator is to help to develop each human being to his highest potential total self—physically, emotionally, and intellectually.

CONNECTIONISM

This theory, which results largely from the work of Thorndike and his associates at Columbia University, stresses that human beings, as well as animals, will voluntarily select things which bring them the most pleasure, satisfaction, and best fill their needs. Although this is similar to the theory of conditioning, connectionists contend that learning must be on a higher plane, for the purpose of education is not to create human vending machines who will give back to the teacher an answer upon demand, but to develop educated citizens who can solve their own problems as well as help solve those of groups intelligently in many ever-changing, complex situations.

Simply, this concept, which is known also as the "S-R-bond theory of learning," means that when a stimulus (S) brings a response (R) which is accompanied by satisfied feelings, the connection between that stimulus and that response is reinforced or learned (bond). The intensity of these positive feelings can produce either an advancing, positive response (choosing it again, joy, satisfaction) or a retreating, negative one (avoiding it again, anger, disappointment, frustration).

According to this theory, the greater the motivation and inner pressure for learning, the keener and more productive are the attempts to satisfy this need and relieve this pressure. All human beings, children and adults alike, have certain common needs. These drives make up the underlying cause of all human behavior:

1. Physiological needs (food, water, air, temperature regulation, rest, exercise).
2. Love needs (sex, mutuality, belongingness, affection).
3. Need for esteem (recognition, mastery, approval, status, adequacy, self-respect).
4. Self-actualization (desire to succeed at tasks for which one is best suited).

5. Need to know and understand.
6. Need for ambiance (balance between love and hate, desire to destroy and build).
7. Need for adventure (to seek ever-greener pastures).

A skillful teacher can and does capitalize upon these drives common to all people of all ages. She, like a minister, can help the learner discover the many wonders created by God and man, as well as awaken in him a desire to contribute to the betterment of humanity, and to find joy, meaning, and purpose in life itself.

FIELD THEORY

This concept, developed first by Koffka and Koehler and later advanced by Hartmann and Wertheimer, stresses that one learns best by grasping whole concepts. It holds that one learns by trial and error plus "insight" or suddenly "seeing" or "catching on" how to do something. Anyone who has ever tried to learn to ride a bicycle usually was battered and bruised before he suddenly found he could do it. The novice swimmer learning the crawl stroke has a great moment of triumph when he finds he can synchronize his arm, leg, and head movements and can move rhythmically through the water using all of these coordinated actions. Insight is "getting the hang" of anything we are learning; it can only be the result of previous trial-and-error attempts. The task of the teacher is to encourage the learner to keep trying and to profit from his mistakes until this thrill of accomplishment does come. Here again, she must take care not to nip learning struggles in the bud by being too much of a perfectionist, overly critical, or impatient. Every pupil learns in his own unique way. There is no such thing as "group" learning. Some grasp ideas more quickly and tend to forget them, others take longer and retain materials more permanently.

This concept of learning, known also as "Gestalt psychology," places the emphasis in any learning experience upon the learner and stresses that he knows more about his own self, values, desires, capacities, and preferences than the teacher. The instructor should help the learner to (1) set his own goals, (2) determine his plans, and (3) judge the results. This does not mean that the teacher is unnecessary but does imply that her main task is that of guiding and directing. Students gain much more from such skillful leadership than from being told what to do, for there will be less friction and more rapport, fewer failures and more success, less boredom and far more excitement in learning.

If the main purpose of education is to help each person increase the number of socially approved things he can do well which are beneficial to him and society, teaching is more than either an art or a science, for it is a combination of both. A master teacher will (1) provide the best kind of learning atmosphere—warm and friendly, yet controlled; (2) motivate pupils to desire worthy goals by making them as attractive as possible; and (3) make even disagreeable tasks seem agreeable and interesting to a bored, uninterested learner by changing negative attitudes to positive ones; and (4) help the learner develop finer and deeper appreciation of himself, others, and what he is doing. A poor teacher treats all students alike, gives them all the same assignments, and tends to favor those who do what she tells them to do.

Gestalt psychology also stresses that the best learning will result when the learning environment is used to its fullest extent. It means, too, that the learner can and will learn only when he has a need to do so, and that he will learn best when he can do so under the friendly, consistent guidance of a firm teacher who regards him as a unique human being. It also contends that learning will come about faster and be more lasting when large blocks of material are mastered. Educators call this the "whole-part-whole method" of teaching and learning. They agree that it is superior to piecemeal learning attempts, for it will bring desired results more quickly by stressing relationships. Thus, it is easier to learn a whole poem than to work on isolated lines, one by one, or that one can learn to hit a ball correctly by trying to hit it, not by first learning to act out the bat swing, correct hand and feet positions, and the proper shifting of body weight from one foot to the other.

THE ROLE OF MOTIVATION

Learning is an individual and progressive experience that is closely associated with goal-seeking. Every human being learns in his own way and at his own rate of speed. Pupil and teacher goals are too often widely separated and different. The best educators are those who help each child select for himself ever higher, broader, obtainable, and more meaningful goals through the use of the right kind of motivation. Since motivation is the basis of all learning, teachers must be aware of and skilled in using a wide variety of ways to interest all children in wanting to learn, for what will fill one child full of a burning desire to master a task will leave others stone cold. Motives which can spur or check a desire to learn include:

Wants and needs	Habits and skills
Interests	Knowledge of progress
Purposes	Previous experiences and failures
Emotions	Attitudes
Group recognition	Rewards
Individual behavior traits	Punishment

The teacher's main job is that of motivation. However, she must be careful that children do not become overly motivated, especially in the areas of health and safety, for there are dangers in causing children to become too health-conscious or fearful. There are great dangers also in overemphasizing competition, for only the child who feels he has a chance of winning responds to competition. In our schools there are thousands of children who have had nothing but repeated failure in school. They think they are failures, so "why try?" is their attitude. The best form of competition is self-competition, in which each child tries to improve upon his previous record. Punishment, whether it be by isolation, physical measures, or ridicule, must be used with great caution. Teachers should realize that praise is far more effective than blame in motivating pupils to learn. Does not our folk saying that you can catch more flies with honey than with vinegar actually mean just this? However, undeserved praise or praise given too frequently has little, if any, educational value, for if everything is labeled good, nothing is really better than anything else.

Children can be effectively motivated to learn more about health and safety through classroom teaching when they:

1. See meanings and relationships in what they learn. Overviews of study units or other materials can quickly accomplsih this, as will skimming through a book before reading any part of it.

2. Are assigned tasks which are not beyond their abilities.
3. Know and understand what is expected of them in the way of assignments, behavior, or in other areas.
4. Can see clearly that what they do each day in class will bring them closer to their goals.
5. Participate in activities which are meaningful and important to them and which they help plan and select.
6. Are guided into developing good work and study habits.
7. Gain recognition for their accomplishments, no matter how small.
8. Like and respect their teacher and know that she, in turn, likes and respects everyone in the class. There is a team effort felt and made by both.
9. Can relate what they are learning with what they are doing each whole day at school, at home, and in their community.

A child's natural urges of curiosity, to communicate, to take part in dramatic and physical play, and to create present an "open sesame" for learning. The purposes, ambitions, drives, and values of each child should be channeled to help him develop along his natural abilities. Teachers must help children value well-earned achievement. Marks and verbal rewards, as well as reproofs, for some, can play a powerful role in what the child does and the development of a child's concept of himself. It is imperative, then, that the teacher knows each child and that she discovers what motivates each best, what most whets his curiosity and sustains his efforts until he does succeed at reaching his own desired goals. For every child, motivational techniques, teaching methods, and goal-setting are an individual thing.

The following principles will assist in motivating pupils to positive action:

1. Become familiar with each child's drives and plan learning experiences that will arouse his interest.
2. Motivation is more potent when the learner sees the relationship between what he is learning and his own goals.
3. Motivation is more effective when the children are involved in setting goals.
4. Pupils should be encouraged to set both short- and long-range goals for themselves as well as to help formulate group goals.
5. Negative motivation (fear of punishment) usually retards learning, whereas positive motivation (anticipation of reward) elicits more favorable responses.
6. A child learns to do best what is the most satisfying to him. The teacher should help boys and girls gain satisfaction from right responses and right conduct.
7. Children are ready to learn when they are healthy, well adjusted, mature enough, and interested.

Every learning situation abounds with character-shaping and value-developing opportunities. Since character can often be best "caught" rather than taught, the behavior patterns and attitudes the teacher displays at all times are of paramount importance, and especially so in the area of health, for children are great imitators, but they copy only those they most admire. Leadership through example is the best way to help young children to develop positive attitudes and learn to behave in socially accepted ways.

It is of vital importance that each child have a favorable and realistic attitude toward himself, his teacher, family, friends, and life in general. Children learn attitudes in many places and from unpleasant as well as pleasant things which happen to them. The school can do much to develop in children desirable attitudes toward their own sex and classmates, as well as the valued concepts of fair play, friendliness, and cooperation. The teacher can also help children develop desirable attitudes toward school, work, teachers, and toward the value of having a good education in their own lives. Those who develop good health attitudes and practices build a strong foundation upon which lifelong positive health beliefs and habits are built.

LEARNING PRINCIPLES

Basic beliefs or action guides are known as principles. They result from experience, the opinion of experts, research, and education. The best learning will result if the following principles are used as springboards for action:

1. *Children learn experimentally with their whole bodies.* Trial and error plus insight produces changed behavior, or learning. In this process, mistakes are necessary and success comes from failure. The whole child is involved in learning, not just his mind alone. Just as all of Johnny goes to school, the whole school educates Johnny.
2. *Learning is doing.* Discovery results from searching. We learn mostly from doing, not from being told, or from watching others perform. In order to learn one must try out things for oneself and through one's own experience gain skill, understanding, concepts, and appreciation.
3. *The learner controls the learning situation.* If the learner feels secure and confident, he progresses faster. He will be handicapped when dominated or told by adults what, when, and how he is to learn. Knowledge of his progress in relationship to that of others can be both an asset or a liability, depending upon the amount of self-confidence the learner has.
4. *Each pupil learns in his own way.* Every learner goes about learning tasks differently, and each develops his own learning progress pattern which leads to victory or defeat over what he is attempting to do. For the majority, this pattern shows a sharp rise at first, tapers off to a plateau, then rises again as the pupil becomes increasingly aware he is reaching his desired goal. Learning is a personal experience, and every person has his own unique method of learning.
5. *Overlearning results in longer retention.* Practice of the correct pattern until what is to be learned is mastered or becomes automatic will keep it longer in the body's memory storehouse. The more a learned skill or concept is used and reviewed, the more valuable it will become. Just as unused silver tarnishes quickly, so do once learned things. Practice must be done correctly if it is to produce mastery. Practice makes permanent, whether for doing things the right or wrong way.
6. *Emotions retard or accelerate learning.* Learning occurs more rapidly if both the pupil and the teacher are enthusiastic about and see purpose in what is being learned. Fear and insecurity are clogs and dam up desire until it stagnates; confidence and encouragement plunge learning on.
7. *Short practice periods are more productive than long ones.* The length of each practice period should be determined by the interest level and potency of desire to accomplish the learning task that the pupil has. Practice will be fruitful only if it brings satisfaction to the learner and is recognized as a basic task necessary for improvement. A "cooling-off period" is needed before a renewed and recharged learning pursuit can become potent enough to lead to final victory, for a learning pause can bring real refreshment, as well as desired results more quickly. Learning attempts must be balanced with play, for the latter is a "battery" recharger.
8. *Transfer will occur when situations are recognized to be alike.* The transformation of anything learned in one situation to another will take place only when the learner sees similarities in the two situations and continues to do

in the second one what he did in the first. Mastery of health facts will have no relationship to health practices unless the learner sees the togetherness of what he has learned to what he does. The child who can name the parts of a tooth, recite in "squeezed-sponge" fashion the rules of proper mouth hygiene, but does not brush his teeth has failed to transfer meaningless information into practice. Teachers must be ever aware of opportunities to help pupils recognize existing relationships which exist among all things being learned. Knowledge is for use, and the real goal of education is improved action.

9. *Learning can be an exciting, challenging adventure.* One has only to watch the happy face of any youngster who first discovered that he can swim, recite the multiplication tables, or sing all the way through any song without a single mistake to see the truthfulness of this principle. The child who wants to learn what he has chosen to master can have a glorious time doing so. The real teacher is one who can inspire him to want to make many new and thrilling learning discoveries, and can guide him to where these treasures are.

10. *The learner reacts to a cluster of stimuli.* The teacher must eliminate those which are distracting.

11. Since the learner is motivated by his urge to explore, act, create, and grow, *the setting must provide freedom* to explore, create, solve problems, and to find new and better ways of working, playing, and learning.

12. *The learner is both an individual and a social being.* Consequently, he must be allowed to work on learning projects which are of vital importance to him as a unique person as well as participate in and contribute to a class group.

13. *The learner should be taught to see relationships* and aided to understand the whole process before he begins to drill on any specific parts.

14. *A child can only learn when he is ready to learn.* Such readiness varies in every grade and in every activity taught at each level.

15. *Recognition works as a powerful motivator to children.* Every pupil should receive approval for tasks well done or attempted, to build his self-confidence. Only when praise is seldom given does a child prefer criticism to being ignored.

16. *Evaluation is an essential part of learning.* Improvement and evaluation are inseparable, for one can only improve when he sees his mistakes and cares enough to avoid them. It is a difficult task for the teacher to know when to stop muddling learning attempts and how to go about it, for doing so at the wrong time and in the wrong way may destroy the pupil's zest and zeal to reach his desired learning goal to such an extent that he will give up trying, or quit. There is truth in Alexander Pope's wise statement that "only fools rush in where angels fear to tread."

FINDING OUT WHAT CHILDREN WANT TO LEARN ABOUT HEALTH

Children are curious! They want to learn about many things. Like hummingbirds, they move quickly from one thing on to the next. They want to taste, feel, smell, push, pull, and do all kinds of things in order to learn how to use their bodies and about their world. By the time the child first goes to school, what an abundance of things he has already learned! He taught himself to talk, walk, and use every body muscle and body sense. Now he wants to find out much, much more about himself, other people, and the world of which he is such a vital part. He wants to *know!* His problem is that his teacher wants him to learn what she thinks he *ought* to know. She, having control of the situation and being bigger, gets her way and all too often Johnny and what he really wants to know are pushed aside or ignored.

Actually, good teaching results from combining what the child *wants* to learn with what the teacher and society think he *must* learn if he is to contribute to the growth of the society of which he is an important part.

Teachers can find out what children want to learn in a number of ways. By simply asking them and writing down their answers; by observing what kinds of things they are already interested in and can do; by watching their behavior at play; by studying their drawings, stories, and choice of books, clothing, and friends; by talking with their parents and by all other ways a dedicated teacher discovers for doing so.

Children have many questions related to health;* all are both simple and complex. In a sixth-grade science and health class in Dallas last year a teacher motivated her pupils to want to find out more about their own minds and how feelings and emotions influence, help, or hinder human behavior. The class listed the things they wanted to learn about their "thinking selves." They sought the answers to such questions as:

1. How big is the human brain?
2. How do nerve impulses make the brain react so fast?
3. What causes us to remember some things and forget others so quickly?
4. What happens to the brain when we go to sleep?
5. What causes us to have dreams and nightmares?
6. Why don't we dream in color more often?
7. How can a person be hypnotized?
8. What is brainwashing?
9. Do animals think?
10. What are mental images?
11. Where is our conscious mind?
12. What are daydreams?
13. Why do some people learn more quickly than others?
14. What causes "mental" illness?
15. What is shock treatment and how does it make a person react?
16. What can we do to have good self-control; how does our brain help us have it?

Although the teacher herself did not know all the answers to these questions, she and the class working and sharing together had an unforgettable learning adventure. The group leader, who had already decided to become a physician and follow his father's profession, brought medical books into the classroom. Even though these materials were far beyond the comprehension of most of the children, certain individuals did glean some needed information from them. The class divided up into committees, with each working on certain of their group questions, others voluntarily accepted library assignments and consulted reference materials, and still others made visual aids in the form of a papier-mâché brain, posters, and charts. The teacher's fiance, who was in his third year at medical school, was invited to speak to the class and share needed information with them that they were unable to find. All in all, this exciting learning adventure was, for many, one of the most challenging educational experiences they had had in school that year. From it they learned far more than mere facts about the human mind, for they also learned to

---

* For further examples read the interesting book *The Questions Children Ask*, by Murray Polner, published in 1964 by The Macmillan Company, New York.

work cooperatively and that each individual in the class could make his own unique contribution to their group endeavor. These children were fortunate to have a teacher with enough insight to draw from them things they wanted to know about, and with enough skill to organize their efforts according to the learning goals she helped them bring clearly into focus.

WAYS OF FINDING OUT WHAT CHILDREN NEED TO LEARN

There are many ways of finding out what children need to learn. These include:

1. The results of dental, visual, hearing, and posture screening tests and physical examinations.
2. Teacher's observation of children at work and play.
3. The results of health surveys, accident rates, and other studies.
4. Local, state, and national health problems and safety hazards.
5. Studying courses of studies and health bulletins others have made for students in their school.
6. Finding what textbooks and teaching aids are available—all of which have been written because of researched health needs.

The home and the school play the major role in the health education of children. The church and youth-serving agencies, such as the scouts and community recreation centers, contribute much in this area. What is now needed is more of a coordinated effort of these groups in order to discover what should be taught to children about health, and how to best help children learn what they want and must learn in that area, if they are to survive in and contribute to our highly complex and competitive society of today.

Discussion Questions

1. Explain what is meant by the statement that each pupil learns in his own way. Give an example of this principle from your own learning experiences.
2. In what way is evaluation an essential part of learning?
3. Explain the differences between conditioning, connectionism, and the field theory of learning.
4. What are the four significant elements in the learning process? What other word might be used in place of the word *drive*, in relationship to the other three steps in this process?
5. What role do the senses play in learning speed and retention?
6. Since the learner teaches himself, why are teachers necessary?
7. Teachers have in the past given gold stars to children to paste on a chart for brushing their teeth. Why do you think this practice is no longer considered wise by present-day educators?
8. Explain and give examples of the "whole-part-whole method" of teaching and learning.
9. What are the basic drives or needs which make up the underlying cause of all human behavior?
10. Motivation is the key to all learning efforts. What are the various ways teachers can motivate each individual child?

Things To Do

1. Teach a young child any physical skill such as how to catch a ball or to turn a cartwheel. In what ways did trial-and-error attempts lead to skill mastery?

2. Make a list of things you are conditioned to do, and compare this list with the things children are usually conditioned to do in the first grade at school.
3. Ask four or more children what they would like to learn more about in the area of health education. Report your findings to your classmates.
4. Observe a physical education class for any elementary school grade. Write a short paper on what the teacher did or did not do at various teachable moments to relate physical education to health education.
5. Write a one-page paper on your reaction to the suggestions given in the article, "Listen to Your Children," mentioned below as one of the suggested readings for this chapter.

Suggested Readings

Brearley, Molly: *The Teaching of Young Children.* New York: Schocken Books, 1970.
Durkin, Dolores: "Listen To Your Children." *The Instructor.* February 1972.
Evans, Dale: "The Super Market—A Consumer's Classroom." *The Instructor.* October 1972.
Harrelson, Orvis: "Health, The Effective Approach." *The Instructor.* October 1972.
Lillard, Paula: *Montessori, A Modern Approach.* New York: Schocken Books, 1972.
Oberteuffer, Delbert, Harrelson, Orvis, and Pollock, Marion: *School Health Education.* 5th ed. New York: Harper & Row, 1972.
Pulaski, Mary Ann: *Understanding Piaget.* New York: Harper & Row, 1972.
Sharp, Evelyn: *Thinking Is Child's Play.* New York: E. P. Dutton Co., 1969.

CHAPTER 6

children: their growth, development, and characteristics

All children react to others according to their own growth patterns. They cannot be seen as unique individuals, unless the teacher truly *sees* and *treats* each one as unique. Every child needs through the help of adults to find his own secure niche in groups as well as to develop skills he can do better than anyone else among his peers, whether this be being the only one in the class who can operate the projector when health films are shown or to be the one to make the most creative health poster. As it is true that each child is an individual, then we must teach each one individually and recognize the potentials as well as limitations in each precious one of them. George, age six, may be the class clown and slow learner, but his social and mental growth by his tenth year, when compared to behavior patterns of the previous four years, may show remarkable progress. Unfortunately, teachers rarely can see these growth miracle results which can be clearly seen several years later after they have had children in a certain grade. As a twig is bent, so grows a tree, but there can never be a tree without a seed, roots, and twigs.

Growth is influenced by many environmental and physical factors. Proper development can be retarded by sibling rivalry, constant criticisms, and rebuffs, by lack of praise for things done well or even tried, or by feelings of guilt from being called "bad" or "naughty." Lack of love and security or the right amount of proper foods, and not enough sunshine and rugged outdoor play can hold a child back from developing along lines in his own unique growth channels. Increasingly, parents are wearing their children out by pushing them into many activities. Boys and girls who are going to school have room in their already full lives to work and play for one or, at the very most, two additional activities a week. Foolish is the parent who has her child taking dancing, music, and figure-skating lessons plus other outside activities during the busy school year, for childhood is the time for few responsibilities and the high adventure of discovery.

Growth might be compared to a ladder, each rung representing a developmental stage. Each child must progress up three such ladders, one marked "physical growth," the second "social growth," and the third "mental growth." Every boy and girl must climb up to, and pass, each developmental rung in order, for there can be no skipping. The best-adjusted youngsters are those whose progress up all three growth ladders is relatively even. Thus, adults will claim that a child reacts like most other 10-year-old children if that child is 10 years in physical growth, socially advanced to levels of behavior characteristic of the average 10-year-old child, and can learn materials suitable for his mental age. Other youngsters may be 5 in chronological age and physical development, may be 8 from the standpoint of mental age, but only comparable to the average 3-year-old child in social development. It is imperative that all teachers study the special needs and growth patterns of each individual child. Although growth cannot be forced, it can be encouraged, for children, like plants, grow best in a warm, favorable environment. Both plants and children suffer from neglect and overnourishment. Skillful, wise handling can aid all growing things to find the best that life contains.

Teachers need to learn more about each pupil, his family and environmental background, rate of development, and where he is in his own developmental stage. Chronological age of a single year's space is of little help. Age groupings that include a two- or three-year span may be more accurate and meaningful. Although it is relatively easy for the teacher to distinguish between boys and girls, black and white children, it is more difficult to see maturation levels. Thus, not all children in the first grade can and will learn to skip correctly even though a majority may do so. The child who has difficulty may not learn to skip until he reaches the third grade, but meanwhile he may learn to perform other skills better than anyone else in his class. It is imperative that the teacher discover with each child activities in which he can succeed and gain positive peer recognition. This will yield more fruitful results than if she concentrated on trying to bring all pupils up to an unobtainable average in a chosen activity. Each child needs to be helped to accomplish the best he can do according to his own ability. Teachers should study each one carefully to discover what his maturation levels are as well as his differences, for these provide the basis upon which a rich personality may be built. A sign of a well-taught class is the number of varied personalities of the pupils who have been allowed to develop as each one is—unique and individual.

The age span during which most children attend the elementary school is a difficult one to study. In seeking greater independence, children often become hostile toward adults or listen more to their peers than to their parents. Motives for actions are often concealed. From their point of view, children are more removed from any other age groups than their own. Mere babies are children a year younger; adults are but one or two years beyond. Faced with the dichotomy of "acting like a man" and being treated as a baby, of being "too big to cry" and not being trusted out of sight, children are more confused than we adults realize we have made them. Although grown-ups, including the teacher, may count for little in the eyes and world of the child, adults must provide much more guidance and help him grow in his own sight and his own world. Greater knowledge is needed about *when* to help children in their stages of confusion and *when* to keep hands off. Teachers, if they

4

are worthy of the name, push children gently away from them—they do not keep them clutched to their breasts. Man cannot fly if he is chained in an abyss—learning how to fly can only come from learning how to stay aloft, from having tried.

It has often been said that the difference between an adult and a child is the difference between *being* and *becoming*. This implies that one must grow into adulthood, and that children change into adults slowly and often painfully. Above all, the teacher should help all children develop their own strengths and uniqueness. Studies show that children placed in an environment wherein they are expected to learn will learn the most. Consequently, *every teacher must have a high degree of expectancy in each pupil*. How the teacher regards each learner and her own temperament is as important, if not more so, as her skill to teach children in the many areas of the school curriculum, for in the final analysis what any good teacher really teaches is a reflection of herself and her love for life, learning, and other human beings.

Research discloses that inconsistent teachers are more damaging to children than not strict, bossy ones. Today we desperately need in our schools teachers who are eager to learn and who love to learn about many things in our exciting, ever-changing world. Such teachers will bring joy and individual challenge back into the school curriculum.

SIGNIFICANT FACTS ABOUT TODAY'S CHILDREN

Although all children are basically alike each is as unique and different as every grain of sand or every snowflake. In order to be a successful teacher of youth, the teacher must know as much as possible about each pupil, his rate of development, where he is in his own developmental stage, his family background and living environment conditions, as well as his own special needs, interests, desires, and problems. Likewise, the teacher must know (1) the characteristics of all children according to their class in school and what to expect of them as a group, (2) what materials to teach each grade, and (3) what methods are best to use to educate each pupil and the entire class most effectively.

There are many changes in recent times that drastically affect children today.[1] Our population is shifting and growing drastically. It is estimated that by 1985 our population will be 300 million. School enrollment will continue to zoom upward on all educational levels. The individual child, the older student, and often the brightest in the class will continue to be lost in the crowd. Although at the present time 36% of our total population is composed of those below the age of 18, this percentage will increase rapidly in each new decade. The present trend is toward smaller families—2 or less children. Our child population is being concentrated into fewer states, however, and seven states (New York, California, Texas, Illinois, Michigan, Ohio, and Pennsylvania) now have 44% of the total number of children under the age of 18. Although mobility rates are highest among nonwhites, our cities are not growing as fast as our suburbs, in spite of the fact that larger numbers of our people are moving from one main geographic area to another. Home ownership is at an all-time high. We have more mothers working outside of the

---

[1] Materials condensed from the publication *Children in a Changing World* (A Book of Charts), prepared by the Interdepartmental Committee on Children and Youth for the 1970 White House Conference on Children and Youth, Washington, D. C., 1970.

home than ever before in our history, and our greatest increase of all working mothers (83%) has been among those with children under six years of age. More children are being placed in nursery schools and day care centers. Among older youth, many more teenagers are now in school, yet approximately *one million youth drop out of school yearly*. Many more come to school physically but have "dropped out" mentally, and although they occupy school space are not learning because of boredom or disinterest in school. This occurs far more in rural than in urban areas. Family income is rising with family spending patterns showing higher living levels. People are working fewer hours and today have more leisure than any Americans have ever known, yet this is only the beginning of tomorrow's new age of leisure, which will only be golden when those of all ages have been educated to use this free time in positive, creative ways, in contrast to the violent, passive, and mediocre leisure-time use found among Americans of all ages today. Likewise, fewer people are church members and go to Sunday and Sabbath schools. More people are living longer, for the life expectancy for the female today is 70+, for the male, 68+. By the end of this century, it is estimated that the life expectancy will be 76.8 years for the female and 71.2 years for the male. In each decade for at least the next 30 years we will have more people who will (1) live longer, (2) have more leisure, (3) have better health status, and (4) be in and stay in school longer on all educational levels. In turn, we will have more serious problems in our homes, industries, the medical field, and especially in our schools. Today's children are now living in a world of speed and luxury that their grandparents could not even imagine. Science will bring even greater and more rapid changes in the next few decades.

Living in this time of sudden change, today's youth are being pressured by their parents and other adults both at home and at school in our tension-filled society. Actually, most of the major problems that so drastically affect children today grow out of the fact that there are just so many of them. The increasing number of elementary pupils attending school too often results in larger classes and diminishing personal relationships. Children today, living in a permissive yet pressure-filled atmosphere of the school as well as the home, are often insecure, undisciplined, "bratty," and rude. Their sense of security is further weakened by the ever-growing bigness of school, church, and community. Most rarely have time alone, and most are lost when faced with free time for leisure pursuits, for they do not know how to create their own fun rather than be passively entertained. Children belonging to nonwhite or other minority groups are faced with serious problems of insecurity and hatred.[2] Many of these youngsters face special physical, mental, and emotional problems; others have economic and educational ones related to the geographic area in which they struggle to exist or compete. In this time of rapid change, there are far more broken homes, yet the number of births is increasing. Today in America almost half of all mothers of illegitimate babies are below 20 years of age, and too many are under the age of 15 years (significant facts for those who endorse and conduct family life education in our schools). Juvenile delinquency, a social cancer, is spreading at an alarming rate in rural as well as urban areas.[3]

[2] Richard Cole, *Children in Crisis*. New York: The Macmillan Co., 1971.
[3] Bernice Moore: *Juvenile Delinquency: Research, Theory and Comment*. Washington, D. C.: Association for Supervision and Curriculum Development, N.E.A., 1970.

Manpower shortages in public health and welfare departments are serious. A few families require a large amount of community service. City slums, an unsolved problem, continue to be a hotbed for the increase in disease (e.g., tuberculosis and venereal disease), infant death, robbery with the intent to kill, and homicide. The poorest housing from the standpoint of healthful sanitary facilities is found in our rural areas and small towns.

On the educational scene, although all but three states have compulsory school attendance laws, under many of these laws children may be excused to work in agriculture. Three out of every five children of migratory workers are found to be in grades far below normal for their age. Children who drop out of school are mostly likely to become common laborers or service workers, for unemployment now is, and will continue to be, highest among young workers with the least amount of schooling. The demand for highly trained workers is increasing rapidly; persons with a college degree have the widest and best chance for advancement.

Today in all public and private schools, shortages of skilled teachers are serious. A few children receive a better education than the majority, depending largely upon which state or city area the child was fortunate enough to be born in or now lives in. Although mortality rates are improving, those for nonwhites are still high, and for Indian children the situation today is similar to that of the general population 25 years ago. Accidents and cancer are the most common causes of death among children. Far too many children on all economic levels have poor diets. Regardless of our many advances in education and science, the number of children with mental and serious emotional problems is increasing steadily.

It is only when each teacher realizes the seriousness of these startling facts and is determined to help each child who is affected by them gain the fullest kind of a more meaningful education that our country can maintain the moral, economic, and political leadership it now holds among the nations of the world. Just as little drops of water and tiny grains of sand do, indeed, make a mighty ocean and a mighty land, the contribution *each* teacher in every school could make through the real education of *each* of his or her pupils could contribute tremendously towards the maintenance of that leadership.

All teachers should capitalize upon each child's eager curiosity to find out all he can about himself and the exciting world in which he lives. Above all, adults must do their utmost to *give childhood back to children*, for they are being robbed of this precious, slow but wonderful growth period so basic to their development as a socially sensitized adult and a contributing world citizen.

BASIC NEEDS OF ALL CHILDREN

Needs basic to all children are: (1) physiological, (2) social, and (3) ego or self needs. If children are to grow in the friendly, warm, healthy environment of school, gymnasium, and playground, answers to these inward pressures must be met. If and when these needs are ignored, submerged, or thwarted the child becomes disturbed, rebellious, and delinquent. Although ideally the home, community, and school should work together as a team to provide for these inward urges, there are some cases of alarming neglect from any or all of the three in many of our public schools. When home or community factors exert negative influence the school must assume greater responsibility. Teachers need be better informed of the background of each pupil than they are; only then can behavior otherwise unexplainable become understandable.

Physiological Needs

Food, elimination, rest, exercise, and fresh air are the center of all human needs. Proper balance between rest and activity is of great importance to the health of the elementary school youngster. Daily children must have from four to six hours of big-muscle activity that involves running, jumping, and hopping. They need eight to ten hours of sleep nightly, plus one hour daily of quiet, restful activity. Many elementary schools provide cots or pallets for mid-morning and mid-afternoon naps. Little if any homework should be assigned so that the children are free to choose what they want to do in their leisure time after school. It is important that children use this time to explore, roam, wander, and play games with their peers in which there are no set rules or anyone giving them directions. Children who play well together away from watchful adults grow as individuals and as group members. It is the lonely isolated child suffering from deep fears of insecurity who often is frail and sickly. Such "loners" are costly to society, for many end up in prisons or mental institutions.

Social Needs

These needs are especially strong among people of all ages. We all need to (1) belong, (2) feel secure, (3) gain recognition, and (4) be loved. These inner pressures are often intensified among children.

Behavior patterns are laid down early in life. Personality problems among adults usually are traced back to early home or school conditions or incidents. Children, regardless of age, need to belong, to be a part of a group. Those who have few, if any, friends, who are always alone, or are the last ones chosen, who are crowd-fringers rather than joiners are greatly in need of a friend. The teacher can best help such a child belong by aiding him to develop extra skills and abilities. She can push the youngster gently forward in the eyes of the other children. Care must be taken that the child does not cling to the teacher friend, but gradually is weaned away.

Children must feel secure in what they are doing if they are to do their best. Two circumstances contribute greatly to insecurity: (1) feelings of not being wanted, and (2) a disturbed home life. Instability resulting from either or both can wreck a boy or girl or an adult.

Day-by-day relationship with adults can build feelings of security. Teachers must, like parents, be consistent in methods of dealing with youth. One cannot laugh on one occasion at conduct that may bring punishment or disapproval two days later. Insecure adult teachers who vacillate between being a friendly advisor and a hostile enemy confuse children. They cause those who are already insecure to be more so. Nonverbal communication through voice tone and facial expressions and in other ways can do much to help children feel more secure both at school and in their homes.

Studies show that children favor teachers who are firm, strict but fair, who do not show favoritism, and who are friendly and really like them. They dislike most teachers who are bossy, who do not know what to do in a situation but try to bluff their way out of it, and who are careless in their own appearance.

Children crave to be noticed, to be "first," and to be singled out. When this need is thwarted and they fail to gain such recognition legitimately, they will get it by negative methods. Deceitfulness, tattling, bragging, stealing, or other such measures may be resorted to in extreme cases. "I can run further than *you*" and "my Dad can lick *your* Dad" are expressions of this normal need. Recognition should be given to all not only by the adult but by the other children as well. This can be made in the form of simple phrases such as "Johnny, you are really getting that step now" or "Mary did the best in this group today," or "Alice learned how to do this faster than anyone yesterday." It can also be given by posting on bulletin boards names of those who won class honors and class events, or squad members who played most cooperatively for a two-week period. Children are not as interested in elaborate awards, such as cups or pins, as they are in receiving earned praise from adults and their peers. Although older youth crave the approval of adults, still more they crave recognition from their friends.

Children also need love—the kind that says "I trust you," "I know you can do it," "Let's figure out how we can do that better," the kind that is consistent. Boys and girls need the security of knowing that adults will be available for help if they need it. They need to feel that the adult cares about their welfare and their pressing problems. Adults need to remember that love or friendship is not a weapon, a big stick, or a favor to be used, denied, or removed when "Johnny is bad." In our society today we need to love each other truly, using love in the religious sense and not as in the popular songs or radio advertisements. Love, the highest emotion of the human being, is too often expressed by our cheapest phrases. Thus, foreigners find it difficult to understand how we can *love* that flavor or *adore* that book.

The American school has neglected too long to answer these basic needs of pupils. Too frequently, little balance between activity and rest has been maintained: often only superior children or the poorly coordinated are singled out for praise or ridicule; all too often the extreme pressing concern of the pupil for the approval of his classmates is overlooked; all too readily we like children only when they do what *we* want them to do or perform according to our adult standards.

Children are *not* miniature adults. They are children who can and will grow into adults. As teachers we can help them or we can be their stumbling blocks. We can aid them by providing for their basic needs. We can retard them or even be their albatross when we teach games, sports, or facts, and not primarily teach children *through* these activities. Educators must realize the great importance of helping all children have as many kinds of successful learning experiences as possible.

Ego or Self Needs

The need to be loved, to feel wanted, and to have a sense of security, which is pressing among all children, should be met in the school as well as the home. Children must also develop a sense of pride in themselves, a type of self-respect without egotism. They will acquire this self-respect from others according to their achievements. Teachers are morally responsible to see that each pupil receives praise for what he has accomplished each class period.

Youth must be aided to accept and make necessary compromises with life. They must know how to accept limitations and how to work, play, and live effectively within these boundaries. Those who are physically handicapped need to learn early in life how to compensate for their handicap and how to work around it.

In order to have good mental and emotional health every child needs to feel and know that:

1. He is loved and matters very much to someone.
2. His parents and other adults will always accept him, even though often they may not approve of the things he does.
3. He belongs to a group or a family and that there is a place where he truly belongs.
4. Adults are there to help him when he faces strange, unknown, and frightening situations.
5. He has a set of socially approved moral standards to live by.
6. He has grown-ups around him who show him by example how to behave and get along with others at school and elsewhere.
7. He must learn self-control, and although it is all right to feel jealous or angry, he cannot be allowed to hurt himself or others when he has these feelings.

CONFLICTS THAT ARISE FROM UNFILLED NEEDS

Physical, egotistic or self, and social needs fuse together and become closely interwoven to cause behavior. If a child's needs are gratified, he is a happy, well-balanced individual; when they clash, become thwarted, or submerged, atypical behavior often results unless the child can be taught to sublimate or rechannel these drives into socially approved patterns. Regression, introversion, segregation, rationalization, dissociation, and projection are escape mechanisms through which the child may avoid self-realization or insight.

Regression means returning or going back to childish behavior. First-graders who do not get their way with their playmates often resort to foot-stamping, temper tantrums, or other antics characteristic of three-year-olds.

Introversion frequently results from deep fears of inadequacy from which the child may escape through excessive daydreams. Children unskilled in play techniques often wander off from the group and sit watching others have fun. Basically such children often want to join their peer group but are held back by fears of failure.

In all children there is the ever-present possibility for the flood waters of pent-up feelings to gush out when ideas and emotions clash. Unless they have mastered the fine art of self-control, mere trifles that exert pressure upon an emotional sore spot can send them flying off into a rage. They become upset, broken up, or dissociated at tiny incidents that previously left them untouched. They may not only "fly off the handle" but strike back at classmates verbally and otherwise. A pupil who is teased by his peers because he is afraid to be at bat in a baseball game may suddenly turn on them and lash out at these tormentors. The child may or may not be aware of his fear of batting but also of many other things as well. Because he wishes to hide his "horrible secret" from others, he may suddenly charge at them like a wild animal. This action expresses a form of dissociation common among children.

At school the child who deeply distrusts or resents the adult teacher may be afraid to show these feelings. He feels safe, on the other hand, in releasing his pent-up frustration upon his classmates. They, not the teacher, become the butt of his pugnaciousness. Prejudice, intolerance, excessive criticism, and cynicism are closely related to projection. One becomes adept in discovering those discrepancies others display that he knows are also his own, regardless of age.

Wise is the teacher who recognizes sudden antisocial behavior in pupils as an expression of a need for adventure. Allowing the child to get away with it is not the answer if the actions are repeated. However, the child has had the thrill of trying and usually passes on into his next growth pattern stage. Here again the teacher's attitude toward the child is the most important. It is suggested that the other children find how they can help the offender solve the problem.

RECOGNITION

This wish is apparent in all age groups. Some gain it in socially approved ways; others find it through exceptional or antisocial behavior. In class some children will gain peer recognition early by being fair or by cheating in their play, physically adept or poorly coordinated, willing followers or rebellious leaders. This drive to display or improve skill mastery is intensified in some children. Pupils must receive recognition and praise legitimately from adults and their classmates. Every child can do some things better than anyone else, and should receive recognition for that ability provided it is socially approved.

DISCIPLINE TECHNIQUES

Many school discipline problems are really caused by the teacher or the teaching techniques. There are times when children deliberately disobey and should be punished. Techniques for doing so vary with each one. Some, who are more sensitive, will wilt before disapproving glances or general statements directed to the whole class, while others who are bolder and used to physical punishment understand only harsher treatment. Suggested ways for handling group disciplinary problems include:

1. *Isolate the child.* This will be most detrimental to those who are already group isolates or scapegoats and is not suitable for them. It works best with status-secure individuals or group show-offs.
2. *Increased activity.* Although this is often used with most students, it is a waste of energy and time or serves largely as a means of increasing individual and group antagonism. Children as well as teachers often "gang up" against each other. The punished one is usually strong enough in popularity to gain a protective cluster of rebellious followers who will join in defying the adult leader.
3. *Send the child to the principal.* A technique that is wise only if the superior is wise, or if he is far more skilled in handling children than the teacher.
4. *Denial of activity.* This works only if the youngster is given opportunity to have rugged play and exercise later that same day. The boy who is kept indoors every recess play period for a whole week as punishment has a teacher ignorant of the basic physical activity needs of all growing children.
5. *Individual conferences.* Two offenders should be separated and spoken to singly, for together they gain needed support. *Having a high degree of expectancy in each child* pays off in numerous ways, especially when the teacher says, "I am disappointed in you," and the child senses that she really is.

CHARACTERISTICS OF CHILDREN

The Physical, Social-emotional, and Mental Characteristics of Children in Grades 1 to 3

Physical Characteristics

Can use big muscles of the body best. Hand-eye-foot-eye coordination poor.
  Period of rapid growth. Imitative play patterns.
Lose baby fat if heavy; also lose weight if thin.
Acquire communicable diseases easily; fatigue easily.
Enjoy rugged big-muscle activities.
Motor skills are important for acceptance and leadership.
Acquire respiratory diseases easily.
Show more daring exploratory behavior.
Less attentive to cleanliness.
Postural difficulties become more noticeable by age of 8.
Lungs relatively small; heart rapidly increasing in size; pulse and respiration
  rates are increasing.
Show gradual increase in speed and accuracy; have better hand-eye coordina-
  tion by the age of 8.
Average gain during this period is $5\frac{1}{2}$ pounds and 2 inches in height.
Slow reaction time.
By age of 6 can throw medium-sized balls with full arm swing; can bounce
  and catch a ball and kick a ball on the run.
Ready to learn to swim.
Girls better at stunts and tumbling than boys.
Boys show superiority to girls in throwing and batting.
Boys like combative games more than girls do.

Social-emotional Characteristics

Ego-centered.
Sensitive.
Fearful of being left alone, of failure, and loss of adult approval.
Seek and give affection.
Cry easily; those most insecure bite nails and grab at themselves.
Have emotional outbursts.
Seek approval for more aggressive behavior.
Poor group spirit or learn loyalty better by age of 7.
"Acting out" by saying cruel, taunting things takes the place of physical
  aggressiveness.
"Play" being tough characters to gain confidence and power.
Own sex role more easily identified by 8 years.

Mental Characteristics

Curious.
Creative.
Like definite directions.
Inattentive and talkative.
Take school seriously.
Imaginative.
Not a marked sense of humor.
Short attention span but have a good memory.
Girls develop reading and writing skills more easily than boys.
Boys grasp number concepts more easily than girls.
Have short-range mental goals.

The Physical, Social-emotional, and Mental Characteristics of Children in Grades 4 to 6

Physical Characteristics

Developing rapidly with danger of damage to heart which is slowly increasing in size.

Rapid increase in strength, especially in boys.

Robust, active, noisy.

By 11, have better coordination and skills are becoming automatic.

For many the beginning of the ugly-duckling, pimply stage by the age of 11.

Have growth spurts, with early physical development for some.

Some girls begin menstruating, and pubic hair and breasts appear; have imaginary and far-removed romantic attachments; show developing interest in opposite sex and want to know about boys and men; show increasing concern for their complexion, appearance, and figure.

Boys have abundant energy and huge appetites; limited skill in sports; slowly developing skill in the use of the small muscles of the body.

Steady increase in size, arms and hands growing longer and bigger.

Around the age of 9, girls are taller and heavier than boys.

Small muscles becoming more developed; large muscles growing.

Most are long-legged, gaunt looking, and always hungry.

Most are in good physical condition, a few fatigue easily and should be watched for overactivity.

Poor posture becomes more apparent and should be corrected.

Eyes focus well near and far; nearsightedness develops in some.

Locomotion is steadier and children move with more grace and skill.

Sex differences becoming more pronounced.

Speedy recovery and increasing resistance to disease.

Average gain in weight—7 pounds; in height—2 inches.

Long bones and hips susceptible to injury.

"The golden age of skill development."

Boys and girls perform equally well in many activities.

Social-emotional Characteristics

Emotionally unstable.

Show less attachment to adults.

Have strong peer ties; in the gang stage.

Seek independence.

Often have personality complexes.

Enthusiasm often exceeds wisdom.

Becoming increasingly conscious of others.

Have an ideal man and woman and copy the actions of each.

Still look to family for security when in a tight spot.

Sensitive to criticism.

Inquisitive about human relationships.

Slowly developing interest in opposite sex and in sex life.

Have independence and security conflicts.

Importance of peer acceptance paramount.

Like responsibility and to be considered trustworthy.

Period of increased worry.

Quick to detect insincerity.

Like self-challenges.

Period of hero worship.

Increased need for independence and recognition.

Easily discouraged and excited.

Adult influence marked.

Sulking and resentment increase at home; anger develops quickly at parents rather than peers.

Loyalty and belonging a vital need.

Girls form close cliques; boys join adventurous and often destructive gangs.

Short-lived and widely varied interests.

Value good sportsmanship, loyalty, moral conduct, and strive to do the right thing.

Mental Characteristics

Interested in the world and the community; want to improve both.

Restless; discouraged easily at learning attempts.

Show initiative; are creative and curious.

Idealistic and like to read about great people.

Enjoy learning new things; short interest span.

Concerned about adult approval of school work.

Concerned with justice.

Read and think a lot.

Preoccupied often with thoughts of sex.

By 11, most outgrow laughing at others; intellectual growth parallels developing sense of values and humor.

Boys like to fight, yell, and tease; girls more sedate.

More comfortable with adults; like to talk seriously with favored ideal.

Developing strong feelings of right and wrong and of loyalty.

Not all children will fit into the growth characteristics listed above according to age. However, the majority of them will. The teacher should realize that a child of five to seven is undergoing a most important transition. Because of his boundless energy and never-ending curiosity as a "doing" creature, adults must be on the lookout that he maintains a careful balance between active and passive play.

As children grow in age, skill, and ability to play with others, they should not engage in competition with children less advanced. The transition from early childhood to adolescence is one of remarkable progress. In schools, children should have increased opportunities for real responsibilities, as well as increased freedom to select, do for themselves, and evaluate their own progress. Growth, like education, is a long, tedious process.

The characteristics of a healthy child are an abundance of vitality, bright, clear eyes, lustrous hair, good muscle tone, clear skin, good teeth, a hearty appetite, and freedom from defects. Such a child gains progressively in weight and height. A healthy child is happy: he radiates and sparkles. An unhealthy child tires rapidly, is irritable, seems and is dull.

Although today's children are one to two years more advanced in many ways, including their awareness of current happenings than those of a generation ago, their interests are still wide ranging and their need for instructional help in learning how to use their total capabilities well in work and play is perhaps even more intense.

The Six-year-old

Six-year-olds are eager to learn! They are often overactive and tire easily. Although they are less cooperative than they were at five, they are beginning to learn how to use their whole bodies. Often they are boastful and eager to show others how well they can fight. Interest periods are relatively short but are gradually increasing in length. Acting things out and all other such forms of spontaneous dramatization are favored pastimes.

Children of this age need increased opportunity to take part in big-muscle activities of many kinds. Teachers can best work with them by giving them indirect supervision with minimum interference. Increased opportunities for making decisions might well be provided.

All need encouragement, ample praise, warmth, and much patience from adults. The importance of the kindergarten and first-grade teacher in the life of a child is vast. Some psychiatrists believe that if a child does not like his first-grade teacher or sense love, acceptance, and security in her presence, he is a potential school dropout. Since all children of this age need a wide variety of activities involving the use of the large muscles of the body, as well as much freedom to explore, adult supervision with a minimum of interference is best.

The Seven-year-old

The seven-year-old suddenly seems to become sensitive to the feelings and attitudes of adults. Fear of their disapproval causes him to be less anxious to try many things than to do a few well. Fairy stories, rhymes, myths, nature stories, and comic characters bring delight to him. Although he is becoming increasingly more capable of some abstract thinking, he learns best in concrete terms and through activity. Boastfulness and exaggerated cocksureness show that he often prefers the word *fight* to fighting.

Both teachers and parents should help the seven-year-old find the right combination between independence and dependence. Warm, encouraging, friendly relations between the child and the adult are imperative.

The Eight-year-old

Although the eight-year-old regresses to becoming dependent upon mother or teacher again, he also is gradually becoming more interested in others. Gang life becomes a part of his play pattern. Although he may appear to adults to be noisy, aggressive, and argumentative, he tends to favor adult-supervised activities. Collections of all kinds fill his pockets, his bedroom, or den. He may have more accidents than the seven-year-old because of his increased daringness.

Special needs of the eight-year-old include receiving much praise and encouragement from adults. Wise supervision from friendly grown-ups can help him belong to groups. Opportunities to develop control over small intricate muscles should be provided. Wood carving, making model airplanes, sewing, sketching, and other forms of arts and crafts can furnish channels for needed creative urges.

The Nine-year-old

By the age of nine most children have formed a reasonably strong sense of right and wrong, although they may argue long and loud over fairness in games or decisions of referees. Prolonged interest and carefully laid out plans become increasingly apparent. Stories of other lands and people and love for his country cause him to desire to become a good citizen, to do a good deed daily. Much time is spent with gang members discussing people and events in his own environment. Active rough and tumble play keeps the nine-year-old on the go.

Children of this age need to be given frank answers to their questions about sex. They need to belong to a gang they can be loyal to, and should have increased responsibilities in the home, school, and community. Training in the advanced skills, such as learning to kick a ball or hit a target in the correct way, should gradually be included in the physical education program for both sexes.

The Adolescent

Although there is a wide range of individual differences in maturity levels among this age group, certain generalizations can be made. The adolescent prefers his gang to his girl friend and will be often more loyal to this gang than to his own parents. Although there is a marked interest difference between the sexes, both tend to like best team games, pets, television shows, radio programs, and comic books. Teasing and other forms of antagonism between boy and girl groups are a favorite pastime. Although the majority of adolescents tend to be overcritical and rebellious, and have a "know-it-all" attitude, some do not display these characteristics. Nailbiting, daydreaming, and often impudence show a regression to habits characteristic of younger children. Fear of ridicule, of being different, becomes a nightmare.

The adolescent needs to know about and understand emotional and physical changes happening within him. A sense of belonging to a peer group and increased opportunities for independence are paramount. Adult guidance that is friendly and unobtrusive enough not to threaten his need for freedom is necessary. Increased opportunities for the adolescent to earn and spend his own money, pick out his own clothes, and set his own daily routine should be provided. Membership in clubs that work toward a "worthy cause" should be encouraged.

Skill mastery is one of the great desires of youth. They long to surpass others in strength, speed, and accuracy. Strict physical training to gain team membership is willingly accepted and should be encouraged and capitalized upon in health education.

ATYPICAL AND EXCEPTIONAL CHILDREN

The majority of children attending public schools are normal. However, there is a small percentage who suffer from physical, emotional, and mental handicaps. These children require additional attention. Because all children should take physical education, no student should be excused from his class because of defects. The social values of play are greater than adults have formerly believed. A neurotic, psychotic, or disturbed child first shows evidence of emotional illness when he withdraws from the crowd and refuses to play. Yet psychiatrists tell us that, oddly enough, the first sign of recovery from emotional involvement among all ages is the sudden desire to be active, to play with others. Physically handicapped children can profit often even more than normal youth from the social aspects of physical activities. The crippled child needs to be accepted. His chances for being taken into groups will be increased through the play approach. Every child can and should be taught to master some type of physical activity. An individual program should be tailored to fit his physical case should he deviate from normal.

Signs and Symptoms of Social or Emotional Maladjustment

Most teachers have children in their classes who have behavior problems. Those needing special assistance and often professional help will show the following signs of maladjustment:[4]

---

[4] *What Teachers See.* New York: Metropolitan Life Insurance Company.

Overtimidity; seclusiveness.

Overaggressiveness; constant rivalry and quarreling with others.

Excessive daydreaming; persistent inattentiveness not due to any discoverable physical cause.

Extreme sensitiveness to criticism expressed or implied; feelings hurt easily; cries easily.

Difficulty in reading or reciting not due to any discoverable physical cause.

Failure to advance in school at a normal rate in spite of good physical health and adequate intellectual capacity.

Extreme docility or anxiety to please.

Excessive boasting or showing off—anything to attract undue attention.

Resistance to authority; constant complaints of not being treated fairly, of being discriminated against, "picked on."

Poor sportsmanship; unwillingness to engage in group activities that might result in losing and so in loss of face; not playing fair, or cheating in group games.

Undue restlessness; habit tics, stammering, nailbiting, or lip-sucking not due to any discoverable physical cause.

Frequent accidents or near accidents.

ENLISTING THE COOPERATION OF OTHERS

Teachers sometimes need help in understanding each child more fully. Cooperation with the parents, teachers, and other pupils can often prove fruitful. Frank discussions should be held with parents, for they know far more about their own child than the teacher does.

Discussion Questions

1. What techniques should a teacher develop in order to see and treat each child as a unique individual?
2. Why do children need teachers? In what way can teachers be of great help or hindrance to them as they strive to learn?
3. Discuss five factors which accelerate growth; five which can retard social-emotional development.
4. What are the differences between physical, social, and mental growth? Give illustrations of children you know who have the physical and mental characteristics normal for their age but are lacking in social development. How can teachers best help these children?
5. What is the significance of the statement that the difference between an adult and a child is the difference between *being* and *becoming*?
6. Why do approximately one million children drop out of school yearly? Discuss the importance of schooling in early years in relationship to this problem.
7. What are the basic physiological, social, and self or ego needs of all children and adults?
8. What kind of behavior patterns are laid down early in life?
9. How can teachers best help children who are "loners?"
10. What are the signs of emotional maladjustment? Where could a teacher in your community go to seek help in learning how to cope better with emotionally disturbed pupils in her class?

Things To Do

1. Bring newspaper clippings to class which illustrate any of the facts presented in this chapter about children.
2. Read the book *Your Inner Child of the Past*. Write a short paper describing your early childhood behavior in relationship to your behavior

today (a) in school, (b) among your peers, (c) with your parents, and (d) with members of the opposite sex.
3. Teach any child a physical skill such as how to throw and catch a ball or build a model aeroplane. Report what you learned about the child through this experience.
4. Make a chart showing the physical, social-emotional, and mental characteristics of children in grades 1 to 3 and in grades 4 to 6.
5. Role play each of the five discipline techniques given in this chapter. Tell your classmates which technique you believe will be most successful with a certain type of children or problem.
6. Visit a child-guidance clinic, hospital for children, juvenile court, or detention home in your community. Give a five-minute oral report on what you learned from this experience.
7. Make a bulletin board display or a poster using cartoons to show the many kinds of problems children face today.
8. Have a class debate on the question of whether or not our schools and teachers are among the causes of juvenile delinquency.
9. Watch any television program for children, such as *Sesame Street*. Discuss in class the various teaching techniques used in the program and your reaction to them in contrast to what a child's reaction might be.
10. Visit a slum or migratory workers' area in your community. Talk with as many children and adults there as you can in order to learn what they like or dislike about school. Report your findings to the class.

Suggested Readings

Breckenridge, M. E., and Vincent, E. L.: *Child Development: Physical and Psychological Growth Through Adolescence.* 5th ed. Philadelphia: W. B. Saunders Co., 1965.

Brisbane, H., and Riker, A.: *The Developing Child.* Peoria, Ill.: Charles A. Bennett Co., 1971.

Byler, Ruth, Lewis, Gertrude, and Totman, Ruth: *Teach Us What We Want to Know.* Hartford, Conn.: Connecticut State Board of Education, 1969.

Espenschade, A.: *Physical Education in the Elementary Schools (What Research Says to the Teacher).* Washington, D. C.: N.E.A., 1963.

Jenkins, G.: *Helping Children Reach Their Potential.* Chicago: Scott, Foresman and Co., 1961.

Lear, M.: *The Child Worshippers.* New York: Crown Publishers, 1963.

Loughmiller, C.: *Wilderness Road (The Story of the Salesmanship Camp for Emotionally Disturbed Boys).* Austin, Texas: The Hogg Foundation, University of Texas Press, 1965.

Missildine, H.: *Your Inner Child of the Past.* New York: Simon and Schuster, 1963.

Smart, Mollie, and Russell, David: *Children, Development and Relationships.* New York: The Macmillan Company, 1967.

CHAPTER 7

what to teach children about health

The school curriculum encompasses all the many kinds of experiences which children have under the guidance of the school. The curriculum can be different for each child and affect each one differently. Essentially it is living and learning in a democratic problem-solving educational environment. In its broadest sense, the curriculum refers to the whole life and program of the school. Seen in the narrowest aspect, it refers to school subjects taught or to a course of study. Modern educators contend that the curriculum can be found only in the actual reality-centered experiences of children and not in a textbook or on a piece of paper. To them a course of study has about the same relationship to the curriculum that a road map has to taking a trip. The modern school is primarily concerned with the development and direction of the interests and abilities of each pupil toward his active and full participation in the life of his school, community, nation, and world. The curriculum in such a school is no longer subject-centered, nor is it child-centered, but it is lfe-oriented. The problems studied at such a school revolve around developing new and better ways to improve living for the present, as well as for the future.

Curriculum planning in an elementary school should be a continuous, cooperatiive experience shared by the teachers, state and national educational authorities, parents, and the children themselves. The final results should be a definite course of action to be used for the primary purpose of achieving the objectives of the school; it should be subject to continuous study and modification. The following principles may well serve as useful guides for those engaged in constructing a curriculum. The curriculum should

1. Coordinate the efforts of all teachers and avoid duplication or repetition.
2. Provide a well-balanced school day wherein children will find opportunity to work cooperatively in groups as well as alone. Work activities should be balanced by carefully selected play activities which have educational value.
3. Be based on graded content and standards which challenge and encourage each child to master the skills and knowledge necessary for effective living in a democracy.
4. Be organized to orient the child to the life and world in which he lives.
5. Provide broad, meaningful experiences which cut across all subject lines.
6. Provide for the development of the fundamental skills and subjects, plus social living and health.
7. Provide for pupil participation in curriculum planning.

Education is largely a process wherein learners are guided to choose wisely, are directed toward higher appreciations and values, and are aided in discovering how to act wisely according to social and ethical customs and mores. The total school health program should be centered around the goal of helping each child develop his ability to make wisely the many decisions and choices which relate to his own health. The real aim of any health education program should be to help others develop positive behavior patterns which will enable them to live well, scientifically, efficiently, economically, and happily. As Oberteuffer says, "Action is the thing. To live healthfully, to practice what one knows, to do the scientific thing, and to be creative—these are the principal objectives for which teaching exists." The real purpose of any health education program should be to help each person learn (1) how to promote and protect his own health and general well-being, and (2) have the desire and knowledge to become a healthier and happier individual and group member. The test of any teacher's or parent's effectiveness as an educator is what the child does when away from his sight, warning cries, and protection.

The interrelated and reciprocal objectives of any health education program should be to help others develop (1) positive health habits, (2) acquire correct knowledge concerning the development and maintenance of good health, and (3) favorable attitudes concerning good health. The emphasis placed upon obtaining each of these goals varies with each grade level, as do the teaching methods used to secure them. Primary pupils respond well to any health program which helps them develop good health habits and independence, such as learning how to brush their teeth correctly or wash their hair often. Proper health attitudes gradually will develop (but not automatically, for they must be carefully shaped). Simple sentences repeated frequently for emphasis will help children grasp the reasons behind taking a bath (to feel clean and to wash off the germs), getting enough sleep (to help you grow and feel good), or drinking milk with every meal (milk helps children grow faster). Major stress in the lower grades should be placed upon developing good health habits, with secondary emphasis on positive attitudes toward health, oneself, and others, and with still less emphasis upon health facts. During early formative years, children are most receptive to conditioning and will find security in receiving praise for repeating simple, habit-forming daily tasks, such as always washing their hands before going into the school lunchroom. Carrying out these routinized habits should be accompanied by adult recognition and approval, for this will not only bring satisfaction to the child, but will also help him to realize more quickly the relationship of his own actions to his own welfare and what admired adults want him to do.

On the upper elementary level, emphasis in the health instruction program should be placed primarily on the development of proper attitudes, secondarily upon reinforcing previously learned practices and developing new ones, and thirdly upon gaining new knowledge. During this period children have numerous problems which revolve around the changes taking place in their own bodies and have an increased need for positive attitudes toward their own rapidly changing selves. As each pupil progresses in school, he should develop more firmly grounded health habits coupled with an appreciation of the value of good health. As he matures he needs to know increasingly more about the meaning of life and his role in the world. Consequently, the teacher of this group should utilize the desire of these older pupils to know and understand the scientific facts of health, as well as help them grasp the significance of this knowledge in relationship to their daily lives. As each pupil grows up it is important that he knows why it is necessary for him to safeguard his own health, as well as to have the desire and skills necessary for doing so. As great educators throughout the ages have declared, the real purpose of education is not acquiring knowledge—it is action!

GRADE PLACEMENT

Since the scope of learning in health education is as all-inclusive as life itself, it is the duty of the school to include in the health education curriculum the study of children's problems, interest, and needs relating to growing up. It is the task of educators to select which interests, needs, and problems are most pertinent and suitable for each grade to study. Above all, duplication of course content should be avoided, for children have the right to an exciting adventure in health education directed by a skilled, enthusiastic, and capable teacher who can take them to new "places" or make many new kinds of discoveries in areas previously only partially explored.

Although most states and large school systems have recommended courses of study in health education for each grade on both the primary and secondary levels, there is no standardization of these courses, nor should there be, for such materials should be used primarily as guides. Each teacher should be aided by health education experts and a curriculum guide devised for her school to discover what major health areas she should cover and what are the sources of the supplementary materials and aids, suggested teaching methods, and activities she should use. In order to avoid duplication, any recommended course of study for all the elementary grades should be carefully studied by teachers from each grade, and changes should be made in the original plans when necessary. Many schools use the block plan for health instruction, in which certain major health areas receive stress during alternate years. Thus, nutrition may be emphasized in Grades 1, 2, 3, 4, and 5, and community health and sanitation in Grades 1, 2, 3, and 6. Table 7–1 shows the distribution of course content for the health instruction program used in Oregon:

TABLE 7–1. FOUR-CYCLE PLAN OF HEALTH INSTRUCTION
IN OREGON SCHOOLS, GRADES 1–12

Areas	Health Units	Cycle 1 Grades 1 2 3			Cycle 2 Grades 4 5 6			Cycle 3 Grades 7 8 9			Cycle 4 Grades 10 11 12		
I	Structure and Functions of Human Body	x			x			x			x		
II	Personal Hygiene[a]	x			x			x			x		
III	Physiology of Exercise		x			x			x			x	
IV	Nutrition		x			x			x			x	
V	First Aid and Safety Education		x			x			x			x	
VI	Choice-use of Health Services Health Products		x			x			x				x
VII	Communicable Diseases[b]		x			x			x				x
VIII	Community Health and Sanitation		x			x			x				x
IX	Mental Health[c]												x

[a] This unit also includes instruction in the area, "Effects of Alcoholic Drinks, Stimulants, and Narcotics."

[b] This unit also includes instruction in the noncommunicable diseases.

[c] On the three lower cycles, appropriate instruction in mental health is included in the units on "Personal Hygiene." The unit on "Mental Health," recommended for grade 12, also includes instruction on "Family Life Education."

Source: Handbook of Health Instruction in Oregon Elementary Schools. Salem, Ore.: State Board of Education, p. 14. (Reprinted by permission)

Some state and local courses of study recommend that the health instruction program be built around broad areas such as Nutrition, Safety, Family Life Education, Sleep and Rest, Drug Education, Care of the Special Organs of the Body, Mental Health, Exercise, Personal Hygiene, and Growth and Development. They also suggest that each of these major areas be included in the program on all grade levels, but that the materials under each area become increasingly more difficult and broader in scope. Outstanding courses of study are available for use as patterns for curriculum development from Oregon, California, Ohio, Indiana, and North Carolina, and from the cities of Los Angeles, Nashville, and Seattle.

TIME ALLOTMENT

Although this varies with each state, all schools must set aside a certain amount of time for instruction in health. Some schools, in order to comply with the law, do devote the time to health but fill it with a makeshift and poorly taught program. Still others combine it with physical education and conduct classes in health on rainy or alternate days during the week. Since no one can be sure when the weather will be bad, teachers are often caught unprepared and have no health lessons prepared, with the result that the students read aloud to one another from a health textbook. In a certain school system when the weather is bad, the children who eagerly look forward to their physical education class are appeased by a doting teacher who lets the disappointed class read comic books, even though the class understands that they will "have health" instead of physical education on such days. In such a city, health education is a farce and rightly held in contempt by the pupils, as well as by their parents. On the other hand, many schools have a definite time allotted daily or weekly to a well-planned health education program.

Authorities are agreed that daily meetings for a shorter time are superior to sharing health instruction time with physical education, with health classes being held either once or twice weekly. In every grade of the elementary school a definite time should be set aside each day for health instruction and children provided with meaningful opportunities to learn about health, discuss it, and take part in health education activities which will increase their understanding, as well as shape desirable behavior and attitudes toward this subject. Starting in the seventh grade and continuing on through the twelfth, all students should have an opportunity to have at least one full semester of health education. Such a program necessitates careful planning and skillful teaching in order to avoid repetition of course content and dullness.

A suggested time allotment plan for school health instruction is detailed in Table 7–2.

TABLE 7–2. TIME ALLOTMENT FOR DIRECT HEALTH TEACHING

Grade	Best	Next Best	Least Desirable
1 2 3	1 period a day	1 period twice a week	1 period once a week
4 5 6	20 minutes 3 times a week	20 minutes once a week	20 minutes once a week
7 8	1 class period a day for the year	1 class period 3 times a week for a semester	1 class period once a week for a year
9	1 class period a day for a semester	1 class period 3 times a week for a semester	1 class period once a week for a year
10 11	1 class period a day for a semester	1 class period 3 times a week for a semester	1 class period once a week for a year
12	1 class period a day for a semester	1 class period 3 times a week for a semester	1 class period once a week for a year

Source: Oberteuffer, Delbert, et al.: *School Health Education.* 5th ed. New York: Harper & Row, 1972, p. 72.

CURRICULAR PATTERNS

There are four types of curricular patterns found in today's schools. These are (1) the subject curriculum, (2) the broad-fields curriculum, (3) the core curriculum, and (4) the experience curriculum. Each employs subject matter and makes use of experience, and in each content is stressed, pupils take part in some kind of activity, the needs and interests of the learners are taken into considerations, and teacher-pupil planning should be utilized.

The Subject Curriculum

This is the most widely used of the four types. It is the oldest, and somehow withstands the attacks made upon it by modern educational leaders. In this pattern, each subject exists as a relatively independent and isolated teaching area. The chief purpose of this type of curriculum is for the pupil to gain factual information and to understand it. Lecturing to more adult students and explaining or "talking" to young children is the chief method of instruction, although more and more instructors are using problem-solving units and laboratory experiments. Since most adults are familiar with this type of curriculum, it receives strong support among insecure and frightened parents who want to return to the "good old disciplined days" they knew as youngsters because it represents a familiar and safe period (much glamorized by memory) in their lives. Critics of this type of curriculum claim that much of the subject matter taught in any given field is too often meaningless, compartmentalized, and fragmentary, presenting out-of-date and inaccurate information, and that the teaching of the subject to the child may become more important than the teaching of the child himself. Advocates of this type of curriculum declare that good teachers will overcome these faults, and they have only scorn for those in their own group who assign "the next ten pages for Wednesday." Perhaps the greatest criticism which can be made of this type of curriculum is that it chops learning up into isolated segments, each of which can become overly important or totally disregarded by a "talking" teacher who does all the planning and carrying of what is to be learned, and in so doing robs children of an educational adventure.

The Broad-fields Curriculum

This pattern is not new, for it dates back 80 years. In most of the public schools using this plan today, such a curriculum usually contains Social Studies, General Science, Language Arts, Health and Physical Education, General Mathematics, and the General Arts.

The chief purpose of this type of curriculum is to systematize, reinforce, and bring together related subject areas so that teachers can spend more time on any one of the larger areas, and pupils can be aided in seeing relationships in what they are learning so that it becomes more meaningful to them.

Three practices are commonly used by educators in this type of curriculum to help pupils see relationships within what they are learning. These are (1) correlation, (2) fusion, and (3) integration.

Correlation is often used as a means of bringing out reciprocal relationships among subjects. Health and science are often correlated, as are American history and American literature. Although there are advantages to this practice, it also has many limitations. When the teacher correlates science with health education, often too much emphasis is placed upon the science, and students end up learning about the bones in the feet without knowing about proper foot care. Often, too, some of the major health areas are given brief attention or no attention at all by the instructor. Science teachers tend to be too scientific when teaching about health, just as classroom teachers tend to know too little about science or its relationship to health and so, consequently, are unable to help children learn about or understand this relationship. In order that correlation of health education with another subject be fully used by two or more teachers it is necessary that (1) they be well enough versed in both areas to do justice to each as the materials are presented; (2) each be willing to work hard to make such a program successful; (3) an in-service training program be given in both areas so that each instructor becomes fully aware of the materials to be presented, their relationship, and importance; and (4) conferences or workshops be held periodically so that all involved in the program become cognizant of new materials and of problems which have arisen.

Health can and should be correlated with all the basic academic areas as well as with all other subjects in the curriculum. Readers in health are widely used in all elementary grades. These can be not only a means of developing reading ability and comprehension, but also inform children about the body and how to keep it well. In the language arts, pupils should be encouraged to make oral or written reports about health topics which interest them, or about field trips the group has taken, in order to learn more about any aspect of individual or community health. New words, such as "nutrition" or "relaxation," can be introduced and children taught their spelling, use, and meaning. There are also numerous opportunities to correlate health with art, for making of puppets, posters, health-record charts, or coloring fill-ins delights as well as teaches children.[1] Music can also be used, although care must be taken that children do not create nonsense jingles set to popular tunes which have no value except to entertain them. Keeping accurate height and weight charts and making bar graphs or charts to illustrate special class reports can help children master the mysteries of mathematics, as well as give them opportunities to practice their newly acquired arithmetic skills. The field of geography abounds in opportunities for children to gain an understanding of other peoples in other lands and their health habits, such as learning about the children of India and their nutritional problems, or how and where the boys and girls of Africa live. Likewise, history contains much of interest to children, especially those of the upper elementary level, who are in the hero-worshipping stage and delight in reading about the life of famous heroes like Florence Nightingale or Louis Pasteur. Nature study can easily be correlated with health education for children are intrigued by caring for animals, learning how birds build their nests, or watching plants grow. In fact, any and all school subjects can easily be correlated with health by a creative, imaginative teacher who is determined to share with youth unusual and meaningful experiences.

Fusion combines and condenses several previously separated, but naturally related, subjects into one course. A common practice under this plan is to merge government, economics, and sociology into a course entitled "American Problems," or to offer a biology course composed of a combination of zoology and botany. In health education separate courses in first aid and home nursing are often fused into a course entitled "Emergency Care and Safety Education." It is also possible to fuse or telescope units within a subject by combining closely related areas or topics. One advantage of such a plan is that unnecessary materials can be discarded. Its chief disadvantage, however, is that since "something will have to give" to fit materials to be covered into a reduced time schedule, that "something" may

---

[1] The Continental Press, Elgin, Ill., has excellent preprinted master carbon units for coloring and use on any liquid duplication equipment for health instructional purposes in each elementary grade. Children using these materials should be asked to explain what each picture means to them.

be vitally important to certain students who were victims of the teacher's final decision to "skip lightly" over this, but to "tread heavily" over that. Too often, under such a plan, health education is eliminated or briefly mentioned by an unknowing teacher who too often assumes that the children are not interested in health, especially since they all seem to be happy, healthy, normal children. Actually, every child has a great need for accurate health information.

Integration is a plan whereby subject matter boundaries are nonexistent or ignored. It is a unique rearrangement of materials devised to help the learner recognize and profit from closely linked subject areas. It is both a state (completeness) and a process (a means of bringing about a harmonious working unit made up of separate parts). Integration, then, is a mosaic created out of many tiny pieces which have been carefully fitted together into a clearly recognized pattern.[2]

Integration in health education is used to organize learning and concentrate efforts on large problems or areas. For the elementary school these may be:

1. School living
2. Health and safety
3. Leisure and play
4. Consumer problems
5. Personal development
6. Family living
7. The control of disease

Fragmentation, or the old-fashioned method of teaching health by day-to-day assignment, such as posture one day and the care of the eyes the next, is rapidly becoming an educational antique that is being replaced by the newer, more functional concept of integration. As a result, children are both seeing more meaning in what they are learning, and mastering more worthwhile materials.

The Core Curriculum

The chief characteristic of this type of curriculum is its emphasis upon the present-day needs of America and the world. It is centered upon life today. Its advocates contend that schools should deal with socially significant content—namely, problems which revolve around living in a democratic society. They stress teacher-pupil planning and purpose, rather than "turning the school over to the kids" or "keeping them busy." This type of curriculum is sometimes called "areas of living," "integrative core," or "centers of interest." It contends that the school must assume greater social responsibility if democracy is to survive, let alone extend itself in the world.

In the elementary school, core programs are organized around units, problems, or areas of living, such as (1) protecting life and health, (2) living at home and school, (3) conserving and improving material conditions, (4) cooperating in social and civic action, (5) earning a living, (6) securing an education, (7) seeking religious

---

[2] The Denison Publishing Company, Minneapolis, now has five new books available outlining daily integrated lesson plans in reading, writing, arithmetic, social studies, health, physical education, library time, etc., for grades 1 to 5. They are entitled The First Grade Log, The Second Grade Log, etc. These splendid materials will prove valuable to all teachers as patterns for integrating subject matter.

beliefs, (8) enjoying and expressing beauty, and (9) engaging in leisure-time activities. In this type of curriculum, stress is placed upon that which is realistic to both the pupils and teachers, upon teacher-pupil planning, and the sharing of many learning experiences. As applied to health education, the core curriculum means a theme or a unit made up of many facets or problems. Frequently, such a core program reaches beyond a single period and extends into the major portion of the school day or into several school weeks. The library is one of the main resources used at school or in the community by students to discover the answers to problems arising in each major unit. Constant evaluation is necessary in order that the learners and the teacher see how much progress they have made toward reaching their goals. The use of resource people, such as the nurse or dietitian in the school or the mayor or firemen in the local community, is a means of providing children with opportunities to become acquainted with a wide variety of people from different ages and occupations in order to help them see that one can learn much from life and persons in it, instead of just from reading books or by listening to teachers. The instructor is of paramount importance if the core curriculum is to be used successfully. She must be a democratic leader who can skillfully guide and channel the enthusiasm of the children, as well as create in them an eagerness to learn about unknown and interesting things, direct them to many learning resources, help them devise workable plans, see meaning and purpose in what they are doing, aid them to relate what they are learning to their daily lives, and finally, assist them in learning how to evaluate their efforts objectively.

The Experience Curriculum

This curriculum is built primarily around the needs and interests of the pupils. Since each group is different, each curriculum must be unique. Consequently, major emphasis should be placed on pupil interest. Planning by pupils, under the guidance of the teacher, is considered essential and receives great emphasis, as do teaching methods which center around problem solving, group activity, and laboratory experiences. Weaknesses of this type of curriculum are that often teachers cannot discover the real and lasting needs of children, and that a careful study of the present and future problems of children is too often neglected. Then, too, the interest span of children is fleeting, so that although they may be engaged in many different kinds of activities, they often do not get very far, educationally speaking. The mere expenditure of energy cannot result in progress unless the work done is meaningful and has educational value.

CURRICULUM PLANNING

Many people should determine what children learn at school. As Willgoose states, "The curriculum is part and parcel of the society, the local community, the pupils, and teachers."[3] Basic factors which must be taken into consideration by all curriculum committees are the health needs, interests, individual capacities, and the stage of development of each class group, for what is to be taught as well as when it will be taught must be determined if each class is to profit from taking part in a carefully planned program. Firstly, all such planning groups should be aware

---

[3] Willgoose, Carl: *Health Education in the Elementary School.* 4th ed., Philadelphia: W. B. Saunders Co. 1974, p. 125.

of those with whom the materials will be shared. Secondly, they must take into consideration state laws and the recommendations from the state department of education, as well as the objectives and the purpose of their own particular school. Thirdly, they must be cognizant of national needs, recent curriculum trends, and the scope and sequences of major materials which should be included in the school program. Total participation in such planning can be made possible by representatives from those to be taught and those directly and indirectly concerned with education within the school, community, and state. Short- and long-range planning should be done in both the broad subject areas and the special subject fields.

Regardless of which type of curriculum pattern is developed as the result of careful planning, the focal point of such a plan must be the pupils. From these curriculum plans, the teacher and children should determine their own objectives and course of action in the pursuit of knowledge in all learning areas. In schools using the core curriculum, group planning among teachers should result in suggested ways in which the health program can be incorporated in the core content. Where a department type of organizational pattern exists, activities selected by teachers engaged in group planning of the curriculum should focus upon the needs and interests of the children, and the allocation of health educative experiences to home rooms or departments. The teachable moments which occur during each day should be discussed, and plans drawn up for how best to utilize them. Health education can be taught most effectively by some teachers using the direct method, while others create marginal and indirect learning experiences. Both techniques are recommended; it is not a question of which method is superior, for this depends largely upon the group being taught and each individual in it.

There are many ways to discover the needs of pupils, the knowledge of which is a necessary prerequisite of good curriculum planning. These include the following:

Steps in Studying Needs

Collect facts related to	through
the pupils' health status behavior	teacher group planning
the pupil environment, including the home, school, and community	teacher-pupil group planning and activities
	student council and committee activities
	community group activities
	individual activities

Awareness of pupil interests and needs is basic in planning health education programs. No list of needs should become static, for it should, like the children, grow and change with the passing of time and with each new pupil and each new group of children. Following the discovery of needs, pupils should be guided to think, plan, choose, judge, take initiative, develop knowledge, appreciation, and skills, and evaluate and draw conclusions through assuming an active role in the learning areas which they help develop. They must come to realize that taking part in desired activities is vitally important to them for their present and future well-being.

Every teacher must be actively and wholeheartedly involved in the school health program. In a real sense, each must feel a responsibility for it and contribute to its success. Each must become a health educator, regardless of whether she is the music or art teacher or any other kind of specialist teaching at the school, for no part of the health instruction program should ever become the responsibility of one person, or only of the professional health educator. Every teacher must be involved to the extent that she will do her utmost to help young people find the way to live abundantly, productively, healthfully and happily.

Curriculum development is a continuous, ever-changing, and growing process. Some school systems supply teaching guides and aids that not only assist the teacher in planning the health education program, but suggest ways to interpret the program to the parents and general community. Such guides often contain:

A statement of the relationship of health education to general education.
A statement of the purpose, philosophy, policies, and scope of the school health program.
Suggested standards, policies, and procedures in the school health service program.
A survey of current health programs and major health problems in the community.
An outline of the scope and content of the school health education program.
A study of the health needs and interests of children.
Suggested resource units.
List of available resources for health education.
Suggested units in health problems in related areas of learning.
Suggested student references in health education.

If the health education program is to become meaningful and dynamic to all concerned with the education of children, each must have a vital part in shaping and reshaping a devised program. In order to achieve this goal, all teachers must believe that health education is as important as anything else taught in schools, whether it be reading, science, or mathematics. There are those who claim that the development of good health is the foundation upon which a sound educational program for the individual and the nation must be built.

PRINCIPLES OF CURRICULUM PLANNING IN HEALTH EDUCATION

Guiding principles for the development of a schoolwide health education program might include the following:

1. The health education program should be an integral part of the total school curriculum.
2. All school personnel should share in the planning for the school health program as well as for health instruction.
3. Representatives from the community as well as the school should play a major role in planning the health program.
4. Pupils should share in planning the program through committees and as individuals.
5. Planning should be continuous, and gains made through experience should be utilized.
6. Leadership for planning should be provided by the school administrator, classroom teachers, and professionally trained health educators within the school and community.

7. Planning should result in a workable, reality-centered course of action which is to be put into practice as quickly as possible.
8. The curriculum for all grades in the elementary school should cut across subject matter lines and core areas in the overall school curriculum.
9. All subject areas included in the health instruction program for the elementary school should be carefully arranged in a graded health education program.
10. Each classroom teacher should assume the major responsibility for carrying out the results of coordinated planning for a health education program and tailor it to fill the needs, interests, and abilities of her pupils in each class.
11. Representatives from parent groups, teachers, the board of education, pupils, and school administration should study, improve upon, and approve the planned health education curriculum.

UNIT TEACHING IN HEALTH

A teaching unit is a plan that is drawn up jointly by the teacher and the pupils. It should be built around life-centered learning experiences and should cut across subject lines. Likewise, it should be based upon the personal and social needs of children, and provide them with opportunities for growth as individuals and group members. Although there are many ways to organize a teaching unit, basically each should contain a title, an overview or introductory statement, objectives to be reached, content guides and possible approaches, teacher and pupil activities, suggestions for evaluation, as well as references for the pupils and instructor.

In the primary grades, children should be given many opportunities to learn how to live healthfully and safely at home and at school. Health for this group should be taught informally and indirectly. Emphasis should be placed upon the development of good health habits and the learning of simple health concepts. For this group, teaching units should largely consist of meaningful and challenging activities. On the upper elementary level, each unit must be planned in greater detail and in relation to broad experience areas. All state departments of education have devised handbooks or guides for health instruction. Naturally there is a wide variation in these materials, as is shown in the three sample units included below, which have been selected from widely separated geographical areas and illustrate various ways in which health units can be presented:

Grade 1:   Getting Ready For School[4]

Suggested Approaches
1. Conduct an informal discussion on what pupils do in order to get ready for school, who helps them, and things they can do for themselves.
2. Read story to class relative to getting ready for school.

Problems and Pupil Interest
1. How much time do you need in order to get ready for school?
2. What kind of clothes should one wear to school?
3. How do you fasten your clothes properly?
4. How and why should you brush your teeth?
5. How do you comb and brush your hair properly?
6. What do you need to do in order to keep clean and look nice or well groomed?

[4] *A Guide for the Teaching of Healthful and Happy Living to Children in the Elementary Grades.* Columbus, Ohio: Department of Education, 1971, pp. 10, 11. (Reprinted by permission)

7. Why is it important that you eat breakfast before coming to school? How much time is needed for breakfast?

Suggested Group Activities

1. Investigate the amount of time it takes to get ready for school, to eat breakfast, and to get to school from home.
2. Discuss and illustrate with cut-out pictures proper clothing for different kinds of weather.
3. Dress dolls in seasonal costumes according to weather.
4. Discuss what to do to keep clean and look nice.
5. Discuss the importance of the following:
     Using individual towels and drinking cups.
     Washing, combing, and brushing hair frequently.
     Taking baths frequently.
     Hanging up clothes removed at night.
6. Demonstrate a good manicure.
7. Demonstrate proper way of combing and brushing hair.
8. Secure one's own toilet articles for use at home and at school.
9. Demonstrate how to brush teeth properly.
10. Make drawings or cut-out pictures showing children getting ready for school.
11. Read stories relative to personal appearance and cleanliness.
12. Plan suitable dramatizations on "Getting Ready for School."
13. Bring pictures of children to class and discuss which ones are ready for school.
14. When playing with dolls, get dolls ready for school.
15. Have pupils tell about experiences of sisters and brothers in grooming animals for fairs or pets for pet shows.
16. Make individual charts on essential items for getting ready for school and have pupils check daily for a period of two or three weeks.

Application For Teachers

1. Encourage pupils to bring to school their own toilet articles, such as comb and handkerchief.
2. Provide time for washing hands after play periods and before the noon lunch.
3. Place a mirror at convenient height for the pupils in the room. It will be conducive to good grooming.
4. Provide facilities for shining shoes and for cleaning shoes before entering the building.
5. Provide hangers for coats, with clothespins attached for overshoes and mittens.
6. Prepare mimeographed letters to parents suggesting things essential for preparing children for school.
7. Discuss problems of this unit with parents in individual conferences and at Parent-Teacher Association meetings.

Teaching Aids

Pupil References
     See the list of basic textbooks in the Appendix.
Teacher References
     Johns, Edward, Sutton, Wilfred C., and Webster, Lloyd: *Health for Effective Living.* New York: McGraw-Hill Book Co., 1954.
     Nemir, Alma: *The School Health Program.* Philadelphia: W. B. Saunders Co., 1969.
Visual Aids
     Filmstrips *Getting Ready for School.* New York: Popular Science Publishing Co.

Miscellaneous
Articles for demonstrating manicure and the brushing and combing of hair.
Pictures of children getting ready for school.
Individual charts for recording and checking items related to getting ready for school.

Grade 3:   *Fighting The Germ*[5]

Objectives of This Unit

One of the major health problems of the elementary school level is the prevention and control of communicable diseases.   While the fundamental responsibility for prevention and control should be centered in the child's home, the school must assume a certain amount of responsibility in preventing and controlling the spread of disease. Health instruction concerned with communicable diseases plays an important role in this program.

The purpose of this unit is to build an elementary understanding of germs and how they are spread, with special emphasis given to the common cold. This unit should help the children realize their responsibility for helping prevent the spread of disease.   The students should be familiarized with conditions that encourage the spreading of germs and what can be done to limit or control these conditions.

More specifically, the objectives of this unit may be stated as follows:
1. The children should learn that many germs enter the body through the mouth.
2. The children should learn that such articles as pencils, money, books, or other foreign objects may carry germs to the mouth.
3. The children should learn to cover coughs and sneezes with a handkerchief to avoid spreading germs.
4. The children should learn that sickness can usually be avoided by staying away from sick people.
5. The children should learn to stay at home when ill.
6. The children should learn to report first signs of illness to parent or teacher.

Teaching Suggestions

A. By the teacher:
1. Talk about cleanliness and its relationship to preventing the spread of disease germs.
2. Discuss doctors, nurses, and dentists as being our friends who work to keep us from getting certain diseases by immunizing us.
3. Discuss the dangers of picking up disease germs from friendly pets.
4. Discuss with the children some of the ways of preventing the spread of colds and some ways to care for colds.
B. By the pupil:
1. Demonstrate the use of the handkerchief to cover coughs and sneezes and relate why it is important in the prevention of diseases.
2. Demonstrate the proper use of the drinking fountain.
3. Do an experiment to show that washing with warm water and soap is the best means of removing dirt. Wash something with cold water, then with warm water, then with cold water and soap, and last with warm water and soap.
C. By all pupils:
1. Work out a dramatization showing how germs will not associate with clean boys and girls but follow those who have dirty hands or put dirty things in their mouths.

---

[5] *Idaho Study Guide for Health Education, Grades 1 to 6.* Boise, Idaho: State Department of Education, 1969, pp. 25–27. (Reprinted by permission)

2. Demonstrate in a skit the ways cold germs may be taken into the body —trading bites of food, putting objects in mouth, handling objects handled by persons with a cold and then putting fingers in mouth, etc.

Basic Content

A. What germs are
   1. Size of germs
   2. What are bacteria
      a. Helpful
      b. Harmful
B. How germs are spread
   1. Coughing
   2. Personal contact with dirty objects
   3. Improper use of public facilities
      a. Drinking water
      b. Washrooms
   4. Food and water
C. How we can control the spreading of germs
   1. Vaccination-immunization
   2. Quarantine
   3. Avoid ill people
   4. Don't spread germs you may have

Evaluation

A. By the teacher:
   1. Do the children know that many germs enter the body through the mouth?
   2. Do the children realize that pencils, money, books, fingers, and other foreign objects carry germs to the mouth?
   3. Do the children know the distinction between germs and bacteria?
   4. Do the children know that germs are spread through food and water?
   5. Do the children know what causes a cold?
B. By the pupil:
   1. Do I appreciate the doctors and nurses who can help me stay well?
   2. Do I appreciate the sanitary conditions of school, home, and community?
   3. Do I accept a personal responsibility for helping to prevent every possible disease?
   4. Do I realize the importance of pure food and water supplies?
   5. Do I know how cleanliness helps prevent the spread of disease?
C. By all pupils:
   1. Do we report the first signs of illness to our parents or teachers?
   2. Do we avoid people who are ill?
   3. Do we stay at home when we are ill?
   4. Do we cover our mouth when coughing and sneezing?
   5. Do we keep foreign objects out of our mouth?
   6. Do we respect quarantine regulations?
   7. Do we avoid using others' personal objects such as towels and wash cloths?
   8. Do we drink properly from the water fountain?

Grade 5: Safety and First Aid[6]

Desired Outcomes

Children know
   1. How to help the corridor and playground patrols prevent accidents.
   2. How to prevent fires.

---

[6] *Handbook of Health Instruction in Oregon Elementary Schools.* Salem, Ore.: State Board of Education, 1972, pp. 56–58. (Reprinted by permission)

3. How to extinguish fires of all types.
4. How to enjoy vacations without being hurt.
5. How to keep from being hurt at home.
6. How to keep wounds from becoming infected.
7. How to acquire a tan without being sunburned.
8. How to identify and use safe places to play.
9. How to use a saw, hammer, pliers, and similar common tools without being hurt or hurting others.

Activities

1. Make a survey of the school building. Check amount of traffic at inter-sections, along corridors, and on stairs. Make floor plan of building showing each floor. Study floor plan to determine whether pupil traffic should be divided, rerouted, or in some cases eliminated in part. Draw up plan to handle pupil traffic most effectively.
2. Field trip to fire station. Find out what constitutes the different types of fires (wood, chemical, electrical). Learn best means for extinguishing each type. Use commercial and pupil-made fire extinguishers to extinguish the different types of fires.
3. Make a survey of school building noting location and type of each fire extinguisher. Make floor plan showing location of each fire extinguisher in red. Study floor plan to determine whether or not the right type of extinguisher is in the right place. If not, contact principal with suggested plan for relocating fire extinguishers. Note date of last inspection of extinguisher.
4. Make a list of accidents and their causes common to different types of recreation engaged in by the pupils. Indicate on a chart which ones pupils have experienced, which ones people in the community have experi-enced, and plan ways to prevent such accidents.
5. Make a survey of pupils' homes to determine whether or not potentially dangerous situations are present. Plan how to correct undesirable situa-tions. Report later on extent of correction achieved.
6. Have teacher, nurse, or doctor set up microscopes showing sterile and con-taminated slides. Find out way in which wounds become contaminated and the resulting dangers. Practice handling sterile gauze and covering minor wounds.

THE CONCEPTUAL APPROACH TO HEALTH EDUCATION

In this method, concepts or "big ideas" are the central theme around which objectives, content, methods, and materials are built to help children develop their own concepts regarding health.* For example, "each family grows and lives out its own unique life cycle" and "body functions cause changes in living things, facilitating or retarding growth and reproduction" are such concepts.

Problem areas around which concepts may be developed include: accident pre-vention, aging, alcohol, disaster preparedness, disease and its control, family health, international health, nutrition, and smoking. Many state and local guides use their conceptual approach through which a child can learn about health in more meaningful ways.†

---

* See the suggested units on Alcohol Education and on Smoking Education, Chap-ter 16, to learn how this conceptual approach is used to develop a teaching unit.
† For more information, see *Health Concepts: Guides For Health Instruction.* Washington, D. C.: American Association For Health, Physical Education and Recreation, 1967.

THE USE OF STATE COURSES OF STUDY

State courses of study and health teaching guides should be used only as starting points for curriculum individualization. Just as a dress designed and made for a chubby ten-year-old girl living in Des Moines would be totally inadequate and unsuited for a frail little lass in the first grade in Dallas, no state course of study or health teaching guide will "fit" all children even in the same grade in the same school in that state. An ideal health instruction is one specially adapted to each class in each school in every locality throughout the land. Such a plan should be a flexible and elastic one which is just right for each child in each school grade. No two instructors, children, or teaching situations are identical. Consequently, no one plan is best for all concerned. Courses of study do have value, but only when used as a suggested pattern or course of action. Skilled teachers will create new and better plans from these suggestions and ideas found in all such materials obtained from the state education department or a local school system.

Every teacher is a builder. Each constructs her own educational house. The superior builder, realizing that such a dwelling is to be erected for the education of children, will quickly enlist the cooperation and capabilities (both apparent and half-hidden) of the youngsters to help build a wonderful place of their very own. Such a master builder will use an already-devised blueprint only to check on minute details which will prove helpful to the group's own creative efforts, and to avoid sure-to-fail attempts along the way. The house, when it is completed, will be a place of pride, joy, and wonder wherein many magical experiences can take place for all who live and learn there. The average builder will stick closely to a preplanned blueprint made by and for somebody else, and she will build just another house, which cannot and will not last long, or become a learning landmark worthy of anyone's remembrance. The poor builder, alas, will not even know that somewhere a blueprint does exist, or that it could be used as a starting point, so her house is never built, and the busy children who were longing to accomplish something merely mill around instead, and leave the incomplete foundation in search of adventure and meaningful accomplishment elsewhere.

Educators, unfortunately, seldom capitalize upon their gains. They could do so, however, by using what has already been achieved as a starting point. Existing, obtainable courses of study, teaching guides, and other such materials are such starting points.

THE RESOURCE UNIT

The resource unit is an organized, preplanned collection of materials and suggested teaching methods developed by one teacher for her own use, or by a committee composed of several instructors and health specialists. These units are also often devised by school health education specialists on the state level and are made available to educators upon request. Such a unit should contain a list of books and other printed references, teaching aids, and people or other community resources which could become most helpful to a project and could share valuable educational experiences with the children. Such units may be built for each health unit included in the subject-centered curriculum, or they may be planned to fit health into a broad-field, experience, or core curriculum. Professionally trained health authorities, including the health supervisor or coordinator, can be of invaluable help to any group of teachers engaged in developing such units of work. All completed unit projects should be kept in a central file so that many teachers may profit from this work done by their co-workers or predecessors. Each instructor should be aware, however, that she must bring life into such a plan that exists only on paper by modifying it to fit her own particular group before using it. Likewise, the teacher or the working committees should revise and keep such units up to date, so that children might benefit from current materials. The pupils should assist in the development and revision of such units. A resource unit might be patterned after the following one:

A Resource Unit in Communicable Diseases for Grade Five

Visual Aids
    "The Story of Dr. Jenner." (10 min.) Teaching Film Custodians.
    "I Never Catch a Cold." (10 min.) Coronet Films.
    "Your Health: Disease and Its Control." (11 min.) Coronet Films.
Pamphlets
    "The Control of Communicable Disease in Man." American Public
        Health Association, 1958.
References for the Pupils
    Jones, Edwina, and Morgan, Jane: *Keeping Healthy.* Laidlaw.
    Schacter, Helen, and Bauer, William: *You and Others.* Glenview, Ill.:
        Scott, Foresman and Co.
    Ways to Keep Well and Happy. National Tuberculosis Association.
    Winter Enemies. Boston: John Hancock Mutual Life Insurance Company.
References for the Teacher
    Health Education. Washington, D. C.: American Medical Association
        and National Education Association, 1961.
    The Science Book of Wonder Drugs. New York: Pocket Books, 1959.
    The Control of Communicable Diseases in Man. American Public Health
        Association, 1958.
    Turner, C. E.: *Personal and Community Health.* St. Louis: C. V. Mosby
        Co., 1960.

Discussion Questions

1. What is the place of health education in the total school curriculum?
2. Define what is meant by "the subject curriculum," "the broad-fields curriculum," "the core curriculum," and "the experience curriculum."
3. What are the advantages and disadvantages of each of these four curriculum types?
4. According to Oberteuffer, how much time should be given for direct health teaching in grades 1 to 3; in grades 4 to 6; in grades 7 to 9; 10 to 12? Was this much time allotted for health education in your elementary, junior high, and high school? What were the strengths and weaknesses of your health education program in each of these schools?
5. In what way should the purposes of health education program differ on the primary and upper elementary levels?
6. Give an example of how any subject in nutrition can be correlated with any five other subjects taught in most schools.
7. Explain what is meant by the words "correlation," "fusion," and "integration."
8. Explain the meaning and significance of the statement that "many people should determine what children learn at school." Give specific suggestions of how this can be done.
9. How can state courses of study in health and health education curriculum guides best be used by teachers?
10. Explain the differences and similarities of a unit plan and a daily lesson plan.

Things To Do

1. Using role play involving the health education specialist and a group of teachers, act out the way plans for the development of a curriculum guide should be made. For contrast, show how the initial planning meeting should not be conducted.
2. Review two health curriculum guides or state courses of study in health education. Report your findings in class as to which one you thought was better and tell the class why you thought so.
3. Interview any elementary school teacher to find out what broad health areas she teaches and how she gathers her materials for teaching the children about health. Report your findings in class.
4. Make a unit plan outlining 10 lessons in nutrition for each of the grades 1, 3, and 5 or 2, 4, and 6.
5. Make a resource unit for any elementary grade in an area of health education. Be sure that you use only materials published in 1970 or later. Discuss in class what you learned about unit planning from this experience.

Suggested Readings

Byrd, Oliver: *School Health Administration.* Philadelphia: W. B. Saunders Co., 1964.

Cornachia, Harold, Staton, Wesley, and Irwin, Leslie: *Health in Elementary Schools.* St. Louis: C. V. Mosby Co., 1970.

Fodor, John, and Dalis, G.: *Health Instruction, Theory and Application.* 2nd ed., Philadelphia: Lea & Febiger, 1974.

Haag, Jessie Helen: *School Health Program.* 3rd ed. Philadelphia: Lea & Febiger, 1972.

Hamburg, Morris, and Hamburg, Marion: *Health and Social Problems in the School.* Philadelphia: Lea & Febiger, 1968.

Schneider, Robert: *Methods and Materials of Health Education.* Philadelphia: W. B. Saunders Co., 1964.

Smolensky, Jack, and Bonvechio, L. Richard: *Principles of School Health.* Boston: D. C. Heath and Co., 1966.

CHAPTER 8

how to teach children about health more effectively

To teach is to guide, lead, inspire, share, discipline, and discover with others. Success in this all-important professional field is due largely to skill in human engineering and to educational development. The best-prepared teachers know *what* to teach and *how* to do it. The latter comes from experience, experimenting, and adapting principles and methods to fit one's own situation. To teach also means to impart information through skilled techniques so that others will learn. To educate means to bring forth latent possibilities and to "lead forth," and these, along with motivating students, are the teacher's real responsibilities.

Good teaching results will accrue more abundantly when each instructor, through the use of teacher-pupil planning, sets desired goals and individual objectives to be reached; selects and sees values in materials to be learned in order to obtain these desired ends; shares planned, purposeful learning experiences; and evaluates the final results in light of the original goals. Through the use of a wide variety of methods, skilled teachers, then, will see pupils improve in skills, make positive attitude changes, develop deepened and broadened understandings, and use the things they have learned by applying them in their daily lives.

TEACHING METHODS

There is no single best teaching method. A good teacher is one who can obtain results by using the best teaching method in a particular situation to reach an educational objective. The use of variety by any teacher will bring spice and life into her work, increased pupil interest, and add to the pupils' eagerness to learn new things. Each instructor who wants to become a master in her chosen professional field must epxeriment, carry on research, and profit from her own learning attempts. A teacher cannot always see all the results of her work, even though these are the many hidden treasures of teaching. All too soon she loses track of her pupils over the years and seldom knows how effective her brief educational contact with each one has been. Many educators create more miracles than they ever know. Behavior cannot change overnight, nor can a tree bear fruit soon after planting; yet the true educator continues patiently to teach others as best she can. Some teaching methods may work wonderfully well with Johnny, but fail miserably with Mary. Consequently, the skilled instructor will not only know a wide variety of ways to reach each pupil, but will also know how and when to use each of them most advantageously. A teaching method is a carefully thought-out plan for achieving definite goals. As applied to health education, method refers to techniques used to provide the best kind of a learning environment possible wherein the pupil's behavior can be shaped, changed, and directed for the betterment of his own health and that of others.

The many methods for teaching health include:

Daily assignments
Lectures
Teacher questions and student
    answers
Special reports
Panel discussions
Teacher or student demonstra-
    tions
Class discussions
Workshops
Informal student-to-student dis-
    cussions
Forums
School camping experiences
Debates
Projects
Role playing
Problem solving
Dramatizations
Arts, crafts, and other constructive
    projects
Analysis of current events
Recitation periods
Student-led class discussions

Surveys
Drills
Workbooks
Field trips
Supervised practice and guided study
Do-and-tell periods
Textbooks and supplementary read-
    ing assignments
Teacher-stimulated and -directed
    discussions
Supervised study
Student reports
Small-group study
Creative dance and rhythms
Educational games
Individual or small-group counseling
Experience units
Small-group buzz sessions
Guest speakers
Storytelling
Research projects
Visual aids
Experiments

Fortunately, health education is rapidly gaining its long-deserved and rightful status in the school curriculum. Luckily, this subject is becoming more than a crash program included in the curriculum, due to the pressure of scared parents, or taught by one forced to do so, in spite of her lack of preparation or interest. There are also many new and wonderfully successful teaching departures now being made by creative instructors in this field from the old-fashioned, unproductive methods used yesterday, wherein students were made to memorize the parts of the body, read aloud to the class from a dull textbook, or repeat a list of hygiene rules. In modern health education, learning activities are centered around helping students solve those vastly important health problems which directly affect them.

Factors which determine the type of health teaching methods to be used include the teacher's skill, time allotment, available equipment and supplies, and the pupil's educational capabilities and needs.

Those teachers who have had little preparation in health education unfortunately too often teach the subject matter straight from the textbook, feeling more secure in doing so. Actually, although the teacher's edition of most elementary textbooks does contain numerous suggestions for covering included materials effectively, all such books should be used primarily as "idea springboards" and should not take initiative away from the teacher. Naturally, in those schools where adequate time is devoted to health education and an interested and skilled teacher is in charge of the class, most progress is being made. In such schools the health curriculum has been carefully planned and made meaningful through the means of a well-selected and well-taught graded program from grades 1 through 6. Although it is wise to have a variety of well-selected visual and other teaching aids, these are not absolutely necessary for a successful program; creative and skilled teachers are far more important than superior materials, equipment, or facilities. Ingenious instructors get students excited about learning about health and how to make their posters, cardboard box movie projectors, and illustrated health films rolled on a curtain rod, or to build a hamster cage for an experiment in nutrition. Having too many commercial gadgets and teaching guides in the classroom can rob teachers and pupils of their creative talents. In schools where health classes are alternated with those in physical education, pupils who were dumped into this latter "catch-all" usually gain little from either experience, for there are often just too many pupils in the former class to teach health effectively, and therefore often too little opportunity to discover the real health education interests and needs of the class. Athletic coaches, who in some schools are saddled with teaching alternate physical education and health education classes as well as producing winning teams, cannot and usually do not do much except coach players who are already above average in ability. All health classes on the elementary level should be kept small enough for the teacher to know a great deal about each of the students enrolled in them. Our best-prepared and skilled teachers must be assigned to teach health before real progress can be made in the improvement of any school health instruction program.

METHODS FOR IMPROVING INSTRUCTION

The best methods for teaching health are the same as those used in the effective teaching of any other subject. The basic aim of any health education program should be to teach people to live healthfully, acquire health knowledge, and develop positive health attitudes for lifetime use. All educators with this aim in mind *will* develop their own best teaching methods. Included below are some ways in which health teaching could become more meaningful and productive for each pupil:

Class Discussions

Class discussions are one of the most effective ways to teach health, but only if students are keenly interested and take part in the discussion, and if it is not dominated by a few bright students. Willgoose suggests the following ways in which class discussions can be made more meaningful:

1. An overnight assignment, which requires some study or searching for ideas at home, will provoke a number of good questions for the next day in class.
2. A list of questions, raised in earlier sessions and distributed prior to the

discussion, helps the student who is a poor thinker. In studying teeth in the third grade, for example, questions such as these tend to generate curiosity: "How many teeth do I have?" "When will I have all my permanent teeth?" "Will baking soda and salt clean my teeth?"
3. A small group discussion or buzz session where the class is divided into small units is often productive.[1]

Although such a method can be used successfully, care must be taken to have the group help select discussion topics on *their* interest. It is wise to rotate student leaders and have each buzz-session subgroup select a pupil chairman to give a brief report to the whole class on what the group discussed. The teacher or a student should summarize the main points presented by each discussion reporter. If the teacher is leading the discussion, she should avoid answering her own questions, for teaching is not a process of pouring in *but rather it is one of drawing out.* Educators have a great fear of silence. Most teachers answer their own questions, sometimes less than seconds after posing them, thus stealing from children their educational right to discover logically the correct answers for themselves, even though this may take up precious class time. One of the first things a child learns early in life is how to get around adults and thus free himself from pressure or work. He will give back to parents or other adults the "right" answers to such queries as "Do you love mommy?" or "What do you like most about school?" etc., in order to please the questioner, not to reveal what he really thinks or feels. Some children even refuse to talk, for they can get what they want from adults they have made into their slaves without making even much effort. Many soon learn in school how to get by with a minimum of effort and are masters of this technique by the time they leave the elementary school.

Field Trips

Although field trips are increasingly being used as a means of teaching, they are often avoided because they are too much trouble. Some schools forbid groups to go on excursions because of the fear of accidents and the consequent legal liability. However, trips can be the bright highlight of an entire elementary school experience. When teachers realize that neither they nor the school have a monopoly on teaching or education, that children often learn more outside than inside schools, and that learning can be accomplished without either a teacher or school, more educators will find ways to provide out-of-school excursions for their groups. Education is not listening, it is not mere reading, it is *doing* many kinds of things in order to learn most effectively. Missing the next regularly scheduled class, if the field trip is to be extended, often is the best thing a teacher can do, for what the children might learn had they gone to class may be trivial in comparison with the gains made possible from a carefully planned, purposeful field trip. Although some parents become alarmed when children leave school for fear they are not learning anything, this attitude can be gradually overcome if such parents listen to the eager narration by their own child of the exciting out-of-class experience at the family dinner table, at a PTA meeting, or elsewhere.

---

[1] Willgoose, Carl: *Health Education in the Elementary School.* 4th ed. Philadelphia: W. B. Saunders Co., 1974, pp. 295–296.

All field trips should be carefully planned, taken with a definite purpose in mind, cleared through the proper authorities, arranged with those in charge of the place to be visited, talked about beforehand, discussed as things are seen, related to materials being studied at school, be safely conducted, and summarized when the group returns to its classroom. Some exciting places to visit in a community are:

Grocery store	Large restaurant
Modern dairy	Veterinarian's animal clinic
Health museums	State health department
Ice cream plants	Fire station
Hospitals	Emergency rooms and first-aid
Bakery	stations
Farm	Children's court for bicycle offenders
Canning and packing plant	Police station
City water and sewage-disposal plant	Zoo
Farmer's vegetable market	Drug laboratory
City health department	Slum area
	Dentist's office

A field trip can become a meaningful experience or a meaningless lark. To have educational value it must be an important adjunct to health problems currently being studied in the classroom. All out-of-school excursions should be taken for a definite purpose which is clearly understood by each teacher and pupil. It is imperative that the trip plans be fully discussed and carefully drawn up before the group leaves school. The classroom teacher should guide pupil committee groups to discuss and make trip plans carefully. Each committee chairman might well be asked to record on the blackboard the answers to such questions as these: "Why do we want to go on this trip?"; "What do we want to learn?"; "What is the relationship of the trip to what we are now studying?"; and "How can we apply what we will learn to our daily lives?"

The following suggestions along with those given above should prove helpful to those who plan and conduct excursions:

1. Take safety precautions at all times throughout the trip; be prepared for accidents and emergencies.
2. Select and plan all trips according to the maturity and comprehension of the class.
3. Discuss the outing with the class upon returning to school and help each pupil link what has been learned outside of the school with what is being studied inside the school.
4. Clear all matters such as parental consent, conduct rules, rest-room stops, meals, and other necessary details before leaving the school. Be sure the principal knows where you are going, when you are leaving, how many pupils you are taking, and when the group will return.
5. Strive to increase the educational values of all future community visits by carefully evaluating each trip taken with the class.

The most fruitful educational excursions are those which enable pupils to learn from many kinds of first-hand experiences those things which cannot be learned elsewhere. Oberteuffer contends that field trips can become more valuable when they are built around surveys or studies in which relationships are stressed, such as visiting a slum area to learn more about the relation of poor housing to disease or delinquency, or evaluating a recreation area in relation to community and indi-

vidual leisure time.[2] Such experiences become a bridge between school experiences
and community life. Some schools have developed procedures for the teacher to
follow when taking children on trips. Such materials help eliminate duplication of
trips through the child's entire school experience, and help the teacher select, from
a list of possible places, those which are best suited to the maturity and intellectual
background of her own particular grade.

A carefully planned and well-organized field trip can:[3]

1. Encourage explorations and interest.
2. Develop pupil curiosity.
3. Cultivate careful observation.
4. Provide careful, accurate, first-hand observation.
5. Clarify concepts and give additional meaning to previous classwork, especially for pupils whose experience backgrounds are limited.
6. Provide opportunities for vocational guidance through direct contact
   with various kinds of work.
7. Promote intelligent citizenship through experiences in social living.
8. Form new ties between the pupil and community.
9. Arouse the interests of parents and other citizens in what the schools are
   doing.

In spite of these worthy contributions, many school systems forbid teachers to
take children on trips outside of the school. However, "where there's a will there's
a way," as all teachers who are determined to give their pupils the richest possible
educational experiences well know. Such educators often contact the Scouts or
other youth-serving organizations in the community and enlist their cooperation in
helping children learn more about their community through Saturday excursions.
Others assign older pupils to visit such places as a recreation center or health
museum on their own time and write a paper which describes what has been learned
from this experience. Regardless of what method is used to make learning about
health an exciting adventure, the community with all its rich resources for learning
should be fully utilized.

Experiments and Demonstrations

Although experiments often prove to be more valuable on the upper elementary
level, primary children can learn much from doing simple ones, too. Their curiosity
can easily be stimulated, for young children especially are eager to find things out
for themselves. Experiments should be kept simple, geared to help children discover
their own answers to the problem around which the experiment has been built,
planned under teacher guidance, and done by the pupils themselves. Care must be
taken in using animal experiments, for although the pupil may learn that a mouse
fed only on unhealthful foods will not grow as rapidly or be as healthy as one given
a well-balanced diet, children know that they are not mice, and therefore what happened to the animal could not possibly happen to them. The teacher must help

---

[2] Oberteuffer, Delbert: *School Health Education.* 5th ed. New York: Harper &
    Row, 1972, p. 141.
[3] *Health Education.* 5th ed. Washington, D. C.: National Education Association
    and American Medical Association, 1961, p. 285.

each pupil see a clear and definite relationship between any experiment or demonstration and his own life and those of others around him.[4]

Experiments and demonstrations which pupils find fun and exciting to do include:

Using balloons to demonstrate how the lungs work in breathing.
Using light meters in discovering which part of the room is best for reading purposes.
Simple food tests for starch, fat, protein, water, and carbohydrates.
Water filtration experiments using layers of sand, gravel, and rock.
Treatment of stagnant water with chlorine.
Examination of bacteria on food and in water before and after they have been destroyed.
Food-intake experiments using colored water and plants.
Using mice, white rats, hamsters, guinea pigs, or chickens to show the effects of good and bad diet upon growth.
Making tooth powder from soda and salt.
Analysis of how bacteria work on bread, cheese, and vinegar.
Food canning.
Oxygen-consuming experiments.
Relaxation demonstrations.
Demonstrations of how muscles work and rest.
First-aid demonstrations, including artificial respiration, snake bite treatment, stopping arterial bleeding at the pressure points, and bandaging.
Posture demonstrations showing how to use the body correctly while lifting, carrying heavy objects, sitting, and moving through space.
Demonstrations of how light and sun affect all growing things.
Reproduction demonstration using fish, insects, eggs, or small animals.
Safety demonstrations, including the conduction of electricity, extinguishing fires, riding bicycles using hand signals, coming and going to school safely, combustibility of materials when improperly stored.

The scientific method used in experiments to prove or disprove a hypothesis embraces a number of other teaching methods, including discussion, problem solving, demonstration, and investigation. Although planning and setting-up experiments are time-consuming and tedious, properly performed experiments do have high educational value. Their correct use will help students develop the ability to follow specific directions, skills in using many new kinds of equipment, an increased appreciation of the scientific method of research, and the ability to see a project patiently through to its completion. Such discoveries are especially valuable to children during their formative years. Now, when there is a marked emphasis placed upon science in our daily lives, youngsters can be guided through the use of the experimental method in the elementary school to gain an understanding and appreciation of its relationship to health. Nutrition experiments to show the value of a well-balanced diet are especially suited to children, as are those in safety, and those which show how the human body, or how any of its systems or separate parts work. The social sciences, geography, reading, and most other subjects taught in the school provide numerous opportunities for the use of both the experimental and problem-solving methods. In schools in which the core

---

[4] See the splendid book which shows how students can do many kinds of fun-to-do simple experiments without elaborate equipment, *Biology Experiments For Children* by Ethel Hanauer, Dover Publications, Inc., New York, 1962.

curriculum is used, group teacher planning is necessary in order to discover and determine the many ways in which health problems can be incorporated and best used in the core content. Where a departmental organizational pattern exists, an important part of curriculum development should be given over to teacher planning based on pupil needs and interests and to the allocation of health learning experiences to the various homerooms and departments.

Problem Solving

Elementary children have a natural interest in solving problems which directly affect them. They can be made increasingly aware that colds and other diseases can be prevented, that personal cleanliness is important, and of other aspects of health education through this method. Actually, the problem-solving method is not an isolated one, for it is used in almost all other methods. The teacher who summarizes the film shown in class by asking pupils questions about what they saw, or who motivates students' interest in conducting an experiment to find out why food decays, or what is the effect of the sun upon growing things, is using this method. The primary objective of the problem-solving approach is to help children develop the ability to think and to appreciate the value of finding things out for themselves through trial and error coupled with discovery instead of merely being told the answers to their questions. Teaching is not telling, as this method so clearly shows. When a child learns to solve problems, he often can better cope with and develop ways to eradicate his own health problems, as well as those of others.

Almost any area of health can be taught through this method. Ideally, the children should be stimulated and guided to set up their own problems and be motivated to find answers to questions they want to know about.

The problem-solving method may be used individually in health counseling or by groups working on a specific project. A careful study can be made of the number of accidents which occur at school, and a program can be evolved to solve this problem. However, any problem which directly affects children can be used.

As Grout points out, the use of the problem-solving method helps children think critically about information, and to collect, organize, apply, and evaluate data in relationship to their own health problems.[5] It also provides children with opportunities to think, plan, participate, evaluate, work individually as well as with others, draw conclusions, show initiative, cooperate, develop good social and group relationships, and develop the valued concepts of behavior so necessary for good growth and development. If the problem-solving method is to be used successfully, pupils should help select those problem areas which are important to *them* for study through teacher-pupil planning. They will only become skilled in using this method and applying it to their daily lives if they are given opportunities to develop skill, and are shown how to capitalize upon their errors in using this technique.

In one school recently, a small group of fourth-graders became aroused (through the help of their teacher) over the lack of good manners among their peers using the lunchroom. Some gulped their food hurriedly in order to get out to the play-

---

[5] Grout, Ruth: *Health Teaching in Schools.* 5th ed. Philadelphia: W. B. Saunders Co., 1968, p. 182.

ground, others pushed and shoved in the cafeteria line, others talked at the table with food in their mouths, and some would even hold their noses or pretend to gag when they saw certain food being served. After considerable discussion in the classroom about this type of behavior, the group agreed that learning how to use the school lunchroom properly was a big problem which they themselves were causing, and they determined to find ways to solve it successfully for the sake of their own health and their reputation as pupils in that school. With the aid of the teacher, the class was able to define the problem clearly, which was that pupils did not fully understand or appreciate why they should eat well-balanced, carefully prepared hot lunches at school, nor the importance of eating slowly and using good manners. The class accepted the challenge this problem presented and decided to solve it. They drew up carefully prepared plans, which included committee assignments, personal interviews, on-the-spot lunchroom interviews, reading reference materials, class reports in which many kinds of visual aids on balanced diets in relation to growth were used, and other kinds of learning activities, including visiting the school kitchen and talking with the cooks and dietitian. When the class felt that they had gathered adequate data concerning their problem, they devised a possible solution to it, which was that the dietitian and two elected students from the class would check each tray of food selected by each pupil and announce daily the names of those who selected the best-balanced lunch and ate it while using the best manners. A student committee composed of two members also selected the pupil who was the most polite in the cafeteria line throughout the entire week. The group also voted upon and accepted the rule that no one could be excused from his assigned table until five minutes before the lunchroom period was over or until everyone else at his assigned table had finished eating. The class also chose a host and hostess for each table group to serve for one month before they were replaced by other elected pupils. A classroom honor roll listed the names of those selected three consecutive times by the dietitian for having chosen the best-balanced lunch and having the best table manners. Committee groups gave reports on what they had found out through library and other assignments about the value of eating a balanced diet. One group acted out an original skit showing the difference between bad and good behavior. Periodically the pupils evaluated their solution to their lunchroom problem and behavior there, and made changes in their original plans several times during the term when they discovered these were needed in order to gain better results.

The teacher plays a major role in helping children become aware of important health problems. As Willgoose reports:

> She often leads the way in discovering such items as community health hazards, causes of accidents and illnesses in school, causes of school absences, difficulties in eating, personal unhappiness, etc. Sometimes the problem is demonstrated by the use of a film.[6]

Throughout each day, school children must make many decisions and choices. The problem-solving method of teaching and learning will, if it has been used well and is clearly understood by the pupils, enable them to make such decisions more wisely, thus increasing their own health, safety, and well-being. It will also help

---

[6] Willgoose, *op. cit.*, p. 301.

them develop desirable habits and attitudes concerning their personal responsibility for the development and protection of their own health as well as that of those in their own family. The wise teacher will utilize the possibilities to health education fully in her daily teaching in each class period. The use of the problem-solving method in health education should result in improved changes in thinking and in attitudes.

The Use of Textbooks and Assignments

Nothing can destroy interest in learning about health faster than merely reading what one is assigned in a textbook. The teacher who says to her group, "Tomorrow we will discuss the materials found on pages 61 to 68 in your text," or the one who spends precious class time having students read aloud to each other is not only a great time-waster, but is being grossly overpaid for the little she accomplishes as an educator. Fortunately, health textbooks are becoming increasingly more fascinating to children, for they are beautifully illustrated and written by experts who know how to appeal to children's natural interests and can help them discover many new and exciting things.*

Effective assignments are those which help children discover the answers to their problems or to questions raised in class. The material in the book should be used both as a reference and an "idea springboard," and as such, need not be studied in the order presented in the book. All possible opportunities should be provided for children to bring to class things like magazine pictures, newspaper articles, or objects from their home or neighborhood which relate to the things they read about. Increasingly, publishers are printing textbooks in a graded series for children on the elementary level, and have done much to assure a logical, wisely selected program of materials. Most teachers can obtain a sample copy of these books upon written request as well as a teacher's edition for an entire series if the book is adopted by the school.

The library should be used in conjunction with outside assignments and as a means of stimulating interest in reading. Children should be encouraged to read widely as well as to develop a scientific attitude about the things read. The school librarian and teacher must work together to help pupils gain skills in using available materials and finding new reference materials. Attractive health education library exhibits, arranged by a student committee assisted by the librarian, often stimulate pupil interest, as will displays of interesting books written for the entertainment as well as education of children in the area of health, such as Munro Leaf's splendid *Health Can Be Fun*, or Jean Walsh Angland's *A Friend Is Someone Who Likes You.*

The teacher should use a textbook in much the same way she does any other instructional teaching aid—namely, as a tool for helping children learn. Although it is common practice to have all pupils use the same textbook, the teacher might well use a variety of textbooks which can be assigned to individual pupils to read and then share additional information about any subject with others in the group. Teachers' manuals, which are usually available, should be modified in order to make them most suitable, for unless the suggestions found in such manuals are made

---

* See the Appendix for recommended health education textbook series for elementary schools.

to fit the needs and interests of each teacher's own class group, they are of no value. Pupils' workbooks should likewise be used with caution; too often such materials merely provide pupils with "busy work" which has no educational value, and can even encourage pupils to copy answers directly from textbooks rather than to help them think about or discover their own answers. Although in some areas school administrators and state committees, rather than teachers, select textbooks, all instructors should have a voice in determining the books best suited for their needs. Those who are responsible for the selection of textbooks might well use the following criteria. The book must:

1. Contain scientific, accurate information.
2. Present graded materials in logical sequence.
3. Have high reader-interest appeal, contain familiar as well as new materials, and be on the comprehension level of the pupils in the grade for which it will be used.
4. Motivate positive behavior and a desire for improved health.
5. Be attractive, easily read, and well illustrated.

Teachers must remember that, although textbooks have a real place in every classroom, there is no textbook which can replace an instructor who plans her teaching materials so that her pupils can have meaningful learning experiences. A text is only a starting point from which teachers and pupils can begin many new and exciting learning adventures together, but it is the teacher who makes such adventures become experiences of real value.

TEACHING ANOTHER CHILD*

Children often can learn more from each other than from adults. Recent studies show that older youth can sometimes teach a younger child more successfully than the teacher. When using this method, the older child and his pupil should choose their own health topics to learn more about. Suggested areas evolve around personal cleanliness, control of communicable disease, and various areas in nutrition, such as eating in order to grow faster or diets for athletes.

NEWER AUDIOVISUAL MEDIA

Concept films, tape recordings, transparencies, audio-visual tapes, participation in a radio or television program on closed-circuit networks, the use of slides, home movies or photographs taken by the children, the use of the walkie-talkie and direct telephone communication from a child or the class to a health authority can all be used effectively in teaching health and can help children learn to develop positive health habits as well as to become more aware of the factual reasons behind the necessity for doing so. It is also suggested that all teachers take advantage of a "Monthly Health Specials Calendar" approach. During Easter Seal Week safety education could be stressed in order to prevent children from being made crippled as the result of an accident, during Fire Prevention Week stress could be placed upon home and school clean-ups as a means of preventing fires, or at Halloween

---

* To discover how well children can teach their peers see the provocative book by Gartner, et al.: *Children Teach Children*. New York: Harper & Row, 1971.

time children could be cautioned not to go trick or treating alone or avoid wearing a face mask which obscures vision, etc.*

EXHIBITS AND MUSEUMS

An exhibit is an excellent means of showing others what has been done by a class group, and of stimulating pride of accomplishment in each pupil. Grown-ups who take their youngsters to visit the camp they went to as children often feel great pride and have real identification with that particular place, for it is here that they helped build the camp chapel or a swinging bridge across a deep ravine. School children need to develop such feelings of pride and to have close identification with their school. A well-planned temporary exhibit or a permanent display in a show-case in the school lobby can do much to produce such feelings, if the things collected for others to see and admire have been made by the children themselves.

All exhibits should convey a message and are best when built around a specific theme or fact, involve little reading, can be easily understood, and are eye-catching and hold the interest. The entire exhibit should be done by the pupils under the guidance of their teacher. Although she can plant ideas for the theme and the content of the exhibit, if the project is to be an educational one, the specific planning and execution of the project must be done by the class. Such exhibits should convey a special message to the viewers. Consequently, each pupil or committee group

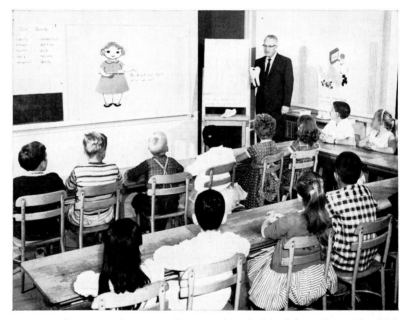

Figure 8-1. Guest speakers can share much valuable information with children. (Courtesy of Los Angeles Public Schools)

* For other suggestions of how to capitalize upon this suggested calendar approach, see the article by Stephen Schnessweiss and Ralph Jones, "Time-Linked Problems: The Monthly Health Specials Calendar Approach for Use in Grades K-6," *The Journal of School Health*, October 1968, pp. 524–27.

making each separate exhibit should determine what specific information they want to get across by means of the exhibit.   This, in turn, will make the development of each project a rich educational experience.

A visit to a health museum such as those in Dallas and in Cleveland, the Children's Museum in Fort Worth, the Museum of Natural History in New York can do much to intrigue children about health.   If the class group is taken on a visit, the trip should be well planned, and the children not hurried along.   The teacher, as well as a museum guide, should help the class understand the things at which they are looking, and make every attempt to broaden and increase each child's interest in and knowledge of health.   Unfortunately, many localities do not have such museums, and many children are denied the rich learning adventure found from visiting them.   Fortunately, the American Medical Association, the Cleveland Health Museum, and several commercial firms have traveling exhibits and miniature museums for loan or rent.   The teacher should make every effort to visit outstanding health museums and bring back ideas to share with her group for making their own miniature museum.   Ideally, each elementary school should have its own health education laboratory, health education room, or have a permanently assigned space for housing permanent health exhibits, displays, and current class projects.

DRAMATIZATIONS

Many free health plays written for children are available from the American Theatre Wing Community Plays, 351 West 48th Street, New York; Human Rela-

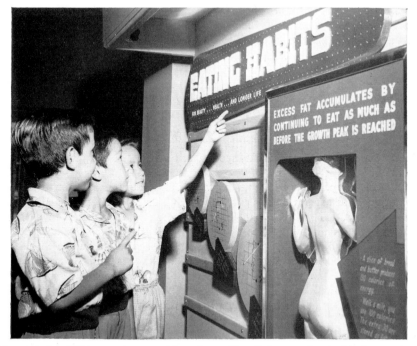

Figure 8-2.   Children gain many ideas for making their own visual aids for a school health exhibit from seeing examples.   (Courtesy of Dallas Health and Science Museum)

tions Aids, 1790 Broadway, New York; National Safety Council, Chicago; Junior Red Cross, Washington, D. C.; National Boy Scout Headquarters, New York; National Girl Scout Headquarters, New York; and Campfire Girls National Headquarters, New York. The best plays, however, are often those written, directed, and acted by the children themselves.

Children delight in dramatic activities. Their small world is largely one of make-believe and imitation. In order that they use this favorite pastime profitably while in school, however, the teacher should be cognizant of the following limitations of dramatics as a method of health teaching as pointed out by Humphrey.

1. Unless the cast is frequently changed, all pupils will not receive the benefit of direct participation.
2. It is possible that entertainment will be substituted for education.
3. Certain forms of dramatization may not warrant the expenditure of time that it takes to prepare and present them.
4. Literary values may be overstressed, with little or no value for health and safety.
5. The lines may be largely "preachment" of health facts.
6. The dialogue might develop into the mere memorization of health facts.
7. There might be an insufficient amount of action and an overabundance of dialogue.
8. There is a possibility that pupils may be considered only as dramatis personae. Despite Shakespeare's immortal words, the play is *not* the thing; the learner should receive the greatest consideration when the dramatic method is used.[7]

Amateur shows in which original plays, songs, or poems can be presented to the class are exciting educational experiences for children. Health plays are more meaningful when written, acted in, and directed by the pupils themselves, as are their own miniature television series in which an individual or family can be shown solving a series of health problems. The use of puppets and shadowgraphs can also be an effective way to teach health to children. The very young enjoy simple finger plays and wall shadows that "talk" and can be made in the form of bears, rabbits, dogs, or other animals. Puppets made from discarded junk materials are far more fun for children to use than expensive store-bought marionettes. Those made of paper bags, socks, tennis balls, brushes of varying sizes, papier-mâché, vegetables, fruits, hedge apples, boxes, corks, spoons, or sawdust can be quickly made and cost nothing.[8]

Tableaus and pageants can be utilized well in elementary schools, for each grade group can be assigned a specific part in a production involving all the children in the school. A definite theme should be selected and attempts made to integrate materials from many subject areas. Role playing and sociodramatic activities are especially well suited to the upper elementary grades. Those using these media of expression should first show, through unrehearsed and spontaneous expression, how people do behave in certain situations, and then how they should behave. This second portrayal should reflect the reactions and suggestions of the actors and the class for improving behavior or eliminating problems which do arise in certain situations.

---

[7] Humphrey, James: *Elementary School Health Education.* New York: Harper & Row, 1962, p. 304.
[8] Vannier, Maryhelen: *Techniques in Recreation Leadership.* Philadelphia: Lea & Febiger. In preparation.

ORAL PRESENTATIONS

Discussions between the pupil and teacher should do more than merely exchange information, for when used correctly, this method has high educational value. Care must be taken that certain bright students do not gain and keep the limelight long enough to cause the already dull to become duller pupils. Carefully devised, concise teacher questions are most effective and yield the most fruitful results. Questions which require "yes" or "no" answers, or the repeating of memorized meaningless phrases should be avoided, for children are not slot machines or parrots, but human beings eager to learn and so solve hard as well as easy problems.

Some teachers can stimulate pupil interest in learning how the human eye works by describing to the class how birds, whales, or dogs see in contrast to how a person sees; others may motivate a class, when introducing a new unit on nutrition, by describing how bird mothers take care of their young. Regardless of whether the pupils are more stimulated by hearing about animals or about children of their own age or those living in other countries, oral presentation can work wonders in arousing pupil curiosity. Likewise, they can help children feel as though their questions are important and help them gain confidence in speaking before others. Through such class discussions children can also learn many other things, such as being kind and considerate to others, or how to express themselves well using good grammar. The instructor should carefully guide class discussions and help each child contribute something of value to this group activity.

Oral reports given by students also have great educational value, for children can learn much from accepting and carrying out responsibility for making such reports,

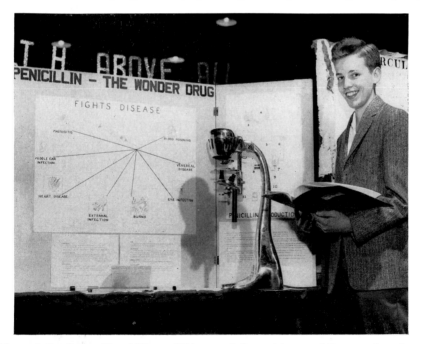

Figure 8-3. Some older children will learn much from giving special reports based on their own research. (Courtesy of Nashville Public Schools)

and gain a feeling of pride that they are contributing something of value to the group. Some develop self-confidence and an interest in speaking before groups which has lasting value; many a politician or lawyer gained a strong desire to select a "talking type" of profession from these early experiences. Pupils giving special reports should be guided into interesting subject channels suited to their capabilities, yet challenging enough to help them develop new interests and knowledge. Each reporter should first give a brief statement of his topic, then report on it, and finally summarize briefly what he said. Experienced public speakers summarize this, "Tell them what you are going to say, then say it, and finally, tell them what you have just said."

The lecture method is considered by many to be the poorest of all methods of teaching, for man's attention span is short, and after a short time the listener tends to hear only snatches of what is said. However, this method, when used correctly, does have great merit. It can be used in the modified form of a story or brief description to motivate elementary children. Illustrated materials should be used and referred to as the teacher talks to the group, for what one both hears and sees can be a potent means of education. A discussion between the learners and teacher following the short talk will add to the effectiveness of this method, as will a summary at the end of the discussion, and a short résumé later, on the following day, or throughout the week. Such emphasis helps children remember longer the things they are learning. Pupils can become active listening participants, but the degree to which they can do so depends largely upon the skillfulness of the speaker and her ability to recapture wandering attention.

What children say and do when out on the playground, at home, or anywhere away from the classroom is the real test of the effectiveness of any educator or teaching method. Any teacher who is determined to help children learn things of value most effectively will experiment, keep trying, and finally, at last, find her own best methods for doing so.

PRINCIPLES OF TEACHING

Good teaching is based upon sound principles. Each instructor must make all class periods meaningful and purposeful, linking what is learned today with what was mastered yesterday. The following principles of teaching are suggested guides which will help eliminate wasting time and energy on the part of both the instructor and the learner:

1. The teacher and learner are working partners who must find purposes, devise plans, share experiences, see relationships in what they learn, and evaluate together what has been accomplished.
2. Individual differences must be taken into account and learners guided toward accomplishments which bring them satisfaction, challenge, and new interests.
3. Each learning and teaching experience should be reality-centered.
4. The primary role of the teacher is to motivate pupils and guide them toward positive actions, attitudes, and values.
5. The teacher should place each student in a group in which he can make the most educational progress.
6. The teaching environment should be group-controlled, not teacher-dominated and be a friendly, encouraging one in which all pupils feel secure and are contributing members.

7. Teaching is helping others discover and develop their latent talents; the role of the teacher is to help the learner do better those things he finds he can do.
8. There can be no productive learning without productive teaching or productive self-motivation.
9. When we help others learn how to do certain things, we can usually do this best by showing how and then helping them analyze and do what we have done.
10. The teacher must discover the causes of slow learning or nonlearning, and find ways to overcome them to improve learning.

Pitfalls to Be Avoided

It is not easy to teach health in schools. Teachers often make damaging and lasting mistakes in their zealous attempts to help children "grow up to be big and strong." Many, forgetting that they are only licensed to teach, not to preach, forecast destruction and doom to those children who do not brush their teeth every night, fail to bathe regularly, or do only a few of the many things they should. Still others overstress competition and rewards in the form of gold stars or other symbols to the extent that they fail to see that the child is washing behind his ears every day in order to have the class see his teacher paste another gold star on his chart, instead of doing so as a means of keeping clean. Other practices which should be avoided include:

1. Contests for the healthiest child.
2. Artificial rewards ("You do this, children, for me and I'll let you out early today," gold stars, and too frequent praise so that success comes too easily and without meaningful challenge).
3. The use of untrue, sadistic, or sensational materials in an effort to shock listeners to become concerned about health.
4. The use of ridicule, sarcasm, or projected frustration upon abnormal, unattractive children who become the adult's scapegoat as well as that of the class.
5. The use of senseless jingles or slogans that are cute and catchy, but educationally worthless.
6. Saying one thing and doing another in regard to health.
7. Making health instruction dull, thus destroying children's natural interest and curiosity to know about themselves and the world in which they live.
8. Causing pupils to become too health-conscious and hypochondriac.

Basic Guides for Teaching Health

Basic guides for teaching health to children in elementary schools include the following suggestions:

1. Place emphasis upon the positive approach toward health.
2. Teach to reach each individual and stimulate his own personal desire to improve his own health, and to value health as a way of life.
3. Teach each child how and why he must take ever-increasing responsibilities for his own health habits.
4. The goal of instruction should be the happy, well-adjusted, healthy child.
5. Base all lessons on the interest, needs, and capacities of children at each stage in their development, yet keep in mind that they will become adults who will be responsible for their own actions and those of others.
6. Relate what is learned in school to the reality in which the child lives.
7. Integrate and correlate learning experiences in health with as many other subjects taught in school as possible.

8. Stress that knowledge gained about health should be applied to one's daily life.
9. Scientific materials from the fields of anatomy, physiology, or other sciences are of value in health education only if they help the pupil understand his own body more and solve his own health problems better.
10. All materials which are taught must be related to helping pupils make right decisions concerning their own health.
11. Present health education as a means to an end, not as an end in itself.

Discussion Questions

1. Which of the teaching methods can best be used to motivate a slow learner; the average pupil; the most intelligent child? Why?
2. Why is there no one "best" teaching method?
3. How should health textbooks be used on the elementary level?
4. In what ways can teachers overmotivate children about health? What are the dangers of doing so?
5. What preliminary plans and actions must be made in regard to taking children on field trips?
6. Why should animal experiments be used with caution when teaching nutrition? How can animal experiments be used in any of the other areas of health education?
7. List 10 problems which children or a class might face which could be solved by the use of the problem-solving method of teaching.
8. How can the school librarian help the classroom teacher teach health more effectively to children?
9. What are the advantages and disadvantages of using workbooks?
10. What are the strengths and weaknesses of using dramatics as a teaching method?

Things To Do

1. Give a sample health lesson to your classmates using the experimental method of teaching.
2. Take a group of children on a field trip in order to learn more about any phase of health. Describe the results to your classmates.
3. Visit the children's department at your local public library. Bring to class the book for children which you would use in a health lesson and describe why you selected that one.
4. Write a critique on an elementary school health textbook series stating the strengths and weaknesses of that series.
5. Conduct an experiment using an animal, fish, or plant in any area of nutrition education. Tell others what you learned from this experiment.
6. Visit a health class in an elementary school. Write a two-page paper on the various teaching methods you saw the instructor use.
7. Give an oral report on any chapter in the list of suggested readings which deals with teaching methods. Tell your classmates what you learned from this experience.
8. Using the problem-solving method, describe one health problem you solved using it. What do you feel are the dangers inherent in overusing this method?

Suggested Readings

Hansen, Ruth and Harlan: "The Child and the Curriculum—Show and Tell. A New Look." *The Instructor*. October 1972.
Harrelson, Orvis: "Health, The Affective Approach. *The Instructor*, October 1972
Morris, Nelson, and Jackson, Sommers: "Using Community Assets For Better Learning." *The Instructor*, August-September 1972.

Read, Donald, and Greene, Walter: *Creative Teaching in Health*. New York: The Macmillan Company, 1971.

School Health Education Study Advisory Committee: *Health Education: A Conceptual Approach To Curriculum Design*. St. Paul: 3M Education Press, 1968.

Stickler, Ruth: "Mini-Instructor—A+ Library Behavior." *The Instructor*, August-September 1972.

Wilbur, Muriel: *Educational Tools For Health Personnel*. New York: The Macmillan Company, 1968.

Zeitz, Frank: "The Emotion Box." *The Instructor*, August-September 1972.

CHAPTER 9

helpful teaching aids

Learning experiences in health can be made more memorable through the use of supplementary teaching aids. Each teacher should have a variety of good instructional materials but should not use them as a crutch or substitute, with the idea that merely exposing the children to them will ensure learning. All such materials should assist in educating pupils and should not be used merely as a means of entertaining them. Schools cannot and should not compete with the amusement world, nor were they ever meant to.

In a sense, all supplementary teaching materials are audio-visual. When properly used, these materials can:

Supply a concrete base for conceptual thinking and hence reduce meaningless word responses of students.
Have a high degree of interest for students.
Make learning more permanent.
Offer a variety of experiences which will stimulate self-activity on the part of students.
Develop continuity of thought; this is especially true of motion pictures.
Contribute to growth of understanding and hence to vocabulary development.
Provide experiences not easily obtained otherwise and contribute to the efficiency, depth, and variety of learning.[1]

All carefully selected visual aids should give a true picture of the ideas they present, contribute more meaningful materials to the unit in which they are used, be appropriate for the class, have good eye and ear appeal, and be well worth the time and effort spent in obtaining and using them.

---

[1] Willgoose, Carl: *Health Education in the Elementary Schools.* 4th ed. Philadelphia: W. B. Saunders Co., 1974, p. 322.

There are many different kinds of teaching aids. Some of the best ones to use in health teaching include:

Chalkboards	Maps	Radio
Scrapbooks	Flashcards	Television
Specimens (live and	Mobiles	Recordings
preserved)	Flat pictures	Models
Pamphlets	Newspaper clippings	Exhibits
Bulletin boards	and magazines	Slides
Flannel boards	Filmstrips	Films
Posters	Photographs	Puppets
Cartoons	Question boxes	Agar plates
Stick-figure drawings	Food samples, labels	Health records
Opaque projector	from cans, etc.	Bicycles
Spot and geographical	First-aid supplies	Small toys or automo-
maps	Mouth mirrors and	biles
Visual materials and	other types of dental	Grooming supplies, in-
records	equipment	cluding a nail file,
Mannikins	Microscopes	hairbrush, etc.
Diagrams	Mirrors	
Charts	Comics	
Graphs	Collections	

SOURCES OF MATERIAL

There is such an abundance of free and inexpensive materials in health that the problem for many teachers is to select, catalogue, and find ways to use those things she has obtained.[2] The wise educator starts her own collection while still a student in college, for such materials will help her feel more secure when she begins to teach. All teachers should subscribe to professional journals, daily newspapers, and several good popular magazines, as well as being ever on the lookout for supplementary materials and teaching aids which they might use in their classes. Going to local and national teachers' conventions will prove beneficial and keep a teacher up to date on new things in her field, as well as acquaint her with new teaching materials which are available.

The children should contribute even more than the teacher in the collection of materials, and will do so if encouraged to bring to class and share things they have found outside of school which pertain to what they are studying. Friends and parents can also contribute many materials but will need to be informed of the type of things needed, for although people are anxious to help others, they are often unaware of how to do so. Recently, the parents of one sixth-grade class also learned a great deal about health when they were asked to help their children collect health education articles from the local newspaper and the magazines. In another school, a group of mothers helped pupils locate old snapshots taken of recreational activities they had enjoyed when they were children. These were used by a committee reporting on "How Our Parents Used Their Leisure Time When They Were Children." Family members of a third-grade class in a school in Georgia recently helped youngsters gather their baby pictures, as well as those taken at yearly intervals. These were used in a written report made by each child entitled "I Am Growing Up."

---

[2] See the Appendix for a list of sources of free and inexpensive health education materials.

The list of suggested readings at the end of this chapter will prove helpful to the teacher who wishes to make her own supplementary materials with her students. Those who guide pupils in creating their own visual aids will share richer educational experiences with their children than those who collect such teaching aids, because the children will profit much more from doing things for themselves.

RECOMMENDED MATERIALS

Each teacher should experiment and discover which type of supplementary materials could be used most profitably with her particular class. For most children, seeing the germs on their own hands under a microscope is a far more potent educational experience than seeing a cartoon entitled "Mr. Germ." Regardless of which type of aid is selected, its use should be made as personalized as possible. Seeing one's own teeth in a magnifying mirror may be excellent for most pupils, but may not be for all in the class. Gadgets to be manipulated, buttons to be pushed, and wooden flaps to be lifted in order to see what they hide are all fascinating to children and should be used in conjunction with their health education class.

Motion Pictures

When correctly used, motion pictures can be one of the finest ways to stimulate interest and motivate changes in behavior in the field of health education. Although it is no doubt true that one picture is worth a thousand words, it must be remembered that one direct, purposeful experience is far superior, educationally speaking, to many pictures. Most state departments of education have a wide variety of health films which are available upon request, and they also are increasingly developing audio-visual aid branch libraries strategically located throughout the state. The majority of our large school systems have their own film libraries and have stocked them with carefully selected pictures suitable for children on each grade level. State universities, private colleges, city, county, and state health departments, youth agencies, commercial organizations, and local libraries also have well-selected health films which are available upon request. The U.S. Office of Education Film Library Directory lists free films which can be obtained for use in the classroom.[3] Most schools request that films which contain advertising not be shown to pupils, and most of them have policies drawn up to guide in the selection of all films.

From research conducted by audio-visual educational specialists, there is no doubt that the use of well-selected films in the schools increases the whole climate of instruction, learning efficiency, and retention, as well as reading ability and comprehension. Certainly, all films should be carefully selected and shown for a definite purpose, whether this be to shape specific attitudes, increase interest in any given area, aid the pupils to gain a clearer understanding by seeing enlargements of things too small to see with the human eye, clarify relationships of events in time, or help pupils gain a deeper appreciation of the wonder and beauty of life and living things.

Factors to keep in mind when selecting a motion picture to show to a class are that it must

1. Be suited to the age level of the group and have high educational value.
2. Contain accurate, authoritative information.

---

[3] See the *Educator's Index of Free Films*, published annually by Educator's Progress Service, Randolph, Wisconsin.

3. Give pupils a more complete understanding of the unit they are studying than they could get elsewhere.
4. Be well organized, clearly audible, and well photographed.
5. Fit the purposes, needs, and interests of the pupils.
6. Be of suitable length.

The teacher should know the correct time in the course of the unit to show the film, for the pupils should see it when they can most profit from the experience. It is important that the teacher preview the picture before showing it so she can best direct the pupils' attention to the important things in it. Likewise, she should give a brief résumé of the content of the film in a manner which will excite the interest of the class. It is necessary to help children know what to look for in the film, so that they will remain alert and interested in what they are seeing. The teacher should summarize the important things learned from the film, or members of the class may do so.

She should be a skilled projectionist; she should know what to do when the film jumps or breaks, or in any other kind of projection emergency. Nothing destroys the effectiveness of a film more than these irritating mishaps, which can become so uproariously funny to youngsters that the whole procedure becomes a farce and an educational waste. Certain pupils in the upper elementary grades will enjoy being taught to operate the projector. This is not only a good means of keeping truancy at a minimum on film days, but also can be a way to provide high-status jobs for those children who are attracted to machines and have a desire to master them. During the showing, the room should be well ventilated, darkened, and the viewers seated so that they can both see and hear well. The teacher should place herself in the best position to watch pupils' reactions to the picture.

After the film, the instructor should review its main points. This may be done by the teacher, by one pupil, by the entire group in response to her questions, or by a simple paper-and-pencil objective test. The film should initiate a wide variety of learning follow-up activities such as experiments, posters, bulletin boards, or creative activities devised around factual materials or concepts learned from the film. The film may be reshown, if necessary, to clarify certain points. Likewise, there are times when it is more advantageous to stop the film and involve the class in a discussion of probable solutions to problems being illustrated, and then, after continuing with the remainder of it, compare the shown solution with that devised by the class. An ingenious teacher will discover for herself effective ways to help pupils use what they have learned from seeing well-selected school health films. Teachers would be wise to make their own film-evaluation file for future planning and reference. Such a file, easily made on index cards, would have notes on each film shown and information which should be given by the teacher in summarizing the main points of the film.

Filmstrips

These visual aids have many advantages over motion pictures in that they are less expensive, more easily shown, and often made to supplement a particular health education textbook series. Many commercial companies have free filmstrips for classroom use.[4] Suggestions given above about the best educational use of motion pictures also apply to the showing of filmstrips and slides.

---

[4] See the Appendix for a list of suggested ones.

Children can make their own filmstrips by cutting up old ones and rearranging the pictures. They can also create their own homemade cartoons by drawing pictures in a series on a long piece of paper, rolling it on a rod, and showing it by using a cardboard carton with a window cut in the front for a projector. Filmstrips allow the teacher more flexibility than movies, for she can more easily adapt the materials to the needs and interest of each class.[5]

Slides

Although there is an abundance of slides available, the best ones are often made by the pupils themselves. Many children have their own cameras and are fairly skilled at taking pictures by the time they are in the fourth grade. Biological supply houses and commercial companies also have slides for either sale or rental at a nominal fee. Pupils will enjoy making their own pen-and-ink sketches on glass slides and seeing their work on a screen. An automatic slide changer is recommended for classroom use, since it can be timed perfectly with any comments the teacher wishes to make about the slide being seen, and frees the teacher from showing the pictures. Slides are ideal for classroom work, for they need not be shown in sequence, and only a few well-selected ones will help teachers get needed information over to children quickly. They are also ideal for presenting and magnifying graphs, charts, tables, or other similar types of information.

The Opaque Projector

Through these inexpensive machines newspaper clippings, charts, graphs, maps, examples of pupils' work, or any other type of written or printed material can be magnified and shown on a screen. Pupils respond quickly to having their own or a friend's best work shown to others in this manner.

As Haag suggests, in schools which cannot purchase human anatomy and physiology charts for health instruction, teacher-prepared slides of drawings from human anatomical and physiological texts can be used.[6] These same drawings can be shown enlarged so that younger pupils may more easily understand or older children may learn important details about the wonders of the human body. In a study of the bones of the body, the teacher might well have each pupil locate each bone shown on the screen in his own body, thus helping the learner grasp the relationship of what is being shown to himself.

The opaque projector has many different uses in the classroom. Pupils should help gather materials to be shown and can, through individual reports, help their classmates relate health and safety concepts to pictures. The teacher should take care that the pupils understand the significance of what is shown and that they do not read their own meaning into what they are seeing; she must always be aware that each pupil understands everything in light of his own past experience. The pupils should be given sufficient time to view each picture in order to gain full value from seeing it. The use of class discussions, question and answers, and asking pupils to identify certain parts in the picture by pointing to it and giving its name are all

[5] See *The Filmstrip Guide*, published yearly by the H. H. Wilson Company, 950 University Avenue, New York, N. Y., for a listing of 13,000 filmstrips suitable for schools.

[6] Haag, Jessie: *School Health Program.* 3rd ed. Philadelphia: Lea & Febiger, 1972, p. 412.

recommended. This could be done especially well in showing a picture of a tooth and asking the class to identify the type of tooth shown, its parts, and care. Any body part and its care could be taught by using this same method. Pupils will especially enjoy learning how to operate the projector, and such experiences can help them build favorable attitudes toward contributing to the class. For some, this type of experience can be a means of gaining group status and helping them build self-confidence.

Television

No other communication medium has grown as rapidly as television. As an educational device, it is powerful and potent—whether for good or evil—for it can produce positive as well as negative results. Increasingly, schools are using television, and children are being given opportunities to see as well as hear master teachers conduct lessons on regularly scheduled programs. The day of educational television is dawning, but meanwhile, teachers who work in schools without sets for classroom use can guide children to watch worthwhile and unique programs in their own homes and report to the group on things they have heard and seen that pertain to what they are studying in health at school.

School-planned television now exists in many of our schools. Such programs are planned and presented by experienced teachers; many show classroom experiences and situations well in advance of each telecast, and a copy of the program schedule and its contents, in the form of teacher and pupil guides, is sent to all teachers so that they can prepare their pupils to obtain full benefit from the program.[7] Educational telecasts vary from one lesson taken from a unit of several lessons on a subject to continued broadcasts of a complete unit shown daily for a week or longer, and to having the studio teacher give basic instruction on a subject to many children in a grade in all the schools in an area. Regardless of which method is used, it is imperative that the classroom teacher in each school "take it from there," and use what has been presented by the studio teacher as a foundation for her own teaching.

It is now possible, by closed circuit, for a class to view demonstrations and experiments in a faraway laboratory. Such experiences, which are less time-consuming than field trips, assure the teacher that all pupils are seeing the same thing, which is not usually the case when they are on an educational outing. Such viewing, however, should only be a supplementary part of the work the teacher is doing in her own classroom.

Since television is a one-way method of communication, its use in the school can only become effective if followed by classroom work such as discussions, questions and answers, written or oral examinations, or other teaching methods which will enable the child to contribute what he has learned and the teacher to gain insight upon what each child has learned and how he will apply it to his own life. The teacher should summarize the main things seen, heard, and discussed at the end of the class period as well as give, or have a pupil or the class give, a review of these things the next day. Such summaries and reviews help children become aware of important things and help them retain this valuable information longer.

---

[7] *Health Education.* 5th ed. Washington, D. C.: National Education Association and American Medical Association, 1961, p. 289.

Radio Broadcasts

In order that children be guided to listen to worthwhile and educational radio broadcasts, the teacher should obtain as much advance information about specific programs as possible. Assigning students to do advance preparation before listening to any particular broadcast is highly recommended, as are follow-up assignments, and class discussions of programs heard either independently or in a group.

In order to retain their licenses, all radio stations must devote a certain percentage of their total broadcasting time to educational programs. Consequently, many local stations are now using school-sponsored broadcasts in which programs are planned and presented by the pupils themselves, assisted by their teachers. Such programs are not only an excellent means for maintaining a high level of pupil interest in health, but do much to arouse parental enthusiasm for the work their children are doing at school.

Like all other audio-visual tools, radio can be used advantageously at school by the teacher and pupils. However, it should be used to bring the world into the classroom and be regarded by the instructor primarily as a teaching aid instead of as an end in itself. The teacher must make every effort to integrate information from a broadcast with the course of study she is using in the classroom in order to help children gain the greatest value from listening to the radio, as well as to assist the pupils in becoming more critical and discriminating listeners. Carefully selected radio programs on such topics as events in history, stories about healthful living, or biographical sketches of health heroes can do wonders in vitalizing health teaching. Just as a reader of a textbook will get more out of his reading if he knows what he wants to accomplish, so the radio listener must also have his purpose well in mind. Consequently, before each class listening period, the teacher and group should discuss and write on the chalkboard their purposes in hearing the broadcast. Each child should then be encouraged to create and make a list of his own listening purposes. During the program, complete attention should be encouraged. By her own attitude the teacher can and should help create attentive listening among the group. Interruptions can be discouraged by cardboard signs, "Please—We Are Listening" or "Do Not Come In—We Are Listening," hung outside the classroom door.

The extent to which radio programs require follow-up activities in order that their maximum educational use be fulfilled is a good way to evaluate the effectiveness of a broadcast. Attempts to obtain more information about a subject, increased creative expression skills in language arts, student participation in their own actual or make-believe broadcasts, increased outside reading at home are only a few of the possible follow-up activities which can be utilized for excitingly valuable health teaching. When radio programs become important to children and they ask their mothers to tune in the same programs at home as those to which they listen in school, it helps to bridge the gap between home and school.

Children should learn to be self-motivated in their actions, and the teacher can help them learn how to become wisely discriminating and critical radio listeners who can select their own programs intelligently. Children should be guided to use their leisure time in and away from school, for this is an important part of their education, too. Teachers should discover what programs children listen to at home and help them select better ones by recommending certain outstanding future programs weekly in class. She can also assign homework listening and follow such assignments by classroom discussions. Older pupils can also learn much from analyzing radio commercials from the standpoint of misrepresentation.

Recordings

Phonograph records and tape recordings can provide learning experiences for children. Records are ideal for classroom work, for the teacher can stop them in order to discuss or repeat certain passages, and they can be played over and over again, can be preheard and evaluated, and can even be made by the pupils themselves, assisted by their instructor. Making a tape recording of a class discussion or panel can be enlightening and thrilling for children, especially when they hear their own voices and each becomes conscious of his need for improvement as a speaker and group member. Recording the talks given by visiting authorities or those heard on radio not only helps motivate pupil interest and makes them more aware of the high regard well-known adults have for the value of good health, but such recordings can be used for the benefit of future classes as well.

As in the case of the use of radio broadcasts or television, the teacher using these communication media should first prepare the listeners for the coming experience, later emphasize the important things that have been heard, and relate them to the actual life of each listening child. There are numerous helpful guides and manuals, issued by leading manufacturers of tape recordings, which the teacher should carefully study before using this type of equipment. Finding the best recording distances and positions in relation to the microphone, having all speak in a clear but natural conversational manner, eliminating background noise as much as possible by recording in rooms where echo can be reduced by drapes, screens, or acoustical tile, and taping the entire program without interruptions will all improve the quality of any recording made at school.

It is comparatively easy to provide elementary children with many kinds of learning experiences in which they can taste, touch, see, or hear, for youngsters in these early formative years are eager to find out everything by first-hand experiences. As they advance in school, such first-hand experiences are harder to find, for they will study history or learn about people in distant lands in geography. Educational recordings of such men as Presidents Franklin Roosevelt and Dwight Eisenhower have done much to bring realism into the classroom and to make history a study of events centering around outstanding, colorful people. Recordings of health heroes can do much to motivate individual desires to enter the medical profession, as well as to help children realize that because of the sacrifices of some people, they live in a healthier world. Such recordings can be taped by either the teacher or students. Excellent materials on health heroes can be obtained free of charge from the Health Education Department of the Metropolitan Life Insurance Company in New York, or from any of its branch offices.

Almost every teacher can make recordings of live events which happen in her classroom. The pupils of the fifth grade in the Horace Mann School recently wrote a play in conjunction with their unit in nutrition education. Although it was a simple, one-act version of imaginary conversations between a supermarket checker and various shoppers who went through her check-out line, the pupils delighted in hearing the tape recording made in class of "their play" and learned much from this experience. In still another school, a group of sixth-graders recorded on tape four panel discussions given in class in a mental hygiene unit on

"How to Be Popular," "How to Overcome Shyness," "When Should We Hide Our Feelings?" and "What Health Habits Can Help Make Us More Attractive?" These were played several times the following week and the pupils were then asked to select the best panel group according to criteria the class used for judging the work: accuracy of facts presented, ability of the panel to stimulate listener interest, and similar standards. In a second-grade class in Texas, the teacher played a tape recording on "Our Eyes and How to Take Care of Them," which she had obtained from the Audio-Visual Aids Department of the Dallas Public Library. In order to help the group get the most out of listening to the recording, she told them briefly about its contents:

> The doctor who made this recording will speak to us about how to take care of our eyes. He will first tell you how our eyes are like a camera, and then he will give you ten suggestions for taking good care of your own eyes. Please write down each suggestion. Let's see which one of you can make the complete list of ten first. We will then divide up into groups of three to act out any of these ten suggestions. Listen carefully to what these suggestions are, and decide which suggestion you would like to act out for the class.

The use of recordings in teaching can only be justified when they bring into the classroom greater pupil interest, and when faster and more meaningful learning can result from their use. The teacher's responsibilities for making such learning experiences valuable ones include prelistening, increasing the listener's vocabulary by teaching pupils the meaning and spelling of all new words, conducting well-thought-out class discussions, evaluating the results of this experience through testing (either verbal or written), and increasing and widening many other kinds of learning activities which revolve around each listening experience.

Pictures and Posters

Pictures and posters must be pleasant to see again and again, and should have aesthetic appeal and power.* There is an abundance of free posters now available for classroom use. Even pupils who are unskilled in art can cut out pictures and use them for a poster, whereas those talented in this area can and should create an entire poster themselves. Traced figures, cut-out silhouettes, montages made from pictures, articles, or newspaper headlines, stenciled or free-hand lettering, the use of pipe-cleaner stick figures, cotton, or other materials pasted on to a poster all may be used effectively. Each child should make some kind of poster during a semester, working on it individually or with a classmate. Those who gain much from this type of experience should be encouraged to develop real skill in this medium of communication.

Commercial posters must be selected with care. Some schools prohibit the use of any visual aids or other supplementary materials which contain advertising. Many

---

* Obtain the excellent record and poster combination, "Let's Sing With Ella Jenkins," available from Scott, Foresman and Co., Glenview, Illinois 60025. The record includes "Juice For Breakfast," "This Is The Way I Wash My Face," "Crossing Streets," "Bedtime," "Did You Have A Glass of Milk?" "I Stop, I Look, I Listen," "A Game: Learning Parts of the Body," and "When We Take a Rest."

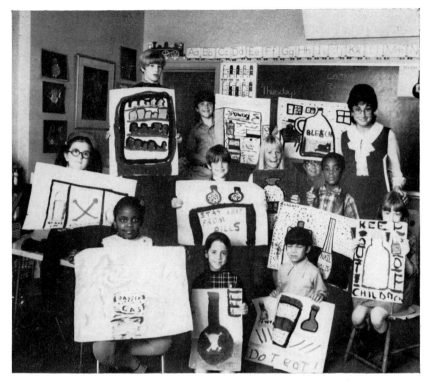

Figure 9-1. All children should learn about products that can cause serious illness or death. (Courtesy of Pharmaceutical Manufacturers Association)

companies that supply free materials have obligingly printed their firm's name in small letters at the bottom so that, if necessary, it can easily be blocked out or covered over by an instructor.

Effective posters, whether they be pupil-created or obtained from other sources, are those which:

1. Contain a simplified idea or message.
2. Create a learning atmosphere.
3. Motivate action.
4. Give accurate, attention-getting information.
5. Emphasize the importance of doing a certain thing or developing a good health habit.
6. Possess eye appeal.
7. Create a lasting impression.

Photographs taken by either the teacher or pupils can provide many meaningful educational experiences. A fourth-grade teacher in Seattle recently discovered that the most effective way to motivate interest and desire to develop good posture among her students was to take individual snapshots of each child in her class as he stood before her facing first frontward and then sideways. A conference was held with each child, and each was asked to look closely at his own photograph as he and the teacher picked out his postural defects. Next, he was shown ways to correct his difficulties. The class later selected pictures of those in their group who had the best posture, and an elected committee group used the photograph for a bulletin board they made entitled "Good Posture for Boys and Girls." Many schools use posture pictures as a means of teaching children the value of having good posture, as well as to show each child what his defects are and how to correct them.

Cartoons, Comics, Sketches, and Stick Figures

Three kinds of simple drawings which can easily be made by most children are those which show faces, figures, and objects. Each should be drawn with the purpose of communicating an important message quickly and effectively. A cartoon should be used to exaggerate. It may show a food gulper instead of a slow and careful eater or stress the value of drinking milk or exaggerate what happens to one's body when one does not eat a balanced diet. In fact, any health concept can be

TABLE 9–1. HEIGHT AND WEIGHT OF CHILDREN

	Boys													
Height, Inches	5 Yrs.	6 Yrs.	7 Yrs.	8 Yrs.	9 Yrs.	10 Yrs.	11 Yrs.	12 Yrs.	13 Yrs.	14 Yrs.	15 Yrs.	16 Yrs.	17 Yrs.	18 Yrs.
39	35	36	37											
40	37	38	39											
41	39	40	41											
42	41	42	43	44										
43	43	44	45	46										
44	45	46	46	47										
45	47	47	48	48	49									
46	48	49	50	50	51									
47	..	51	52	52	53	54								
48	..	53	54	55	55	56	57							
49	..	55	56	57	58	58	59							
50	..	..	58	59	60	60	61	62						
51	..	..	60	61	62	63	64	65						
52	..	..	62	63	64	65	67	68						
53	..	..	..	66	67	68	69	70	71					
54	..	..	..	69	70	71	72	73	74					
55	..	..	..	..	73	74	75	76	77	78				
56	..	..	..	..	77	78	79	80	81	82				
57	..	..	..	..	..	81	82	83	84	85	86			
58	..	..	..	..	..	84	85	86	87	88	90	91		
59	..	..	..	..	..	87	88	89	90	92	94	96	97	
60	..	..	..	..	..	91	92	93	94	97	99	101	102	
61	..	..	..	..	..	..	95	97	99	102	104	106	108	110
62	..	..	..	..	..	..	100	102	104	106	109	111	113	116
63	..	..	..	..	..	..	105	107	109	111	114	115	117	119
64	..	..	..	..	..	..	...	113	115	117	118	119	120	122
65	..	..	..	..	..	..	...	...	120	122	123	124	125	126
66	..	..	..	..	..	..	...	...	125	126	127	128	129	130
67	..	..	..	..	..	..	...	...	130	131	132	133	134	135
68	..	..	..	..	..	..	...	...	134	135	136	137	138	139
69	..	..	..	..	..	..	...	...	138	139	140	141	142	143
70	..	..	..	..	..	..	...	...	...	142	144	145	146	147

illustrated with educational cartoons. Such pictures are especially fine to use with slow learners, especially when the teacher helps them get the point of the drawing. Carefully chosen comics or strip drawings which appear in newspapers or magazines can be used effectively with this group also, for often they can be strongly motivated to develop certain positive health habits because such heroes or heroines as Buck Rogers or Nancy or animated creatures like Scampy or Donald Duck urge them to do so.

Creating cartoons, comics, sketches, and stick figures can also be a valuable classroom activity. The teacher should "draw out" each child as he shows and explains his pictures to others in the room in order to discover if he has clearly and correctly understood the fact or idea that he has drawn, and if he has made the drawing with a definite purpose in mind. The class might well devise criteria for selecting those creations which were the most meaningful. Since cartoons are

TABLE 9-1   (Continued)

Height, Inches	Girls													
	5 Yrs.	6 Yrs.	7 Yrs.	8 Yrs.	9 Yrs.	10 Yrs.	11 Yrs.	12 Yrs.	13 Yrs.	14 Yrs.	15 Yrs.	16 Yrs.	17 Yrs.	18 Yrs.
39	34	35	36											
40	36	37	38											
41	38	39	40											
42	40	41	42	43										
43	42	42	43	44										
44	44	45	45	46										
45	46	47	47	48	49									
46	48	48	49	50	51									
47	..	49	50	51	52	53								
48	..	51	52	53	54	55	56							
49	..	53	54	55	56	57	58							
50	..	..	56	57	58	59	60	61						
51	..	..	59	60	61	62	63	64						
52	..	..	62	63	64	65	66	67						
53	..	..	..	66	67	68	68	69	70					
54	..	..	..	68	69	70	71	72	73					
55	..	..	..	..	72	73	74	75	76	77				
56	..	..	..	..	76	77	78	79	80	81				
57	..	..	..	..	..	81	82	83	84	85	86			
58	..	..	..	..	..	85	86	87	88	89	90	91		
59	..	..	..	..	..	89	90	91	93	94	95	96	98	
60	..	..	..	..	..	..	94	95	97	99	100	102	104	106
61	..	..	..	..	..	..	99	101	102	104	106	108	109	111
62	..	..	..	..	..	..	104	106	107	109	111	113	114	115
63	..	..	..	..	..	..	109	111	112	113	115	117	118	119
64	..	..	..	..	..	..	...	115	117	118	119	120	121	122
65	..	..	..	..	..	..	...	117	119	120	122	123	124	125
66	..	..	..	..	..	..	...	119	121	122	124	126	127	128
67	..	..	..	..	..	..	...	...	124	126	127	128	129	130
68	..	..	..	..	..	..	...	...	126	128	130	132	133	134
69	..	..	..	..	..	..	...	...	129	131	133	135	136	137
70	..	..	..	..	..	..	...	...	...	134	136	138	139	140

Source: Williams, Jesse Feiring, and Wetherill, G. G.: *Personal and Community Hygiene Applied.* 2nd ed. Philadelphia: W. B. Saunders Co., 1960, p. 28. (Reprinted by permission.)

associated with entertainment, care must be taken by the teacher to assure their use for educational purposes. Although many valuable cartoons can be obtained from commercial companies, the most effective ones are those which they make themselves. Those with a good aptitude for drawing and a poor aptitude for reading can be motivated to develop skill in the latter through their interest in cartoons and sketching.

Charts

A chart is a diagrammatic visual rearrangement of materials which is made so that one can see relationships or a sequence of events more clearly and easily. The types of charts used most frequently are *time charts* (traveler's itinerary), *tree or flow charts* (a genealogical tree), *organizational charts* (a personnel chart), and *comparison or contrast charts* (height and weight tables). For classroom use, a chart should be simple, easily read, and clearly labeled. Upper elementary children can make their own charts and show them on an opaque projector. To use charts effectively in teaching, it is vitally important that the instructor help the child see the meaning of the chart in relationship to himself. A fourth-grader who looks carefully at the height and weight chart (Table 9–1) can find how much he weighs and should weigh and how tall he is and should be.

Teachers should file and catalogue all charts so that they are easily accessible. Care should also be taken that only scientifically accurate charts be used in the classroom, and that those which are selected for showing be displayed well so their use be educational, whether this be to motivate interest, stimulate thinking or action, show factual or comparative data, influence pupils' opinions, or help boys and girls develop desirable attitudes and behavior in relationship to their own health.

Pupil-made charts are a valuable means of helping youngsters grasp an understanding of the relationship and impact of figures to themselves. A *data* chart is the most commonly used type of chart in health education. For example, a fifth-grade teacher recently motivated her class to conduct a survey among 99 children from grades 3 through 6, who were selected at random, on whether or not they ate breakfast every day. After the data were compiled, she helped the class make a chart of their findings so that they could not only "see" the facts but could draw their own conclusions from them. Found below is the type of chart the group made:

BREAKFAST INFORMATION CHART
Number of pupils who usually did or did not eat breakfast

	Boys		Girls		Total	
Grade	Did	Did not	Did	Did not	Did	Did not
3	6	5	6	7	12	12
4	5	3	5	12	10	15
5	5	4	4	12	9	16
6	4	4	4	13	8	17

After this study was completed, the children then made another survey to find out what children in grades 1 and 2 usually ate for breakfast and how many of them usually had a good breakfast before coming to school. Such activities were part of a unit on nutrition and the value of eating three well-balanced meals daily. Projects of this type are especially well suited to the field of health education for they offer many opportunities for a teacher and class to correlate arithmetic, art, and other subjects with health education.

A skilled instructor in a sixth-grade class recently showed her group a commercial flow chart to help the youngsters gain a better understanding of the step-by-step process by which flour is made from wheat. Later, she asked the children to choose partners and assigned each couple to bring to class a well-illustrated flow chart they had made which would show how blood circulates into, around, and out of the heart. She was amazed at and proud of the work the children brought and shared with the class. Once again she realized how much more the group and each individual pupil in it learned from making their own charts than they did from seeing the flour and wheat chart she had previously shown them. Consequently, when shortly afterward the class was studying the organization of the local health department, she asked each pupil to select a new partner and make an organizational chart of the local department of health. Such endeavors not only helped children learn about health co-workers in their own community, but also helped them to gain a new appreciation of the work of their own fellow classmates, as well as encouraged each child to widen his circle of friends.

Graphs

Although often confused with tables, graphs are diagrammatic methods of showing *numerical* data which show quantitative comparisons in forms of bars, geometric shapes, or pictorial symbols so that one viewing them can quickly see relationships between figures. There are various ways to help children grasp the significance of numbers when comparing things. These include *bar graphs; figure graphs* containing pictures of human beings, animals, birds, or fish with each one representing a certain number of the same kind; *pie charts;* and *line or curve graphs.* These can be obtained commercially, collected from books or other printed sources, or better still, be made by the pupils.

Dale gives the following suggestions to teachers for the best use of statistical data when showing them in graph form.[8]

1. Each symbol should be self-explanatory.
2. Large quantities should be shown by a larger number of symbols and not by an enlarged symbol.
3. Only approximate quantities should be compared, not minute details.
4. Only comparisons should be charted, not isolated elements.

Elementary children should be carefully taught how to read and interpret graphs correctly, and be taught that these materials can be used effectively to show statistical data, comparisons, and relationships. One of the best ways to do this is to have them make their own graphs using simple stick figures, squares, or lines. Giving each one an assigned task, such as making a series of stick-figure drawings to show how many persons there were in his grandmother's family, in each of his parents' families, and his own family is often a good beginning, and can be used in

---

[8] Dale, Edgar: *Audio-Visual Methods in Teaching.* 3rd ed. New York: Dryden, 1970, p. 334.

units on family education, heredity, and for other purposes. Others will find pleasure in keeping careful records of how many hours of play or sleep they had each day for a week and then showing this on a bar graph to the rest of the class, when the class is learning the value of exercise, sleep, and rest in relationship to growth. Some health education experts believe area graphs give pupils on the upper elementary level an opportunity to integrate health and safety with arithmetic because a circle graph can be used effectively in the study of simple fractions. Such graphs are also effective ways to help students see how much time they actually spend daily in sleeping, going to school, watching television, or at play. To make such a circle graph, the pupils should divide the circle horizontally in the center, and in the lower half of the circle number from 1 to 12, going around the circle right to left. The upper part of the circle should be numbered 12 to 1, from right to left. The circle should then be cut like a pie, showing the hours which a pupil actually spends at this or that activity daily. Such experiences are revelations to many pupils. They often can become more concerned and profit more from this type of an experience than from hearing a teacher "preach" to them about going to bed earlier or playing outdoors more. All will enjoy making pie charts or other types of graphs and experimenting with different kinds of colors and materials, in order best to present accurate information. Such graphs are especially well suited for cost studies, such as how much of the family budget is spent for clothing, rent, food, or medical care.

Maps

Maps can also be used effectively in health education, whether they be commercial ones purchased by the school or those made by the children themselves, for they help children understand special relationships. Maps of the route followed by each pupil as he comes to school, locating playground hazards on a map drawn of the playground, showing railroad crossings, national highways, and city streets in one's own town or within a mile radius of one's home can be both an interesting and profitable experience for children who are studying safety education. Such endeavors will help each see his school, town, or city as a whole, gain a concept of where he lives in relationship to hospitals or fire stations, and become more cognizant of hazards or dangers at school or on the way there. The use of maps can provide many opportunities to integrate a study of nutrition as pupils are studying the states of their nation, their own particular state, or the nations of the world. It is important for children to know where the food products they eat come from, how they are raised and transported, as well as the nutritive values of food.

Bulletin and Other Boards

Modern classrooms have large, colorful bulletin boards on which examples of children's work are attractively displayed. Such boards can be used as a means of bringing new or current things to the attention of the class, showing parents and other adults what pupils are doing in school, and giving children a place in the classroom which is their primary responsibility to use creatively and well. Class bulletin-board projects, which are carefully planned around a health unit, such as "Safety at School" or "The Muscles of the Body," may take several days and much class work by many pupils assigned to various committees. Such an educational adventure should be carefully thought through and the class should have definite objectives in mind as it determines how it can find out what it wants to know. Wide reading, visits to places of importance to that particular project, interviews, and many other kinds of experiences can become vital parts of any well-planned health education unit. A bulletin-board committee should become responsible for displaying new materials or the final work of the class on any such project. Naturally, the success of any such learning experience depends largely on the teacher and her ability to spark student interest. The pupils will need as much guidance and encouragement as possible. Likewise, the teacher should assist them by showing how the bulletin board can be used most effectively in order to reach general and specific learning objectives the group has devised. Shared evaluation, often called "action research," should be used throughout such projects and be viewed as a means of learning where one is now in relationship to where he wants to go. Some educators refer to a well-arranged, well-displayed bulletin board as a "silent but an effective teacher."

Any bulletin board can become a potently effective communicative device if it can

1. Get an important message across through the means of well-selected and well-displayed materials.
2. Attract and hold attention in such a way that it becomes a living and frequently changed medium for reaching others.
3. Stimulate thought and motivate action.

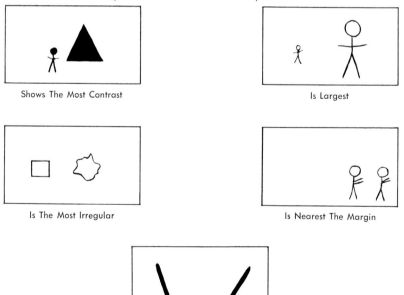

Eyes Will Be Attracted To The Object That

Shows The Most Contrast   Is Largest

Is The Most Irregular   Is Nearest The Margin

Moves From Left To Right

Figure 9-2. Health education can be correlated to art when making posters.

Bulletin boards, or "tack boards" as they are sometimes called, can serve several purposes, including that of displaying announcements, student work, posters, short-term projects, and art work. Here again, since children learn mostly from their own direct experiences, they should keep their class bulletin boards up to date and full of interesting and worthwhile materials which have aesthetic, cultural, and educational value.

A well-planned bulletin board is one that contains information and pictures which can be seen from a distance, has a title to indicate its purpose, well-arranged educational materials, and brief but pertinent informative statements which communicate what it is intended that the viewer learn or do. Such a teaching aid can arouse curiosity, quicken interest, motivate action, and inform.

A cooperatively created bulletin board can provide many kinds of stimulating and satisfying educational experiences to children. It can be used to illustrate steps or phases of a unit as they are developed by the class and teacher together. It can be important as a summary or review device. It can be a versatile and valuable teaching tool.

Suggested ways to make attractive eye-catching bulletin boards for health education purposes are to

1. Use a few well-selected pictures rather than a large number.
2. Capture, center, and focus viewer attention; this can sometimes be done best by providing contrast through a generous use of space, having an irregular shape in a group of similar ones, placing the most important materials nearest the margin of the board, using both large and small pictures, and moving viewer attention from left to right.
3. Use color, remembering that reds and browns or their combinations (warm colors) attract attention better than do blues and greens and their combinations (cool colors).

Regardless of what type of health information is used on a bulletin board, and whether the display is homemade or commercially made, created by the teacher, a pupil, or a committee, the instructor must keep in mind that merely exposing learners to a picture does not by any means ensure that they will gain anything of educational value from this experience. The teacher must bring to the attention of the class the specific importance of each picture or item of information displayed on the board, alert the pupils to definite things to look for, and make sure that the viewers understand and appreciate what they see. Likewise, she should help the pupils develop habits of making a careful scrutiny of all pictures they see, as well as teach them how to gather quickly the general impression a picture gives, and help them develop an aesthetic appreciation of the materials as a whole.

Learning how to set up and utilize a health education bulletin board effectively can be a part of any unit on any level in health education. Suggested activities for a class bulletin-board committee of any one of the five grades studying safety and first aid might well include the following:

1. Have each pupil on the committee bring in several pictures in this area of concern which have been taken from magazines or local newspapers.
2. Help the group select a bulletin-board theme and determine the information they want to get across to the viewers.
3. Guide the committee in their final selection of the best pictures, and help

them learn why some pictures are better than others for their purposes of communicating a message or information to others.

4. Have the group mount the best pictures, stressing the value of different shapes and colors.

5. Teach the committee how to focus viewer attention by using contrast in color and size, regular and irregular shapes, moving the best pictures closest to the margin of the board, and moving the viewer's attention from left to right of the board.

6. Help the group set up and evaluate their display.

7. Evaluate the work of the committee and the display on the board by means of a full class discussion.

8. Assign the committee to prepare a file of future pictures which might be used on another bulletin board later in the year for any other aspect of safety education, such as "Safety on the Playground" or "Safety in the Home."

Since pupils will soon lose interest in bulletin boards which are unattractive, dull, and lack eye appeal, the wise instructor will make every endeavor to learn, either by her own trial and error or from specialists in audio-visual education, how to make attractive displays for the purpose of helping children appreciate health as a valued concept. Such an educator will soon learn the necessity of displaying pertinent, up-to-date materials which have eye and interest appeal plus the power to stimulate thought, understanding, action, and appreciation. In short, then, a bulletin board can only be as effective as the teacher who will use it creatively to help children learn better about health.

The Chalkboard

The classroom chalkboard is fascinating to young children. They are attracted to its magic, for on it writing and drawings can come and go, and can be whisked away by a sweep of the hand. It is a vehicle on which things can become *real*, where visual symbols become important. Today it is most often green in color and when the teacher puts "something on the board," children sense immediately that this is going to be important. It is a big day in every child's life when *he* finally gets to write on the board.

The chalkboard can be used fully as a means of helping children learn if one keeps the following suggestions well in mind:

1. Keep the board clean.
2. Be sure that all can see what is written or drawn on it.
3. Avoid standing in front of it and blocking the full view of the pupils.
4. Use class time to the fullest extent; do not waste it by using half of a period making a chart, but rather do this before the class begins.
5. Get an idea or fact over to the students quickly. Accurate, time-consuming drawings done to scale can be a waste of time if a quickly drawn stick figure can accomplish the same purpose.
6. Prepare an entire board in advance, cover it, and remove parts of the cover as a means of stimulating interest. Use such a trick sparingly, however.
7. Avoid putting too much on the board at one time.
8. Write key words, new ones, or key phrases on the board as you discuss things in class.
9. Have your pupils use the board often and encourage them to discuss what they have written or drawn there for the benefit of the group.

The use of colored chalk will add to the effectiveness of drawings made on the chalkboard, such as a sketch of the body or a diagram of the eye. Since one of the purposes of the teacher is to help children build a vocabulary in order that they can communicate effectively with others, she should clearly print all new words which will be introduced in each day's health lesson, such as "digestion" or "retina." It will help the pupils learn the meaning, spelling, and use of each new word or slogan such as "Play safely," if the instructor takes the time to point out how each new word is pronounced and then have the class repeat it with her several times, have the group spell and write the word, and encourage through praise each pupil who does use a new word or slogan that day in class discussion, written work, or in a question-and-answer period.

Collections and Specimens

Children are pack rats! Their pockets are full of magical things which range all the way from an old key to a lucky rock. Many future world authorities on insects, plants, butterflies, birds, or health now sit in elementary school classrooms somewhere in this nation. Still more future amateur hobbyists and collectors of all manner of strange things are found there, too. Seemingly an interest to gather together, catalogue things, and label them is found in most human beings, but it bursts into bloom as children grow older. Teachers should do their utmost to encourage pupils to become experts in their chosen field of interest, even though this may frequently change, for in so doing they can spur on the desire to learn and encourage an awakening interest. They can help children develop lifelong hobby interests for wise, positive leisure-time use, for studies show that many lifetime hobbies begin in childhood, usually around the age of ten.

Making a collection of specimens is both an interesting and valuable experience in health education for children. They will enjoy bringing to class real objects to supplement pictures found in their textbooks. Since most of our learning comes through the senses, it is important that children touch and feel, as well as see and hear about, the many wonders of creation in their world, such as a baby duck or a milkweed. An understanding of any part of the human body can be quickened through this method of teaching.

It is important that any collection be more than a gathering of dead things, for children can be helped by their teacher, through a fresh and creative approach, to see life and meaning even in a mounted fish or a stuffed owl. As Whitehead points out, a pupil should never be taught more than he can think and wonder about. This implies that the teacher must guide children to well-presented and carefully selected learning aids, which she has tailored to fit their short interest span and comprehension level. Consequently, this instructor, aided by a committee of pupils, should sort through, select, and arrange well those collections and specimens children bring to class which can best serve as educational aids.

The field of health education provides many opportunities for children to bring to class and share with others things they have collected in relationship to their work in health and safety on every grade level. One sixth-grade class recently made a collection of all the kinds of animal teeth they could find (either in actual or picture form) for a comparative study of human teeth. Next, they examined each specimen for evidence of decay. Finally, they discussed what causes tooth decay and how they could prevent it happening to their own teeth. The group also studied the parts of a tooth and the relationship of a well-balanced diet to the prevention of decay. A fifth-grade class studying food buying in a nutrition unit at a school in Florida last year made an extensive collection of empty food containers. The class spent the next two weeks discussing the Pure Food and Drug Law and its application to food-packaging labels. They then learned how to stretch each food dollar further by discovering how much more good nutritive food could be purchased by knowing what constitutes a good diet and why one should read and know the declared weight or other vital information found printed on each packaged food product. Still another group of second-graders who were studying "Happy Families" brought to class pictures they had found in magazines of family groups enjoying themselves together. Even "bad" specimens can be used, as Willgoose illustrates by describing an interesting assignment once given to a group of fourth graders.[9] This class was studying food spoilage and proper food storage. Each pupil was asked to bring to class one good and one spoiled piece of food, such as a good and bad orange, a sound and unsound potato, or a fresh and spoiled tomato. Through the use of the vivid contrasts between healthful and harmful food, the class saw for themselves enough evidence to make up their own minds about the value of proper food storage. They were then highly motivated to learn how to store food in safe and sanitary ways. Such vivid experiences help make learning about health and safety exciting and meaningful and long-lasting experiences to boys and girls.

Models

Models are imitations of real things, and usually are made on a smaller or larger scale than the actual object they represent. A miniature grocery store used in a nutrition unit is a model, as is an enlarged replica of the human heart made of plaster of Paris. Models can be used for teaching pupils many things in the area of health education. They serve chiefly, however, as a means of motivating pupil interest so that they can gain a clearer understanding and appreciation of the things they are studying.

Some pupils can learn quickly about traffic safety through "dry runs" using miniature toy cars on a table, or by three-dimensional representations of a highway and potential hazards a pedestrian or driver might encounter. This type of visual aid is called a diorama and has great possibilities for enriching health instruction. Others grasp the meaning of the red, green, or yellow stop-light signals from seeing these colors flash through a milk carton in which three windows have been cut; a light is turned off and on to shine through at each color. Still others can create many kinds of models which test their ingenuity and creativity. Thus, balloons and plastic tubes might be used to demonstrate how food is digested, or a water gun squeezed and a faucet turned on to show the difference between arterial and venous bleeding.

Many commercial firms now have splendid models available which show various parts of the human body. Some of these are available in cross-sectional form, or in parts which fit together and can be separated so that each piece may be examined singly and relationships clearly seen. Cutaway models or those which show what "the inside" of any body part looks like are also available at small cost.

---

[9] Willgoose, *op. cit.*, p. 374.

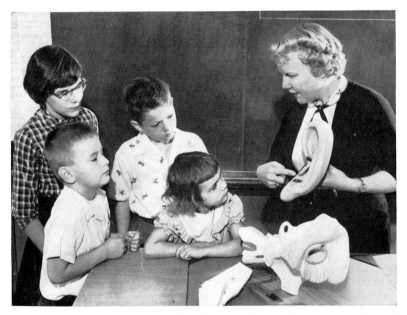

Figure 9-3.   Finding the path to good health is not difficult with the help of this teaching
aid.   Throughout, the teacher explains the functions of different body
parts, and the role that proper health habits can play in keeping well.
(Courtesy of Dallas Health and Science Museum)

Children love to make their own models and experiment with clay, papier-mâché, soap carving, wooden blocks, plasticine, flour-and-water paste, plastics, and an abundance of other materials.   The teacher must encourage them as much as possible in their attempts to gain a clearer, better understanding of health and its importance in their lives, and, if the use of models can assist them to learn this faster and better, they should be used accordingly.   Caution must be exercised, however, for the mere making of a teaching aid can become an end to itself, and "making things for health class" can all too quickly become meaningless busy work. Likewise, the teacher must be sure that the children's attention is directed from the model to the actual thing it was meant to represent, and that they see the relationship of that object to their own lives and general well-being.   Many children have learned how to count money and work together, and about the values of eating well-balanced meals by using miniature box models of food and a toy cash register.   Pupils should have increased opportunities to make things and learn from their own creative efforts as they progress in school.   Far too often such experiences are limited to the first grade, and as the children move upward on the academic ladder, they are given fewer opportunities to do and make things in the classroom.   Often, too, they are provided with fewer opportunities to talk in class or plan their approach toward learning and mastering assigned materials.   In haste there can be much waste, for it is not a question of how much a child learns but how meaningful his learning experiences become to him and are expressed in what he does and how he feels.

IMPLICATIONS FOR HEALTH TEACHING

Learning is a teacher-pupil responsibility. One of the major tasks of the modern school is to help students in any age group to gain an understanding of good health and its importance to the individual and society, along with the skills necessary for developing and maintaining it. As a subject in the school curriculum, health is not easily taught, nor is it generally taught well. Consequently, teachers on all levels must first develop a great and deeply felt desire to become efficient and effective instructors in this important field. Supplementary teaching aids, created mostly by the learners themselves, can and will add much to the worth of any health education program, but only if they are used intelligently for a definite purpose always kept well in mind. Supplementary teaching materials are effective and worthwhile only to the degree that they can motivate behavior and learning. The greatest motivator of all, it should be stressed, is an enthusiastic, capable, and skilled teacher.

As Love has pointed out, a teacher's way of life is her greatest source of inspiration for teaching, because everything she sees and does is viewed through the very special eyes of an educator. These eyes are trained to analyze quickly any situation and take from it that which is meaningful and applicable to teaching.[12] She tells how she used some materials from the comic strip "Peanuts" concerning Charlie Brown's posture problem for the bulletin board, as an illustration in a unit on posture. When she read *The Hidden Persuaders*, by Vance Packard, she gained many valuable ideas on how to sell ideas to others which helped her in all phases of her work as an educator. Although the life of every teacher is a busy one, involving contact with many people of varying ages and backgrounds, plus keeping up a wide range of reading, the best educators are those who always are seeking and utilizing new and better ways to improve their teaching skill. Such inspired and inspiring leaders help children discover the thrill of learning new things every moment of every day in the school year, and at home as well as at school.

Suggested Readings

Burton, William: *The Guidance of Learning Activities*. 3rd ed. New York: Appleton-Century-Crofts, 1962.

Hanna, Lavonne: *Unit Teaching In The Elementary School*. New York: Holt, Rinehart and Winston, 1963.

Klein, Frances Tyler: "Curriculum Boon Or Bane." *The Education Digest*. September 1972, pp. 15–18.

Noar, Gertrude: *Individualized Instruction: Every Child a Winner*. New York: John Wiley and Sons, 1972.

School Health Education Study: *Health Education: A Conceptual Approach to Curriculum Design*. Minneapolis: 3M Education Press, 1968.

Tyler, Ralph: *Basic Principles of Curriculum and Instruction*. Chicago: University of Chicago Press, 1967.

Yamamoto, Karoru: *The Child And His Image*. Boston: Houghton Mifflin Co., 1972.

---

[12] Love, Alice: "Look into Your Daily Living to Find That Extra Something for Your Teaching." *Journal of Health, Physical Education and Recreation*, 322, 21, April 1961.

Suggested Sources of Audio-Visual Materials for Health Education

Dale, Edgar: *Audio-Visual Methods in Teaching*, 3rd ed. New York: Dryden Press, 1970.

Educator's Grade Guide to Free Curriculum Materials. Published annually by the Educator's Progress Service, Randolph, Wisconsin.

Free and Inexpensive Learning Materials. Published annually by George Peabody College For Teachers, Nashville, Tennessee.

Weisinger, Thelma: *1001 Valuable Things You Can Get Free.* Published annually by Bantam Books, New York.

Journal of School Health. Kent, Ohio. Each issue contains a section on "New Teaching Aids."

The Education Digest. Praken Publications, Inc., Box 623, 416 Longshore Drive, Ann Arbor, Michigan. Each issue contains a section on "New Educational Materials."

Discussion Questions

1. What are the advantages and disadvantages of using motion pictures as a health education teaching aid?
2. How can photographs be used in health education?
3. What are the three types of charts mentioned in this chapter? Give an example of each for classroom use.
4. Explain the differences between bar graphs, figure graphs, pie charts, and line or curve graphs.
5. How can maps be used as a teaching aid in health education?
6. In what ways can the bulletin board be a "silent, effective teacher?"
7. What factors should be kept in mind when using the chalkboard as a means of helping children learn about health effectively?
8. What kinds of models could children make in the area of health education? Give an example in each of the major teaching areas.
9. Explain the meaning of the sentence that "learning is a teacher-pupil responsibility." Role play a teacher-pupil planning session.
10. How can collections and specimens be used in teaching health? Give specific examples in three areas of health education.

Things to Do

1. Select a teaching unit in any area of health education such as dental health or safety and prepare a list of teaching aids to use in connection with it.
2. Learn how to operate a movie projector and an opaque projector.
3. Make a health education mobile, and explain how it could be used to teach nutrition.
4. Make and use a flannel board to teach a sample lesson to your classmates in the area of safety education.
5. Bring to class a collection of cartoons and/or comic strips to share with your classmates in any area of health education.
6. Watch any television program for children such as "Sesame Street." What could children have learned about health in this program?
7. Learn how to use an overhead projector. Teach a sample lesson in health education for third-graders using this medium.
8. Look at any issue of *The Journal of Health Education* in the audio-visual aid section. What did you learn from this experience?

Teaching Materials and Guides to Special Media

Beyrer, M., *et al.*: *A Directory of Selected References and Resources For Health Instruction.* Minneapolis: Burgess Publishing Co., 1970.

Educators' Guide To Free Films; Educators' Guide To Free Filmstrips; Elementary Teachers' Guide To Free Curriculum Materials; and *Educators' Guide To Free Tapes, Scripts and Transcriptions.* Randolph, Wisc.; Educators Progress Service. Published yearly.

Free and Inexpensive Health Instruction Materials. Carbondale, Ill.: Southern
    Illinois University Press, 1969.
Instructional Television Materials. 3rd ed. New York: National Instructional
    Television Library, 1971.
Programmed Learning—A Bibliography of Programs and Presentation Devices.
    (Quarterly.) University Center, Mich.: Delta College.

PART FOUR

the program—what to teach children in specific areas of health

Health is a very personal thing (it focuses on the individual)

Health is a very complex thing (the definition embraces physical, mental and emotional processes)

Health is an ever-changing phenomenon (the variables are dynamic, interacting, and interdependent).

> —Kay Tift, "Individualizing Health Instruction."
> The School Health Review,
> November 1970, p. 2.

overview of part iv

Included in this part of the book is a suggested graded program in health education for grades K to 6. It is a pattern which should be tailored to fit into any specific elementary school curriculum. Such a recommended program teaches health from the concept of total well-being, consisting of physical, mental, emotional, and spiritual fitness. It has been based on the typical needs, interests, and characteristics of children in each school grade. A wide variety of learning activities is suggested which will help make health education become an alive, exciting, and important learning adventure for children. It shows how the curricular patterns and the teaching methods, as well as all other previous materials, can best be used for an improved health instruction in all elementary grades.

CHAPTER 10

nutrition

Although Americans are considered by many to be the best-fed people in the entire world, there is an abundance of evidence that many in our land have faulty food habits, are undernourished or obese, tire too easily, are the victims of false advertising, food fads, and starvation diets. Nutrition experts estimate that nine out of every ten Americans are not eating properly. Some are all but starving in our land of plenty. Education in nutrition can do much to improve the food habits of children. In a two-year study, conducted among sixth- and seventh-graders in Kansas City in 1956, the food habits of pupils in five schools were appraised. Children in all schools were found to be eating unbalanced diets and to fall below daily nutritional standards by not eating enough milk, eggs, citrus fruits, butter or margarine, potatoes, and green, leafy vegetables. An intensified nutritional education program was established and by the end of two years noticeable differences were made in food-selection patterns of the pupils as well as their scores on standardized hygiene tests.[1] Recent studies also show that children are not eating as wisely as they should but can learn to do so at school.

Far too many pupils come to school without eating breakfast, in spite of the fact that medical authorities say that this is the most important meal in the entire day for human beings. Some family dinner tables are miniature battlefields, where children are trying their best to eat in a tension-filled, hostile environment, and yet pediatricians and nutritional experts agree that how a person feels *while* he is eating is as important as *what* he is eating. Children with emotional problems often use food as a weapon—some by refusing to eat, others by gorging themselves. Some educators say that we have a "grab-me-gulp" type of educational program in America on all academic levels that is similar to the 15- or 30-minute school lunch

---

[1] Haag, Jessie: *School Health Program*, 3rd ed. Philadelphia, Lea and Febiger, 1972, p. 20.

program conducted in any noisy, packed school cafeteria, from which children emerge dissatisfied, confused, and miseducated. Surgeon-General Thomas Parran has warned that as taxpayers we are wasting our time trying to educate children with half-starved bodies, for they cannot absorb teaching, they hold back classes, and they require extra time of teachers and repeat grades, all of which he claims is pure, expensive stupidity.

The total school nutritional program should and can be an important educational experience for children, so that as they grow older they will become increasingly concerned about maintaining a diet that meets high nutritional standards. Such a program should consist of nutrition education, school lunch and midmorning feeding, nutritional appraisal, guidance for individuals with specific food problems, and the adjustment of the school day for those who are below par physically and mentally.

The general objectives of any program in nutrition education in the elementary grades might well include the following:

1. Help children develop and practice good eating habits.
2. Develop in each child an understanding and interest in foods necessary for growth.
3. Build favorable attitudes toward eating a wide variety of foods, regularity of eating times, and possessing good table manners.
4. Develop school and home cooperation in relation to good nutrition as well as in all other aspects of the health instruction program.
5. Provide for integration and correlation of nutrition and all other aspects of the health instruction program with other teachers and in all school subjects.

The program must be based upon the needs and interests of the pupils. These can be determined by observation of what the child chooses to eat in the school cafeteria or brings from home for lunch, the results of a periodic weighing and measuring program, postural tests, detection of growth deviation by the use of the Wetzel grid, observation of facial skin and hair, health records to check for recurrence of colds, results of dental and physical examinations, attitude and knowledge tests, and conferences and question boxes from parents, as well as other sources.

Nutrition can be a fascinating subject to learn about, for everyone has a need and interest in food in some degree. It can be studied as a part of other units such as growth, or be an integral part of units such as dental health or good grooming. It is imperative that home cooperation be secured if the educational program in nutrition is to become as effective as it might be, especially in the primary grades. Lunchroom experiences can be used to provide teachers with much valuable information regarding how much or how little pupils really know and apply about eating balanced diets. Consequently, they should eat with their pupils frequently.

SUGGESTED GRADED TOPICS

Suggested graded topics in nutrition education include the following:

GRADE 1
1. The necessity for eating three well-balanced meals.
2. What is a good breakfast, lunch, and supper.
3. Why children should drink milk.

4. Washing before eating.
5. Why too many sweets are harmful.
6. Food, sleep, play, and rest, and their effects upon growth.

GRADE 2

1. The Four Pathways to Good Nutrition.
2. Why raw fruits and vegetables are good for you.
3. What sweets are best for health and when they should be eaten.
4. Why you should drink water.
5. Eating new kinds of foods.
6. The best kinds of between-meal snacks for young children.
7. The difference between white and whole-wheat bread.

GRADE 3

1. How food affects growth.
2. What each pupil should and does weigh; how tall each is and should be.
3. The necessity of eating a good breakfast.
4. What are three well-balanced meals a day.
5. How to plan and prepare a simple, nutritious lunch.

GRADE 4

1. Review of The Four Pathways To Good Nutrition.
2. The six classifications and function of foods.
3. Foods which best aid growth and digestion.
4. Grading and pasteurization of milk.
5. Milk products and their values.

GRADE 5

1. How to plan and choose three well-balanced daily meals.
2. Foods essential for growth and good health.
3. Comparative study of milk and carbonated beverages.
4. Sources and functions of vitamins and minerals.
5. Normal and abnormal weight.
6. Advertising and food fallacies.
7. Food allergies.

GRADE 6

1. Foods in relationship to health, attractiveness, fatigue, growth, strength, and the emotions.
2. Interrelationship of weight to health.
3. The digestion and absorption of food.
4. The effects of coffee, tea, and alcohol upon the human body.
5. Sanitation in the preparation and serving of foods.
6. The Pure Food and Drug Act.
7. Social customs and etiquette.
8. A weekly food budget and food selection for a family.

CURRICULUM PLACEMENT

Teachers who work in self-contained classrooms should be aided by the school health coordinator in planning ways in which nutrition education can be correlated and integrated into all subject areas in the school curriculum, as well as what topics in this field should be stressed at each grade. In those schools which are not fortunate enough to have such a specialized person to guide and direct the total school health program or the health instructional part of such a program, all elementary teachers (or chosen representatives from each grade in large school systems) should draw up plans and suggested ways in which nutrition education can be interwoven into the entire elementary school curriculum. Even the teachers in those institutions where the subject curriculum is used and health education is either a separate subject area or one combined with safety education or science should use and be guided in their teaching by graded, outlined teaching units. Each instructor should utilize every available opportunity to correlate and integrate nutrition education with all other subjects she teaches. Regardless of the type of curriculum used in the school, there are many pitfalls to be avoided when teaching nutrition to children. These include "preaching" or predicting doom for those who fail to eat a well-balanced diet *every* day, accepting food fads and fallacies as facts, becoming the victim of faulty and inaccurate advertising, placing too much stress upon the often dry facts of physiology (such as requiring older pupils to memorize the name and function of each digestive enzyme), or stressing one's own food likes and dislikes ("My favorite food is cottage cheese" or "I cannot *stand* liver!").

Nutrition education can best be correlated and become an integrated part of the subject areas given below, in the following suggested ways:

Mathematics

1. Make height and weight charts for recording the monthly weighing and measuring of each child.
2. Calculate daily caloric intake; make a list of those foods which are the highest and lowest in calories.
3. Make graphs showing the results of animal- and plant-feeding experiments.
4. Add food costs.
5. Show in percentages and pie graphs the part of the family budget which should be spent on food, rent, medical care, insurance, clothing, and recreation.
6. Determine the food cost per person in a family of two adults and two grade-school children, aged 6 and 9, for one day, one week, and one month.
7. Show with measured string the length of an average large and small intestine of a child and adult; make a model from clay or papier-mâché showing the exact size of the stomach, liver, heart, or other organs of the body used in the digestion of food and circulation of blood.
8. Discover the difference between the cost of three well-balanced daily meals for one person or a family of four and the price of a doctor's home visit and medication for treating a cold for one person or all four family members for one week.
9. Determine which foods are the cheapest and most nutritious to buy in three of the six main food groups (fats, proteins, carbohydrates).
10. Study food bargains as advertised in the local paper and show how much can be saved by buying the groceries for one week for a family of four by planning well-balanced daily and weekly meals.
11. Prove on paper that advertised "real" bargains which might be available in your city are not money-savers after all.
12. Observe and estimate on paper how much money is lost weekly in one's own home by food waste, spoilage, and improper storage.
13. Discover and prove which is cheaper—eating a well-balanced diet or medical and dental care.
14. Plan and give a party in your home for five friends for one dollar, or do so for your class. Determine the cost of the refreshments per pupil. Make a list of foods which you could have served for this same amount of money, a dollar more, and for half a dollar.

Social Studies

Suggested activities which will enable the pupils to learn much about both areas include:

1. Study local, state, and national food and drug laws. Bring illustrations to class showing how these laws are obeyed on can labels or other ways.
2. Compare the food eaten in other countries with that eaten in America.
3. Learn of the discovery of vitamins and their role in the prevention of such conditions as scurvy, pellagra, etc.
4. Study the geographical areas of the United States which produce certain foods, such as the Corn Belt, and the areas where citrus fruits, sugar cane, etc., are raised.
5. Discover the ways in which foods are transported, packaged, and marketed.
6. Learn of the laws regarding the pasteurization of milk and the fortification of margarine or other food products.
7. Compare the diet of our early pioneers with that of the Indians and of people living today.
8. Study the role diet plays in longevity today as well as in the past.
9. Learn of local co-workers in the health protection of the people in your community in the foods they eat.
10. Compare the methods of cooking used by the pioneers with those of today.
11. Study the varieties of frozen food on the market today and compare these with methods of canning and preserving foods used by the early American settlers.
12. Bring to class current-events clippings which pertain to nutrition.
13. Prepare and give a class party based upon the theme, "The Gold Rush Days."
14. Study the life of the pioneers, their problems, government, music, type of clothing worn and food eaten, games they played, and their work. Illustrate what you learn from this experience by writing and presenting a play or pageant using scenery, props, and costumes made in class.
15. Learn about some of the great health heroes, such as Louis Pasteur or Clara Barton.
16. Study fallacies and fads about food.
17. Learn to what extent the United States "feeds the hungry people of the world." Have a debate on the pros and cons of this action.
18. Study about epidemics and plagues in Europe and America.
19. Have a "tasting" party of each favorite vegetable or fruit brought to class.
20. Have each class or grade plan the school cafeteria luncheon menu for one week or for a special holiday such as Thanksgiving, assisted by the school dietitian. Divide the class into committees, such as publicity, table decorations, etc.
21. Divide the class into groups, giving each the responsibility to plan, prepare, and serve one foreign dish for an all-school International Night party. Have each group present a folk dance or song typical of that nation for entertainment.

Science

There are abundant opportunities for correlation and integration of nutrition and science. Suggested ways in which this can best be accomplished include having the pupils

1. Learn how food grows, and the effects soil conditions and the weather have upon their growth.
2. Conduct animal- and plant-feeding experiments.

3. Test foods for chemical content, such as potatoes for starch or beets for sugar.
4. Make a chemical analysis of milk.
5. Study the influence of the endocrine glands, emotions, and fatigue upon diet.
6. Learn how animals are government inspected for human consumption.
7. Study about food spoilage and its prevention.
8. Learn the relationship of sugar to tooth decay.
9. Study how foods such as prunes or apricots are dehydrated.
10. Study the claims of certain "health foods" and health faddists.
11. Learn the relationship of a good diet to good health and to the prevention of colds, food poisoning, etc.
12. Study the effect of a poor diet upon the skin, hair, and body.
13. Learn of the dangers of being overweight and underweight.
14. Learn how food-allergy skin tests are made.
15. Study the hazards of food additives.
16. Learn how exercise helps in body growth and the digestion of food.
17. Study the effects of coffee, tea, alcohol, and cola drinks.
18. Learn how diet can prevent night blindness or other vision defects.

The Communicative Arts

Reading, writing, and speaking can be correlated well with nutrition education. The following suggestions for doing so include having the pupils

1. Report verbally or in writing on places they have visited which were connected in some way with food.
2. Suggest ways to learn to like new foods.
3. Locate foods in the Four Pathways To Good Nutrition Chart. Tell something important about each food.
4. Discuss ways foods are sold, such as meat by the pound, eggs by the dozen, milk by the quart. Correlate this with the units of measure in arithmetic.
5. Discuss the daily school lunch menu served in the cafeteria, which one pupil can copy on the board. Guide each child in making a wise food selection. Send the weekly menu home, and enlist the cooperation of parents in helping their children choose a wisely selected daily lunch. Also send the Four Pathways To Good Nutrition Chart home to parents who prepare their child's school lunch, and help them plan this meal according to good nutritional standards.*
6. Discuss and list on the chalkboard the relationship of good food to growth and good teeth.
7. Tell how to care for a pet or a baby sister or brother, or how wild animals seek food and what they eat.
8. Make a list of new foods seen or heard about on radio or television, and of new foods each has tasted or would like to taste.
9. Talk about ways to improve eating habits at school, at home, and in a restaurant.
10. Plan a class visit to a grocery store, giving each group a definite assignment, such as having them visit the meat section and find out all they can about it, another the frozen-food section, etc. Have each group compile a written, illustrated report on what they learned.
11. Have individual students report on their experiences in eating at a Chinese, French, or Italian restaurant; invite foreign adults to visit the school and describe or serve a typical meal or type of food from their homeland.

* See the Appendix for a suggested letter to send to parents enlisting their cooperation.

12. Teach the class to prepare simple menus in the school kitchen or out of doors. Experiments with different kinds of cooking such as boiling, frying, baking in pans or in foil. Have the group discuss what they learned from these experiences.
13. Demonstrate correct table setting and experiment with flower arranging. Discuss the importance of atmosphere to good eating.
14. Devise a miniature cafeteria or grocery store. Figure out how much a well-balanced meal costs, or "buy" the groceries for a family of two, four, six, or eight persons for a week on a preconceived budget. Have each pupil write a paragraph on what he learned from doing this.
15. Clip weekly food ads from the newspaper. Discuss how to shop well and get the most from every food dollar.
16. Tape-record skits, special reports, or other types of pupil work.
17. Write and give a playlet, puppet show, or skit to a local P.T.A. group on any aspect of nutrition.
18. Give an oral report on a book, such as Mabel Robinson's *Pioneer Panorama* (Denison), or *Swift Arrow* by Alice Pendergast (Denison). Describe a typical day in the life of the main character of either book.

Drama and Art

Activities which are suitable for correlating with nutrition are numerous. Have the pupils

1. Do dramatizations of good manners at the table; a "mother" buying, preparing, and serving a meal; eating out at a large restaurant.
2. Visit a farm, bakery, dairy, or ice cream plant. Have the class make a list of things they would like to find out about, and make an illustrated poster of their visit.
3. Color pictures of fruits, vegetables, and other types of food, cut them out, and arrange a balanced meal on a desk or flannel board.
4. Make a clock, learn how to tell time, and show the best time for eating each meal, going to bed, getting up, and resting.
5. Play cafeteria, store, or going shopping.
6. Display in the school lunchroom or lobby, children's posters of three balanced, well-planned meals.
7. Make posters showing "Foods I Take in a Lunch Box," "Foods for a Birthday Party," "Cold Weather or Summer Foods," "Foods for Thanksgiving," etc.
8. Create and give a puppet show or playlet revolving around any aspect of how to select a balanced diet.
9. Discuss and list on the board the relationship of good food to growth and teeth.
10. Dramatize the correct way to chew and eat food properly; exaggerate the incorrect ways to do so.
11. Bring magazine pictures of people eating food. Make up and tell a story about the pictures.
12. Make jigsaw puzzles out of colored pictures of food.
13. Present in charade form any activity done in the preparation of food, such as rolling dough or shelling peas. Have the class guess what is being done, and select the best charade.
14. Make models of different kinds of foods such as oranges, corn, steak, pie, etc., out of clay or heavy cardboard. Have each pupil make up a story about any one of these which will stress its nutritional value.

Physical Education

Like science, physical education can be more easily and naturally used for correlating and integrating nutrition education than certain other subjects included in the elementary school curriculum. Suggestions for doing so include having the pupils

1. Learn the relationship of exercise and proper nutrition to growth.
2. Become aware of the dangers of stimulants, alcohol, tea, tobacco, and soft drinks to athletic performance.
3. Learn which are the quick-energy foods and the best foods to eat before playing in strenuous or competitive games.
4. Study the caloric intake of athletes.
5. Learn how to keep well and be in top physical condition.
6. Learn the cause and relationship of fatigue to accidents.
7. Learn the role that poor nutrition plays in poor posture.
8. Know their own body type, proper height, and proper weight according to age.
9. Learn how diet affects the rate and speed of recovery from sprains, broken bones, and other injuries.
10. Know the value of eating a good breakfast as a means of avoiding fatigue and becoming a top performer.

USE OF TEACHING METHODS

Planned instruction in nutrition should grow out of the problems of the daily living experiences of the pupils at home as well as at school, and include many of those of the community in which they live. As Haag points out, each teacher should receive in-service educational programs which will help them to do a better job of teaching nutrition. Such a program might well include:

1. Informing the teachers of the incidence of nutritional deficiencies among their own pupils.
2. Discovering the causes of these problems.
3. Helping teachers realize and understand the interrelationship of nutrition with human growth at all ages of the school-age child.
4. Recognizing the signs of nutritional problems.
5. Emphasizing the role of nutrition in the total school health program.
6. Helping the teachers correct their own food habits.
7. Understanding the benefits of supplementary school feeding programs, and becoming aware that the school lunch can supply one-third of the daily food intake.
8. Giving each teacher a comprehensive set of facts on the elements of nutrition.
9. Encouraging teachers to attend extension courses and workshops in nutrition education offered by departments of home economics or foods and nutrition in teachers' colleges, universities, and schools of public health.
10. Stimulating parent education in nutrition.[2]

It is the task of the elementary teacher to help children (1) develop the attitude that health is important for growth, fun, and appearance, (2) accept increased responsibility for their own health, (3) understand their own health problems in the areas of nutrition, emotional health, safety, promotion of health habits, and prevention of infection, (4) develop desirable practices for healthful living in the areas of physical, social, and emotional health, (5) learn the ways in which they can solve their own health problems. Nutrition education plays a foundational role in the school health education program, for it touches every subject area which should be included in it either directly (as in dental health and growth) or indirectly (as in social adjustment and first aid). Consequently, expert teaching in this important area is necessary. The following suggestions for using various teaching methods successfully in nutrition education include:

---

[2] Haag, *op. cit.*, pp. 208–209.

Problem Solving

Teachers using this method must be skilled in discovering nutritional problems which are real to pupils. Often much class discussion and observation are required before an existing problem can be isolated and defined. Recently, a group of third-graders in a school in Atlanta, Georgia, selected a nutrition problem for further study when they realized (with the help of their teacher) that too many of them were not eating all the food on their plates at the school cafeteria. The class discussed such things as why they should eat a balanced lunch and of what such a meal should consist, what caused likes and dislikes in food choice, how three well-balanced daily meals stimulated growth, and other related topics. The teacher, who noticed that most of the group avoided eating a variety of fresh and cooked vegetables, helped the group plan a visit to the fresh vegetable counter in a large supermarket. There they talked with the manager of the store, who showed and told them about the many kinds of food displayed, where they came from, how they were shipped across the country or state, and many other interesting things. The pupils decided later to divide up into committees and each group chose a specific area to find more information on, and others volunteered to make special reports in class or informative posters on good nutrition. Within a few days the class, as one of their proposed solutions to the problems, suggested that a "Clean Plate Club" be formed and all children who ate all the food on their plates be listed on the chalk-board as members. They also decided to have another honorary list made up of those who ate a new kind of vegetable served in the cafeteria. These learning experiences not only helped the pupils to learn to like many new kinds of foods, and motivated them to eat all the food on their plates, but also helped them recognize a problem which existed which they could solve collectively through the improved actions of each individual.

Group interest in many kinds of nutritional problems may arise from current news items, such as a mass attack of food poisoning at a church picnic, reported in the daily newspaper, or the occurrence of floods throughout the nation and the problem of how homeless people can be housed and their daily dietary and other health needs met. Studying such problems provides many kinds of rewarding learning experiences for boys and girls, and they can be made to feel an important part of our ever-changing world.

Guidance

Individual health counseling can help many pupils successfully solve their own dietary and nutritional problems. It can assist the boy who is worried about being the class "runt," or the one who knows he should have more calcium in his diet but is allergic to milk products, or the sixth-grade girl who is concerned about her oily skin and pimply face, or the third-grader who always brings a jelly sandwich, candy bar, and drinks a Coke for lunch. These are real pupils with real nutritional problems. These children should be helped to solve their own problems with the assistance of professionally trained adults, including their own teacher, and by the things they and their classmates guide them to find out and learn more about at school.

Class Discussions

Class discussions in nutrition education can be a valuable means for helping the teacher find out what the pupils know about the subject, as well as provide her with opportunities to clear up misconceptions, and to learn how the children are applying what they have learned. Care must be taken, however, not to "pry" into the private lives of the pupils or to put them in situations which prove embarrassing. She should not ask direct questions such as "Johnny, what did you have for break-fast?" and then, after hearing his report ask Billy what he had, for the latter, even though he has not even had breakfast that morning, will be most apt to tell her that he had even a better breakfast than Johnny's. Children feel that they cannot afford to "lose face," especially those in elementary schools, to whom the teacher's approval means so much.

Discussion in the area of nutrition might well revolve around the following topics:

1. The importance of eating three well-balanced daily meals.
2. How food helps us grow.
3. Why we should chew our food well.
4. Where does food come from?
5. How can we prevent illness by eating certain kinds of food?
6. How our bodies use food.
7. The importance of good manners.
8. The role of public health in nutrition.
9. Food preservation.
10. Each individual's height and weight chart; his weekly food consumption chart.
11. Eating in a restaurant or cafeteria.
12. The use of color in food serving; table decorations.
13. The emotions and food.
14. Dangers of being overweight or underweight, and how this can be avoided.
15. How to count calories.
16. Self-medication and vitamins.
17. Food allergies.
18. Growing up.
19. Consumer protection and education.
20. Foreign foods.

Special Reports

Research assignments for certain pupils who have specific health problems re-lated to nutrition, such as frequent colds, food dislikes, or bad table manners, often will help them gain new insight into their own difficulty. Some teachers prefer to have pupils volunteer to make class reports on certain phases of a unit which especially interest them. They should remember, however, that often those needing practice in speaking before groups rarely volunteer or want to take advantage of such an opportunity. Certainly no good teacher would want to make the already good become better at the expense of the already weak becoming weaker, and yet this too frequently happens.

Special reports in the area of nutrition suitable for older pupils might well include:

1. Signs of malnutrition.
2. Restored cereals.
3. Menu planning.
4. Religious customs.
5. Trends in American dietary habits.
6. Effects of cola drinks upon dental health.
7. Diets for those who are ill.
8. Foods as disease carriers.
9. How animals are tuberculin-tested.

10. Infections spread by food handlers.
11. How foods are contaminated by rodents and insects.
12. The diets of athletes.
13. Food buying.
14. Vitamin therapy.
15. The use of color and food selection.

Demonstrations

Children will enjoy and profit from doing the following:

1. How to prepare uncooked vegetables for storage in the refrigerator, such as lettuce, celery.
2. Buying food at the class "grocery store."
3. How to cook simple foods, such as frying eggs.
4. How to use a microscope to see germs and bacteria.
5. Good and poor posture and its relationship to diet.
6. Animal experiment results.
7. The effect of lighting upon food, such as blue lights upon milk, green ones on meat, etc.
8. Relaxation techniques and their relationship to relieving tensions before meals.
9. Food tests for the presence of water content in vegetables, fruits, etc.
10. The dehydration of foods such as grapes, plums, etc.
11. Table setting and decorations.
12. Good and bad table manners.

Field Trips

Visits to places within the community which have a direct relationship to nutrition education can often be a more valuable means of educating pupils than many hours of class time spent reading or studying about food and related topics. Suggested places to visit are a farm, bakery, ice cream plant, food-packaging firm, grocery store, food-storage or locker plant, community or farmer's outdoor market, garbage disposal plant, city water department, meat market, fish market, and a flour mill.

Experiments

Experiments can be used effectively for getting the message of the dangers of eating an unbalanced diet across to growing boys and girls. When they see for themselves that one mouse which had been fed only tea or coffee looks and acts sick in comparison to one which had eaten a balanced diet, this experience becomes far more meaningful than merely hearing the teacher warn them against eating unwisely, especially when they realize that what happened to the mouse could also happen to them. Rabbits, hamsters, baby chickens, and birds are especially well suited for such experiments.

Simple food tests such as those mentioned below can be used to help children learn to identify the content of various foods, as well as motivate interest in learning about the classification and function of the six types of foods:

Tests for starch. Crush and soften with water one soda cracker. Place this in a test tube. Add one drop of well-diluted iodine. The material will turn blue, indicating that starch is present.

Test for fats. Place fried bacon, a pat of butter, or pastry on a piece of paper. Remove the food and put the paper on a radiator to heat. Observe the oily marks left on the paper. Compare the amount of fat in whole milk and skimmed milk in the same way.

Test for proteins. Burn raw lean meat, cheese, dried milk, or dried beans over the direct flame of a Bunsen burner. Since proteins are present, the food will give off a smell of burned feathers.

Test for minerals. Place peas, dried milk, or egg yolk on an asbestos metal plate. Burn it over the direct flame of a Bunsen burner. A gray ash will remain, showing that the food contains minerals. Nonmineral foods such as sugar will burn up quickly and leave no ash.

Test for water content. Cut an apple in two. Leave it exposed to the sun for one week. Note how it dries out.

Role Playing and Storytelling

These methods are best suited for younger children. Taking the part of a father, mother, or family member doing the weekly grocery shopping can also help them gain a better understanding of the duties and functions of each of these persons. Such experiences can be used to integrate nutrition with that of family life education. Playing grocery store, enacting the part of the ice cream man, etc., can also help the youngsters develop creativity, as well as give their teacher insight into their knowledge of nutrition, behavior, problems, and family background.

Older pupils will profit from making up and telling stories about what happens to vegetables or fruits from the time they are ripe until ready for market, along with their "adventures" while being shipped to market and at the canning factory. Stories can also be written about people who work on farms or elsewhere and are engaged in the production and transportation of food. Sixth-graders can learn much from their outside reading either for special reports or for pleasure. Such books as Edna Ferber's *So Big* or Mark Twain's *Huckleberry Finn* are especially well suited for this purpose.

Surveys

Surveys made by the pupils of the actual eating habits of people in their own community will help them gain insight upon the scope of nutrition problems and the role each might play in finding solutions to them. Suggested surveys might discover:

1. The number of pupils in each grade who eat their lunch daily in the school cafeteria or bring it from home.
2. The amount of milk drunk daily by each pupil in each grade.
3. Favorite foods of boys in contrast to those of girls.
4. How much a family of four spends, on the average, for groceries weekly.
5. How many food buyers go to market with a shopping list; how many buy impulsively.
6. How many adults in a city block eat breakfast regularly.
7. Favorite between-meal snacks among children, teenagers, and adults.
8. Family rules regarding the amount of candy children can have daily or weekly.
9. How many in the community or a city block have refrigerators and home freezers.
10. How many mothers bake their own cakes, bread, cookies, etc.
11. How often does an average family in a city block eat in a restaurant.
12. How much pupils help with the preparation and serving of food at home; how many have regular dishwashing duties.
13. How many in the community or a city block have their own kitchen sewage disposals and electric dishwashers.
14. Which is used most frequently, canned, fresh, or frozen orange juice by the people living in a community or a city block.

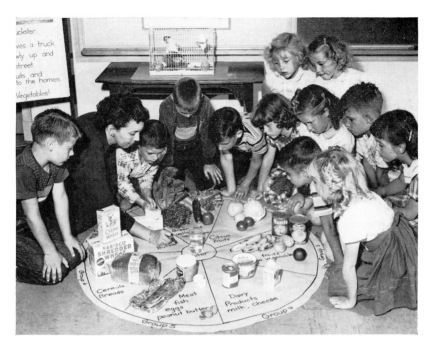

Figure 10-1. Nutrition education can be exciting. (Courtesy of Los Angeles Public Schools)

Regardless of which type of a survey is used, the gathering of data must be of educational value. Likewise, the findings and results of such surveys must become important in the lives of the children.

USE OF INSTRUCTIONAL MATERIALS

Many different kinds of instructional materials and supplementary teaching aids can be used in nutrition education.

Specimens

The different kinds of food in the four food classifications, examples of home canning in contrast to commercial, food packaging and the labeling of contents, food decay, "best" food buys for a given amount of money, carious teeth, improperly and properly cooked vegetables and meats, as well as many others are possible specimens to use. The pupils will profit most from bringing to class things they have collected, and explaining what they are and why each brought in what he did. All kinds of displays can be set up as a result, such as one showing the many kinds of vegetables which are good for growing children. Such experiences not only help certain youngsters to belong and contribute to a group endeavor, but also help to personalize education and give each pupil tangible things to see and do, as a result of factual materials he has learned at school.

Chalk and Bulletin Boards

Suggested "idea springboards" for using the boards including showing

1. New vocabulary words by making a weekly list and adding to it daily.
2. A list of new words seen or heard on television or radio.
3. The names of new foods told about or tasted by classmates.
4. Showing on a big map of the state or nation where certain foods are grown.
5. Questions requiring yes or no or short answers to discover what has been learned.
6. Restaurant menus collected by the class.
7. Illustrated lists or reports of a field trip made by the class showing the main things learned from it.
8. Posters made by individuals or small committees on any phase or subject regarding food or nutrition education.
9. Drawings of the digestive and circulatory systems of the body.
10. Current events pertinent to the subjects being studied in nutrition.
11. Pictures of families enjoying Thanksgiving dinner together, or other family traditions.
12. Illustrated evidence that good food affects good health.

Films

Films, in the classroom, at home on television, or in a movie theatre, should be fully utilized by an alert teacher. There is an abundance of free films on nutrition available from many sources.* Likewise, many television programs can be used, including the morning food shows in most areas and favorite weekly serials. Older pupils can profit from learning to distinguish between true and false advertising, as well as from watching more grown-up programs built around central characters, different times in history, or current and historical events. It is not enough, however, merely to have a class view such programs. They should be given opportunities to discuss what they have learned, as well as be guided to understand fully the meaningful facts and "messages" which have been presented.

Photographs

Photographs collected by the pupils of colorful recipes can be used for outdoor cookouts and picnics. Pictures of how to cook on a large coffee can which can be used as a stove can motivate pupils to try frying hamburgers or eggs on the top of such stoves. These can be made by cutting off one end, making a hole for smoke to come out of near the opposite end, and setting the whole can over a small wood fire.[3] Pupils who are members of the Campfire Girls, Boy Scouts, or Girl Scouts will be eager to share their outdoor campcraft and cooking skills with their classmates. The class going on such an adventure should plan, purchase, and prepare the food they are to have.

The pupils can also bring and display photographs taken of themselves when they were babies and each year thereafter to show others how much they have grown, and describe the role good health habits played in their own development. They can each also make a poster showing what they want to be when grown up, whether this

---

* See the Appendix for specific listings.
[3] Vannier, Maryhelen: *Methods and Materials in Recreation Leadership.* 3rd ed. Philadelphia, Lea & Febiger (In preparation) for directions for making these tin-can stoves as well as outdoor cooking recipes.

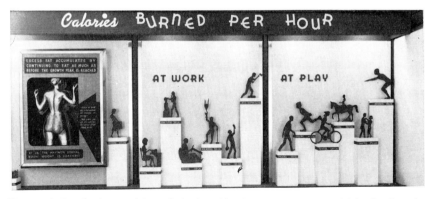

Figure 10-2. Seeing models and displays like these can stimulate children's ideas for making their own visual aids. This exhibit shows the number of calories used in various activities. (Courtesy of Dallas Health and Science Museum)

be a fashion model or astronaut, and list below the picture things they should do to be able to reach this grown-up ambition.

DESIRABLE OUTCOMES

A well-planned and well-taught unit in nutrition education should yield the following results by obtaining desirable knowledge, attitudes, and practices.

In the primary grades the pupils will

1. Eat three well-balanced meals daily.
2. Wash before eating.
3. Avoid eating too many sweets.
4. Know the relationship of good food to growth and good health.
5. Know what the Basic Seven Foods are.
6. Eat slowly.
7. Drink at least three glasses of milk and eight of water daily.
8. Help prepare the food and table at home according to skills suitable to their age.
9. Recognize that each parent has a unique contribution to make in the family, and that the father usually works to buy food and the mother works to prepare it.
10. Not talk with food in their mouths.
11. Know the names of and eat a wide variety of fruits and vegetables.
12. Know what unwise food selections will do to their teeth.

In the upper elementary grades, the pupils will

1. Continue to eat a balanced diet and to try new foods.
2. Wash their hands before eating.
3. Become more cognizant of good table manners, the social graces, and practice them.
4. Know and appreciate that pleasant surroundings are desirable at meal time, and that one should eat slowly.
5. Assist in planning the family meals and in their preparation.
6. Become aware of food nutrients and the functions of growth, energy, and repair.

7. Understand how the body digests food.
8. Understand in more detail the specific values of each type of food to the body.
9. Practice cleanliness when handling food.
10. Know about vitamins and the specific function of each one.
11. Become aware of how food values can be diminished or destroyed by improper storage or preparation, and know that a balanced, nourishing diet need not be expensive.
12. Know how food patterns and social customs differ throughout the world; become aware of the many types of food eaten in America and the countries from which these come.

Found below are suggested teaching units, lesson plans, and other instructional suggestions for teaching nutrition to children grades K–6:

Kindergarten
Objectives
1. To develop a positive attitude toward eating and nutrition.
2. To learn the importance of eating a variety of vegetables and fruits.

Suggested Approaches
1. Bulletin boards
2. Games
3. Demonstrations

Basic Concepts
1. To develop an interest in learning to like a variety of foods.
2. To have a happy attitude about eating.
3. To gain an understanding of the importance of drinking milk and fruit juices.
4. To develop a desire to avoid too many snacks, candies, etc.

Group Activities
1. Bring various fruits to feel and learn about their names and colors.
2. Taste different fruits and vegetables at lunch or snack time.
3. Bring magazines to class, and cut out pictures of vegetables and fruits.

Correlation To Other Subjects
1. Arithmetic
   a. Bring various fruits and vegetables to class and have the children identify and count them.
   b. Count the number of students who buy milk at lunch.
2. Drama
   a. Have the children act out parts in a skit as different vegetables.
3. Physical Education
   a. Talk to the children about how good nutrition helps people grow strong.
4. Art
   a. Have children color and draw pictures of fruit, etc.
   b. Make puppets out of fruits and vegetables.

Evaluation
1. Observe manners and eating habits at lunch.
2. Parent conferences.
3. Observe general health of each child.

Pupil References
   Being Six. Scott, Foresman & Co., 1961.
   The Kaleidoscope Readers. Field Ed. Publ., 1969.

Teacher References
   Cornacchia, H. J., Staton, W. M., and Irwin, L. W.: *Health in Elementary School.* 3rd ed. St. Louis: C. V. Mosby Co., 1970.

Grade 1

Objectives
1. To develop positive attitude toward eating habits.

Suggested Approaches
1. Bulletin boards
2. Games
3. Demonstrations
4. Role playing

Basic Concepts
1. Importance of drinking milk and fruit juices.
2. Need for a variety in food selection for a basic diet.
3. Development of good eating habits.
4. The importance of a good breakfast.
5. Cleanliness in handling and eating foods.
6. Difference between good and bad snacks.

Group Activities
1. Plan a trip to your school's lunchroom and observe where foods and supplies are kept.
2. Discuss how much better fruit juices are than soft drinks and candy.
3. Have children practice having a quiet happy lunch break.
4. Cafeteria dramatization—have the children choose a balanced lunch.
5. Talk about eating at home. Good manners. Helping mother set the table and clean up.

Correlation To Other Subjects
1. Arithmetic
   a. Have the children count vegetables.
   b. Count children's lunch money.
2. Art
   a. Have children draw and color different foods.
3. Music
   a. Play soft music for lunch period.
4. Drama
   a. Have them play the parts of different fruits and vegetables.
5. Physical Education
   a. Have the children pick vegetable or fruit names for teams in activities outside.
6. Science
   a. Discuss how drinking milk helps to build strong bones.
   b. Discuss how certain foods are good for skin.
7. English
   a. Have a spelling contest using the names in the food groups.

Audio-Visual Aids
1. Chalk board
2. Bulletin board
3. Felt board

Grades 2 and 3

Objectives—To teach:
1. The nutritive values in milk, butter, and other dairy products.
2. Use of margarine as a substitute for butter.
3. Variety of fruits and vegetables; their protection and processing.
4. Necessity of protein in the diet.
5. Willingness to try new foods as a means of eating a balanced diet.
6. Importance of a balanced breakfast, lunch, dinner, nutritious snacks.
7. Undesirability of tea, coffee, and cola drinks for children.

7

8. Importance of having a happy, relaxed atmosphere while eating.
9. The importance of maintaining regular habits of elimination of body waste products.
10. Correct use of eating utensils; acceptable eating habits.

Suggested Approaches
1. Make a chart showing how much and what kind of the following foods to eat: vegetables, fruits, meats, cereals, desserts.
2. Discuss the place of sugar and candy in the diet.
3. Investigate the extent of malnutrition in the U.S.

Basic Concepts
1. Good eating habits; types, kinds, and values of different foods.
2. Some people are allergic to certain foods.

Group Activities
1. Visit a farm.
2. Field trip to dairy.

Individual Activities
1. Have children keep a diary of foods they eat and have them evaluate their own diets.
2. Have each child start his own garden and report on it.

Correlation With Other Subjects
1. Art
   a. Create a collage using basic foods as a theme.
2. Social Studies
   a. Discuss the types of crops which are present in certain countries.
   b. Discuss the various foods grown in all areas.

Audio-Visual Aids
"Breakfast and the Bright Life." Cereal Institute.
"How Food Becomes You." National Dairy Council.

Evaluation
1. Do the students have an understanding of the importance of good nutrition and its part in overall good health?
2. Do the students have an awareness of the effects of malnutrition?
3. Have the students learned the 4 Basic Food Groups?

Teaching Resources
Best, C. R., and Taylor, N. B.: *The Human Body*. 4th ed. New York: Holt, Rinehart & Winston, 1963.
Bogart, L. Jean, Briggs, G. M. and Calloway, D. H.: *Nutrition and Physical Fitness*. 8th ed. Philadelphia: W. B. Saunders Co., 1966.
Davis, Adelle: *Vitality through Planned Nutrition*. New York: The Macmillan Co., 1948.
Goodhart, R. and Shils, M.: *Modern Nutrition in Health and Disease*. 5th ed. Philadelphia: Lea & Febiger, 1973.

Grade 4

Objectives—Teach:
1. The students the importance of eating from the four basic food groups every day.
2. That the food you eat really affects how you look and feel.
3. The importance of eating a good breakfast.
4. The values of vitamins to the body.
5. The importance of drinking milk and fruit juices for strong bodies.
6. Regular elimination habits and variations in individuals.
7. The function of food in the body, and the purpose of the different essential elements in the diet.

Suggested Approaches
1. Illustrate a well-balanced diet from pictures cut out from magazines.
2. Discuss the following eating habits: eating between meals; eating alone; eating before going to bed; eating too much.
3. Discuss how the following affect digestion: cheerfulness and happiness; too much exercise; resting before and after eating; general health of an individual.

Basic Concepts
1. Know what foods belong to the four basic food groups and what foods from each group do for the body.
2. Know the values of vitamins for the body.
3. Learn the importance of water to the body.
4. Learn the importance of drinking milk and fruit juices for strong bodies.
5. Good eating habits and personal hygiene while eating; the time and way in which to eat are important.

Group Activities
1. Make posters showing the four basic groups of foods.
2. Let each pupil plan his own diet for a week.
3. Draw a large milk bottle, and list the food values found in milk and their use.
4. Fill 8 glasses with water to illustrate the amount of water needed each day.

Individual Pupil Activities
1. Let each pupil bring to class the 5 vegetables he likes best.
2. Make a list of foods you eat each day for a week.
3. Suggest each pupil visit a food store, and notice the way the store tries to keep the food clean.

Correlation With Other Subjects
1. Social Studies
    a. Read about crops and industries.
    b. List fruits, vegetables, and nuts grown in your area.
    c. Make a list of food eaten yesterday.
    d. The processing of different kinds of meat.
2. Art
    a. Plan a group picture on a food industry of your area.
3. Language Arts
    a. Read story concerning nutrition about foods, other people and nations eat, such as the Indians, Eskimos.
4. Arithmetic
    a. Using artificial fruit, show sets and adding and subtracting.

Audio-Visual Aids
   "Breakfast and the Bright Life." Cereal Institute, Inc. 135 South LaSalle Street, Chicago, Ill.
   "The World of Wonderful Foods." National Dairy Council, Food and Nutrition Board, 2101 Constitution Ave., Washington, D.C.
   "How Food Becomes You." National Dairy Council, 111 N. Canal Street, Chicago, Illinois 60606.

Evaluation of Results
1. Make a test to appraise pupil's knowledge about the food crops in his area.
2. Do students have an understanding of the importance of good nutrition and its part in overall good health?

Pupil References
  Hodges, Margaret: *What's For Lunch, Charley.* New York: Dial Press, 1970.
  Ipcar, Dahlov: *Ten Big Farms.* New York: Knopf Publishing Company, 1969.

Teacher References
  Pilty, Albert: "How Your Body Uses Food." Chicago: National Dairy Council, 1970.
  Why Break the Fast. Kelloggs Food for Thought, Kellogg Company, Department of Home Economics, Battle Creek, Mich.
  "Anatomy for Beginners." *Instructor Magazine.* October 1970.
  Ediger, Marlan: "Upper Graders Look at Modern Farmers." *Instructor Magazine.* August-September 1970.

Grade 5

Objectives
  1. The importance of food.
  2. Meeting new foods.
  3. Where does our food go inside our bodies?
  4. Beginning etiquette.
  5. Socialization with the family at mealtime; togetherness.
  6. Food; the way you look and the way you feel.
  7. Introduction to vitamins and minerals.
  8. Introduction to the digestive process.

Basic Concepts
  1. Provide a general view of the food groups.
  2. Three balanced meals and their importance to the body.
  3. What is fat, and what is muscle?
  4. Why do we eat food each day?
  5. The importance of quiet activity before and after meals.
  6. Contributions to a happy family: meal hours together, helpfulness, good table manners, conversation, sharing.
  7. Fallacies about foods.

Suggested Approaches
  1. Bulletin boards
  2. Role playing
  3. Demonstrations
  4. Dramatizations
  5. Individual and group learning situations.

Group Activities
  1. Visit the school lunchroom; watch clean-up procedures.
  2. Visit a dairy or cannery.
  3. Plan a balanced diet for three meals a day.
  4. Games with teams named after foods, (i. e., SPUD elimination game).
  5. Plan bulletin boards.

Individual Activities
  1. Have individual reports on vitamins and on minerals.
  2. Complete posters for the bulletin board.
  3. Various health projects and reading in texts.

Correlation With Other Subjects
  1. Arithmetic
    a. Play grocery market and assess the cost of the food purchased.
    b. Play with numbers—of fruits.
  2. Geography
    a. Study the main diets and foods of people in other countries and regions of the world.

3. English
   a. Have spelling bees.
   b. Write sentences with the new vocabulary words from nutrition class.
4. Science
   a. Discuss the proper diet and the care needed for a healthy body.
   b. Care for a small animal in class—a hamster, turtle, or mouse. Show how good and bad nutrition affects growth.
5. Drama and Art
   a. A play featuring a family on a farm.

Evaluation
1. Observations at lunch periods.
2. Parent-teacher conferences.
3. Notice general health of each child.
4. Oral discussions.
5. Occasional quizzes on facts.

Audio-Visual Aids
   "Food From Grains." (Coronet)
   "Why Eat A Good Breakfast." (National Cereal Institute)

Pupil References
   Health for All. Glenview, Ill.: Scott, Foresman & Co., 1969.
   Four Corners of the Sky. San Francisco: Field Ed. Publ., 1969.

Teacher References
   Richmond, R. S. and Pounds, A. M.: *Health and Growth—Grade 6.* Glenview, Ill.: Scott, Foresman & Co., 1971.
   Godshall, Frances: *Nutrition in the Elementary School.* New York: Harper & Row, 1958.
   Jelliffe, Derrick D.: *Nutrition Survey.* Geneva: World Health Organization, 1966.
   Four Corners of the Sky—Kaleidoscope—Chicago: Field, 1960.

Grade 6

Objectives
1. To learn to determine health status of each child.
2. Understand that no one food contains all the nutrients in the quantity the body needs, but a varied diet is necessary.
3. How to have a healthy body.
4. Learn the importance of vitamins and minerals in the maintenance of the body.
5. Understanding the digestive processes.
6. Know what malnutrition is.

Basic Concepts
1. Review the basic food groups:
   a. Balanced meals and diets
   b. Foods for occasions
2. The relationship between adequate diets and weight control.
3. Food nutrients help build and repair tissues, regulate body processes, and supply fuel for energy.
4. Six classes of nutrients:
   a. Proteins
   b. Carbohydrates
   c. Minerals
   d. Vitamins
   e. Water
   f. Fats
5. How to get the most nutrients from your food.

6. Digestion and how it breaks down food into usable particles for our bodies.
7. Water—an essential—4 to 8 glasses each day for nourishment, digestion, and elimination.
8. Foods—the best source of vitamins.
9. Diseases due to vitamin shortages:
   a. Rickets—vitamin D—(crooked bones)
   b. Beriberi—vitamin B_1—(nervous disease)
   c. Scurvy—vitamin C (bleeding gums)
   d. Pellagra—niacin (rough skin)
10. What is digestion, and how do our emotions affect this process?
11. The effects of coffee, tea, and alcohol on the body:
    a. They may cause impaired digestion, headaches, or other ailments.
    b. Pure Food and Drug Acts.
    c. Caffeine
    d. Stimulants and their effects.
12. Social customs and etiquette.
13. Fallacies about foods.

Suggested Approaches
1. Role playing
2. Bulletin boards
3. Demonstrations
4. Speakers and guests, such as a nurse or a doctor

Group Activities
1. Newspaper oral reports.
2. Important men in health such as Pasteur.
3. Visit a dairy to learn about milk pasteurization.
4. Taste different types of fruit and cheeses.
5. Plant a small garden in the classroom.
6. Plan a group picnic with a balanced meal; plan together.
7. Periodic "treats" by the teacher; use nutritious foods.

Individual Activities
1. Share recipes.
2. Lunch-ins on rainy days.
3. Contribute to a bulletin board with pictures and articles.
4. Individual meal charts.

Correlation With Other Subjects
1. Arithmetic
   a. Games with calories.
   b. Ratio proportion games with foods and prices.
2. Science
   a. Test two different diets in two rats for four weeks; weigh each rat periodically.
   b. Discuss animals and their health and eating habits; i.e., horses, turtles, fish, dogs, and cats.
   c. Place penny in a glass of Coke, and see the chemical reaction.
   d. Observe the milk to cheese process.
   e. Body needs and the role of food in supplying these needs.
3. Social Studies
   a. Oral news reports on nutrition.
   b. The farmer and his crops on the plains of the United States.
   c. Foods and the place they grow best.
4. Health
   a. Show pictures of children suffering from malnutrition.
5. English
   a. Health words in stories.
   b. Spelling tests and bees.
   c. Games such as hangman, puzzles, and scavenger hunt clues.

6. Drama and Art
   a. Skits and plays; Caddie Woodlawn, country themes, or plays about Thanksgiving traditions.
   b. Learning to paint with water colors.
   c. Student bulletin boards.
7. Physical Education
   a. Relay races passing vegetables.

Audio-Visual Aids

"*Eat For Health.*"   #337.   Encyclopedia Britannica Films, 1150 Wilmette Avenue, Wilmette, Illinois; 44th Street, New York, 17; 5625 Hollywood Blvd., Hollywood, California.
"Run With Food."
"Diabetics Unknown."
"Digestion in Our Bodies."
"Vitamins and Your Health."   New York: Modern Talking Picture Service, 1969.
"Eat To Live."   Chicago: Wheatflour Institute, 1969.
Slides on calcium and its purpose.
Why foods spoil.

Pupil References

Callahan, Dorothy, and Payne, Alma Smith: *Great Nutrition Puzzle.* New York: Charles Scribner's Sons, 1964.
Blanche, L.: *Around the World in Eighty Dishes.* New York: Harper & Row, 1969.
Richmond, R. S. and Pounds, A. M.: *Health and Growth: Grade 6.* Glenview, Ill.: Scott, Foresman & Co., 1971.

CHAPTER 11

dental health

Dental decay and loss of teeth are major health problems among people of all ages in America. It is estimated that nine out of every ten people have carious teeth or more serious dental difficulties. It is the chief health problem among school-age children. In a survey of the health problems of 78,448 pupils in the Philadelphia Public Schools, the number of pupils with dental caries was six times as large as those with the next leading health difficulty.[1] Like all pressing health issues, the solution to this problem lies in prevention, education, and proper care. The school must assume real and increased responsibility in helping to eliminate this vast problem, for eradicating dental disease is a public health responsibility. As Oberteuffer has pointed out, the school is in a strategic position to formulate a complete program in dental health education and to assume leadership in organizing community resources for dental care of all children.[2]

Specific responsibilities of the school lie in health protection, correction of defects, health conservation, and health promotion. In an effort to promote improved dental health, some schools have assumed the following responsibilities:

1. Provide periodic dental health examinations.
2. Inform parents of dental disabilities in children.
3. Refer children for dental treatment to appropriate sources.
4. Recheck for correction of dental defects.
5. Provide a continuous program of instruction in dental health.
6. Give individual dental health guidance.
7. Provide special services where indicated.
8. Establish interest among parents through a program of education and participation in the dental health of school children.

---

[1] Haag, Jessie: *School Health Program.* 3rd ed. Philadelphia: Lea & Febiger, 1972, p. 72.
[2] Oberteuffer, Delbert, et al.: *School Health Education.* 5th ed. New York: Harper & Row, 1972, p. 389.

9. Give adequate financial support to provide a complete dental health education program.
10. Provide sufficient professional personnel to staff the program of service and instruction adequately.[3]

School administrators should work closely with local dentists in order to establish policies which outline the role of the school in dental health and follow these up with a well-planned educational program and dental service for all children. Any periodic school dental examination is worthless unless it is coupled with a remedial program, and unless those needing special attention receive it. Parental cooperation is necessary on all educational levels if health problems among children are to be solved, but it is particularly imperative in the elementary grades, for these pupils by themselves can do little, if anything, to correct existing dental or other difficulties.

A complete dental health program should include:

1. Dental health service—including periodic dental checkups, informing the parents of dental defects, rechecking for corrections, compiling and evaluating findings.
2. Dental health instruction—including the presentations of authentic factual information in understandable units in a graded program through the entire school curriculum from grade 1 through senior high school. Such a program should stress the development of proper knowledge, attitudes, and habits which will promote good dental care.
3. Dental care—although this responsibility rests with the family, if it cannot assume it, this falls upon the community, the school, the state, and the nation.

The role of the elementary teacher in the area of dental health education is of major importance. Children should not only be taught the essential facts about teeth and their care but be motivated and encouraged to put in practice what they have learned, for only then will the development of good habits formed in school be carried out at home. Without the cooperation of parents, little can be done to help solve the great problem of dental disease among primary children, for this disease is caused largely by improper diet and lack of proper mouth hygiene. The content of the dental health program must be timely and carefully planned. Readiness for learning about teeth begins when the child starts losing his deciduous, or baby, teeth. Likewise, when the permanent teeth begin to appear, most youngsters become increasingly curious to know what is happening and thus can be easily motivated to receive favorably information concerning proper mouth hygiene. As children grow older they become more conscious of their appearance and are ready to learn how to be good looking and popular, as well as the importance of having the good teeth necessary for an attractive smile. Children can be motivated to want to learn more about dental health if they are provided with meaningful experiences coupled to an increasing awareness of their own health needs and changing selves. All should be taught that the care of the teeth is a lifelong responsibility.

SUGGESTED GRADED TOPICS

There is no doubt that in far too many schools, instruction in dental health has suffered from lack of continuity, along with any subject area usually included in the

---

[3] Stoll, Frances and Catherman, Joan: *Dental Health Education.* 4th ed. Philadelphia: Lea & Febiger, 1972.

health program. There will always be omission and repetition, as teachers come and go, and not enough of them really care about the physical well-being of their pupils. One way to ensure a meaningful graded program in health education is to have a group of representative teachers from each grade meet to:

1. Prepare an outlined recorded plan stating the objectives and desired educational outcomes for each health topic for each grade.
2. Prepare a complete list of facts and concepts to be included on each grade level.
3. Devise a list of reference materials for the pupils and the teacher in the range of classes to be taught.
4. Make a list of supplementary teaching aids such as films and other audio-visual aids.
5. Revise these materials yearly.

Any teacher worth her salt knows the needs and interests of her class group and of each child in it. This knowledge is invaluable in gaining insight into the degree of readiness of the group. Just as it would be foolish to teach first-graders who are losing their baby teeth about the whole set of teeth, including wisdom teeth, so it would be to teach any group a "canned," prepared lesson found in a text-book which is supposed to be suitable for any class studying any aspect of health. Unless units of instruction represent the joint planning of the teacher and the class, or are made in a flexible outline form, they cannot help children reach the desired educational goal. As Stoll points out, the desire for good dental health should originate within the child, rather than from a demand made by outside influences or forces.[4]

Suggested graded topics and outlines for dental health instruction in each elementary grade are:

GRADE 1

1. Regular good tooth care, and how to brush the teeth properly.
2. Eating a well-balanced diet three times daily.
3. Why sweets are harmful to the teeth.
4. How many teeth a first-grader usually has.
5. The dentist as a friend; a visit to a dentist's office.
6. How teeth can be safely protected in play, at home, and at school.

GRADE 2

1. Review of tooth-brushing methods.
2. Why we lose our baby teeth.
3. The importance and care of the six-year molars.
4. What causes tooth decay and how it can be prevented.

GRADE 3

1. Review of proper dental-care techniques.
2. How to make and use our own dentifrice.
3. What is the best type of a toothbrush to use.
4. Proper care of a toothbrush.
5. Why we should go to a dentist.

---

[4] Stoll and Catherman, *op. cit.*, p. 4.

Grade 4
1. The structure and function of the tooth.
2. How human teeth work like scissors and grinders.
3. A comparison of human and animal teeth.
4. How second teeth form and appear.
5. The best kinds of food to eat in order to have well-fed teeth.
6. The value of chewing food properly.
7. Review of how teeth can best be cared for daily.

Grade 5
1. Study of the basic foods needed daily for a balanced diet.
2. Why sweets are harmful to the teeth.
3. Function of vitamins, minerals, phosphorus, and calcium in the teeth.
4. How poor nutrition affects the teeth.
5. Fluoridation and its effect upon the prevention of decay.
6. Review of the techniques of proper oral hygiene.

Grade 6
1. Review of the role nutrition plays in dental care.
2. Accident prevention in competitive games, with special reference to injuries of the mouth and teeth.
3. Malocclusion—its cause, prevention, and correction.
4. Analysis of advertising and consumer education in the purchase of dental care products.
5. Detailed study of tooth structures.
6. The causes of diseases of the mouth and protection from them.
7. The importance of periodic dental examinations.
8. The use of a dental x-ray in dental examinations.
9. The use of mouth protectors in competitive sports.

CURRICULUM PLACEMENT

It is the obligation of all teachers to provide those educational experiences in the school curriculum which will enable children to learn how to develop and maintain good health, for it is in the formative years that lifelong habits, upon which the foundation of health and happiness rests, can best be built. Opportunities arise every day for the integration and correlation of health with most subjects included in the elementary school curriculum. In the broad-fields, core, or experience curricular patterns dental health education can be interwoven into larger areas of study such as the communicative arts, science, mathematics, and creative expression. In those schools wherein health, safety, and science are integrated in one broad field, numerous opportunities arise for direct health teaching in all health areas.

The Communicative Arts

Reading, writing, and speaking, as well as seeing and hearing, enable children to learn much on their own about dental health when carefully guided by a teacher. Stories about initial dental experiences, such as Burchheimer's *Let's Go to the Dentist*, the reading of scientific facts in library reference materials assigned to the older pupils, and other reading materials can all contribute to the improvement of reading speed and comprehension, as well as serve as a means of dental health education. Increased understanding and use of new words can aid pupils to build a good vocabulary for increased communicative purposes. When each new word is introduced, it should be written on the chalkboard, and the pupils taught how to spell, pronounce, and use it correctly. Skills in writing can be practiced and developed through the correlation of dental health instruction and the communicative arts by having the pupils write about their first experiences at the dentist, how the selection of good foods helps prevent decay, or writing for a make-believe dental appointment or to the American Dental Association for bulletin-board materials or information. Group discussions not only help bring to light how much or how little children really know about dental hygiene, but such experiences can help them learn the value of talking over and logically thinking through a problem, as well as assist them develop skill in expressing themselves verbally. Discussions among primary children might well revolve around such topics as why we have teeth, what happens when we lose a tooth, or in what ways a dentist can be a good friend. Among the older pupils, interest in the improvement of oral hygiene can be stimulated through panels as well as group discussions around such topics as evaluating a dental film seen in class, or modern dental treatment in contrast to that found throughout history. For these older pupils, individual research reports can do much to help them learn to speak well before groups as well as to develop research skills. Younger children, through their "do-and-tell" periods, might well demonstrate the correct way to brush the teeth, how a dentist examines the teeth, and many other kinds of similar experiences. Visiting speakers, such as the local dentist, dental hygienist, or a school dietitian, can all add much to the effectiveness of the program, especially if each pupil is asked to make a list of the most important things he learned, or if there is a class discussion following the speaker's presentation.

Social Studies

There are rich opportunities for the correlation and integration of dental health with social studies which can increase an understanding and appreciation of the fact that dental disease is a community and national problem. Through the study of history, children can learn that ancient people also had this problem, as well as learn how it was handled. The effect of food upon health in our own as well as in other lands is one of many areas in which dental health, nutrition, social studies, and geography can be combined into an integrated learning experience. Visits to places of interest in the community in a unit entitled "Getting to Know Our Health Co-workers in Our Community" might well include a trip to a dentist's office, as well as to the local health department or local dog pound. Listed below are some other suggested activities for correlating dental health with social science:

1. Make a comparative study of the incidence of dental caries on a state-by-state and nation-by-nation basis.
2. Learn the role the state and national government plays in the prevention of dental disease.
3. Study superstitions and fallacies regarding dental care throughout the history of America.
4. Learn about dental care among the ancient peoples in contrast to practices of today.
5. Find out how industry helps promote good dental hygiene.
6. Write a research paper on the value of fluoridation in the prevention of tooth decay. Compare what your city and state are doing in this area with those elsewhere.
7. Debate the pros and cons of socialized medicine, including free dental care.

Science

Science and dental health are closely related, for science provides the facts necessary to help pupils learn more about any part of themselves. Units on nutrition and dental health have frequently been successfully combined. In such units children should learn about the necessity of chewing food well, as well as of eating a balanced daily diet. Science fairs, which can be the work of a school science class or club, are increasing in popularity throughout the nation. Experiments, collections, and projects made by the pupils, either in class or as extracurricular activities, are usually open for the public to see. Although dental health materials made by children can only be a part of such a fair, they can do much to motivate both pupil and parent interest in obtaining better health, as well as help both learn more about how it can be accomplished.

Specific activities which can be used to correlate dental health with science include:

EXPERIMENTS

1. Make tooth powder composed of one-third salt and two-thirds baking soda.
2. Bite an apple and leave it in the classroom overnight. Show it to the class the next day, and have them discuss the cause and prevention of decay in food as well as in teeth.
3. Examine a decayed tooth under a microscope.
4. Conduct an annual feeding experiment to learn the relationship between a poor diet and decay and unhealthy gums.
5. Teeth are fed by blood. Of what is blood made? How does it look under the microscope?
6. Examine the teeth under a magnifying glass, and with a dentist's hand mirror. Discuss.
7. Test for starch. To one-half teaspoonful of cornstarch add a little water and a drop of iodine. The blue color that appears shows that starch is present. Learn how starches and sugars affect teeth.
8. Examine the saliva, or materials from your tongue under a miscroscope. Learn how mouthwash destroys bacteria.

Mathematics

Mathematics also offers good opportunities for the correlation of dental health. However, care must be taken to select topics with the purpose of teaching children about dental health instead of just numbers. For example, if the problem given pupils to solve is to discover how much ten toothbrushes and two tubes of toothpaste costs if the former costs 30¢ and the latter 38¢, often the group will think of toothbrushing in terms of expense instead of as a good habit. When numbers enter naturally into a class discussion is the best time for mathematics to be used. Simple addition and subtraction problems, such as finding out how many have ever been to a dentist or how many teeth are missing from the number children should have at a certain age, enable both the class and the teacher to learn, for the group will gain an understanding of a dental health problem and the teacher will find out another significant fact about each child. Problems which can help children gain a deeper understanding of percentages can be based upon discovering the total number in the class who need dental care, according to the school dental examination, in relation to the total number in each class or grade, or to the total number of students in the school. In the upper grades, graphs and tables can be used to show such things as a comparison of the number of people needing dental care in one state with those in another, the amount of money from the family budget which should be spent on health care and protection, and the percentage which should be spent on dental care. Finding needed information for such problems will also help youngsters learn how to use the library. Dental health also provides many opportunities for drill in learning numbers. However, care must be taken to individualize the meaning of figures; if the children find out that 350 pupils in their school have unfilled cavities in their teeth, there is no direct relationship to each pupil unless each cares for his own teeth properly, and knows and practices ways to prevent decay.

Drama and Art

When used as a means of helping children learn more about dental health, drama and art have great educational value. The use of puppets, one-act plays, mime, mock radio and television broadcasts, etc., can also be successfully integrated and correlated with both the creative and communicative arts. Merely coloring outlined pictures of teeth, however, has questionable value other than giving the young child a chance to improve his hand-eye coordination. Likewise, making dental care posters from pictures cut out of magazines will have no value in teaching dental health unless this experience motivates the postermaker to take better care of his own teeth and mouth, as well as eat the proper kind of foods necessary for maintaining good overall well-being. Free-hand drawings, color choice, the use of finger paints can all help children express pent-up emotions and tensions about going to the dentist or losing their own teeth. Clay, plaster of Paris, and other materials can be used successfully in helping older pupils make their own models of teeth. Such experiences are often more meaningful than merely showing the class a slide or three-dimensional model, for they provide avenues for youngsters to use their own hands in creative ways to express what they know and have learned.

Suggested art and dramatic activities which can be used for dental health education purposes include:

1. Divide the class into committees. Let each group make a poster or present a skit on any aspect of a unit on dental health.
2. Make clay models of teeth, dental instruments, etc.
3. Demonstrate the proper way to brush the teeth by using a large model of teeth and a brush. Have each child brush his own teeth, preferably with a brush, or with his pencil or forefinger, or by using a paper model of a set of teeth and a pencil.[5]
4. Have each pupil draw a picture of a happy person with pretty teeth. Let each make up and tell a story about his picture.
5. Dramatize going to the dentist, getting ready for school, buying a toothbrush and toothpaste.
6. Make a dental health exhibit of clay models, posters, and other creative media.
7. Study drawings and pictures of malocclusion. Discuss the prevention and treatment necessary to avoid disfiguration of the mouth and face.
8. Present mock or real radio or television programs built around any work done in class in dental health.

---

[5] Such models and other free dental teaching aids are available from The Bristol-Myers Company, Educational Department, New York. Also see your local dentist for sources of teaching aids in your area.

9. Make a toothbrush rack for the family bathroom or for a tent group at camp.
10. Black out certain teeth. Examine yourself in the mirror. Explain your reactions to what you see there.
11. Discuss the dental films seen in class.
12. Make your own movie or cartoon about any character and his experiences in learning any aspect of dental health. Show this to the class. Use a curtain roll and a cardboard carton for the film and camera.

Safety

Safety education should teach children to take chances wisely in order to avoid accidents by knowing what the risks are and instilling in them a desire to eliminate them. Children should learn the danger of putting foreign objects in their mouths or biting on them. Stress should also be placed upon playing safely at school and at home, drinking from water fountains correctly, and using other precautions in order to prevent having broken teeth or jaws. On the playground, care should be taken to use the swings, jungle gym, monkey bars, and other equipment correctly, for this type of play can be especially hazardous to young children. Head-on collisions, which often occur in chasing and fleeing games such as "Run, Sheepie, Run" can also be prevented, and injuries to teeth be avoided. It would be foolish to eradicate all hazards from children's play areas; wise instructors utilize dangerous and adventuresome playground games for some of their most fruitful lessons in safety education. Teaching youngsters, who seemingly are ever on the go, the value of taking time out to perform routine health and safety practices should be promoted and praised at every possible occasion. Drinking fountains are especially hazardous to primary children. Consequently, rules regarding pushing and shoving when someone is drinking should be enforced, and those whose horseplay causes a classmate to suffer broken front teeth should be punished. Children should also be taught the dangers of running with sharp or pointed articles in their mouths and biting hard objects such as pebbles or cracking nuts with their teeth. Those who have been taught well and have gained an understanding of the relationship between continued thumb sucking or grinding the teeth and malocclusion are most likely to discontinue these appearance-damaging habits.

TEACHING METHODS

There is little doubt that reading materials and the lecture method of instruction have been used excessively in dental health instruction. Reading a pamphlet on how to brush the teeth correctly has little educational value unless this experience motivates the reader to brush his own teeth properly. There are many teaching methods which can be used successfully for helping children gain needed dental health information and motivating positive and healthful behavior. Such methods might well include the following:

Problem Solving

The problem-solving method is especially well suited to dental health education. However, problems which are selected by the teacher and pupil should be of real and vital concern to them, and more than mere busy work. These may well be problems concerning community health, of which dental health is but a part, but they can also be specific ones, such as studying why and how the community should educate its voters to establish water fluoridation for the protection of its citizens.

A sixth-grade class in Florida recently made an intensive study of their community's health problem. The class was divided into committees and each group chose an area for intensive study—dental health, mental health, etc. The pupils interviewed people, did library research, visited clinics and other places in order to collect as much information as possible. Daily committee discussions brought many interesting facts to light. After the class had studied this problem for almost a month, each committee group reported its findings, and the class as a whole came up with some excellent recommendations of ways in which the health of all the people in the community might be improved. Such projects have lasting value, for those children who were so enthusiastically involved in this type of learning experience gained a new outlook on their own city, and they learned to use the problem-solving method successfully and became better-informed future voters and citizens.

Class Discussions

Successful discussions depend largely upon the skill of the leader to get each pupil to contribute and become an active participant in discussions of a selected topic. The interchange of information during such periods should stimulate thinking which should lead to action and to change. Consequently, the pupils who take part

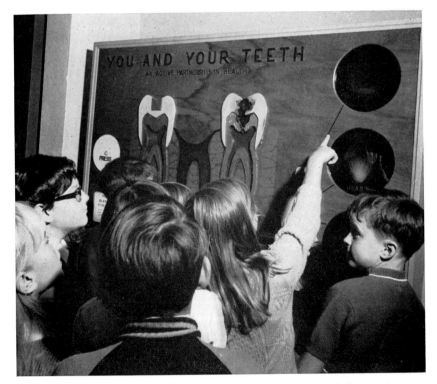

Figure 11-1. Youngsters can learn the many reasons why periodic dental checkups and filling small cavities promptly are important from this exhibit. They learn that early care prevents formation of larger cavities, infection of gums, and loss of teeth. (Courtesy of Dallas Health and Science Museum)

in this type of health education should, through their actions, affect their families and help bring about improved health practices in their own household. A good discussion leader sets the stage for thinking, brings everyone in the group into the discussion without allowing any one person to dominate or dictate group action, helps the group set goals, and finds a feasible solution for the problem at hand. Likewise, such a leader should be skilled in keeping the discussion on the right path and avoiding time-consuming and needless digressions which have no bearing upon the problem at hand. Skill in uniting individual efforts for the attainment of group goals can only be mastered through trial and error. The elementary school should be the place wherein such skills can be developed. Each group member must be an informed participant if the group discussion is to be a learning experience. Topics suitable for class discussions in dental health might well include the following:

1. How serious is the problem of tooth decay and improper dental care in our school? How can we help this problem?
2. Discuss how to prepare young children for the periodic school dental examination.
3. The relationship between good teeth and good health.
4. The harmful effects of food containing sugars.
5. The food habits and dental problems of the peoples in the countries studied about in social science.
6. The cost of early dental treatment versus neglect.
7. Changing concepts in dental health procedures.

Guidance

Often guidance opportunities are individual in nature and involve working directly or indirectly with adults, as well as with pupils, Although most parents want the best for their children, there are many who do not know how to go about getting it; there are some too, unfortunately, who simply do not care. It is then the task of the school administrator and school health authorities to reach these few adults in order to convince them of the value of obtaining corrections of defects. Sometimes this becomes the task of the teacher, or she may be asked to work in cooperation with the school nurse to help reach the parents. In such cases, informal home visits can sometimes accomplish more than having the parents come to the school, although this often has advantages as well. Regardless of where the conference is held or which school representative is involved, it is vitally important that rapport be established and a feeling of mutual concern for the child in question be present. The counselor or teacher should inform the parents of the findings of the school dental inspection, help them understand what these mean, and explain to them why the defects should be corrected. Suggestions of sources of care unknown to them will often prove helpful. Through encouragement, patience, and good guidance, the cooperation of these difficult-to-reach parents can often be gained and, in turn, the child concerned is aided. Teachers, then, should often do more than "just teach children."

Individual and group guidance can also be used effectively to help children find solutions to their own health problems, whether these be uncared-for and dirty teeth or halitosis. Many problems revolving around oral hygiene are delicate and require skillful handling. Since children are often unknowingly cruel in their frankness, the teacher should guide class discussion periods if this is the approach she thinks best to use in any particular situation. In some cases it is wiser to talk over with the class problems which might be delicate or embarrassing, thus controlling what is said.

Drills

Drills can be used effectively for teaching primary children how and when to brush their teeth. Some schools have a tooth-brushing time after lunch, and the children are taught the importance of brushing the teeth within five minutes after eating. Vocabulary drills can also assist these children in learning the meaning of all new words introduced in a dental health unit. No kind of drill can be effective, however, if the children taking part in such an experience merely go through meaningless, routinized motions which have no value to them. Movement does not always mean progress, whether in life or in learning.

Field Trips

Children can learn best many things about dental health from direct experiences. Ideal places to visit in the community include a dentist's office, a firm that specializes in the making or repair of dentures, or a local health museum. The teacher can prepare the group for such trips by drawing from them a list of specific things they want to learn while there, and the purpose of their visit. Likewise, she should ask leading questions of the host in the place visited, for this will, in turn, encourage the pupils to ask also about specific things they want to know. Upon returning to the classroom, she should discuss the trip with the group and have a pupil write on the chalkboard the specific things the class has learned from this experience, for the summary will cause important items to remain in the memory for a longer time. Frequently, trips to such places as a bakery, ice cream or milk pasteurization plant, or farmers' market can teach the youngsters about food, as well as provide the instructor with an opportunity to review or reemphasize facts concerning the relationship between a well-balanced diet and the prevention of dental decay.

Role Playing

Role playing can be an especially valuable method of teaching primary pupils facts and shaping proper attitudes towards dental experiences. They will both enjoy and profit from dramatizing "going to the dentist," "buying a toothbrush and toothpaste," or "how the dentist cleans our teeth." Such experiences will prove to be far more valuable than taking part in professionally written plays, for children find their own skits, which express their own knowledge and experience, far more interesting. Youth needs opportunities to gain legitimate recognition, such as taking part in many kinds of positive learning experiences in their own classroom, or being in an all-school assembly program. Such activities also give them added opportunities to express themselves. In one school recently, a group of first-graders made up their own skit which revolved around using a giant toothbrush. They chose certain of their classmates to act out the story their class made up, and after it was all over, they talked about this experience many times throughout the year. Role playing can also be used to demonstrate the importance of brushing after meals, good dental habits, balanced diets, the work of each type of tooth, safety in play, or other related topics. These little dramatizations and skits can also be used to show visiting parents what their youngsters are learning in school. Following the class presentations, a pupil, the school dental hygienist, the teacher, or the health coordinator might well explain the school dental health program in order to enlist the parents' cooperation. On such occasions, pupils can also prepare simple instruction sheets on the techniques of proper toothbrushing and a list of the food needed daily to build and maintain a strong, healthy body and teeth. Such activities can do more than entertain adults, for they can be especially fruitful in getting the message across to parents that their help is needed in providing good home care for those in their family, as well as for obtaining needed dental treatment for all children.

Surveys

More suitable for the upper elementary grades, the best surveys are those which are part of the child's own world, such as a study made in his own class, school, home, or block, to find out facts such as how many have missing teeth, brush their teeth three times daily, etc. When all these data have been collected, the pupil or committee involved should draw conclusions from the findings, as well as determine how the problem can be remedied or eliminated. The important thing for the teacher who is guiding pupils in such projects to remember is to determine what can be done with the knowledge gained from making such a survey, as well as helping each pupil see the relationship between what he discovers and his own life and well-being.

INSTRUCTIONAL MATERIALS

Audio-visual materials can help pupils learn faster, more, and retain information longer, but only when properly used. They are not meant to take the place of the teacher, but instead can add to her effectiveness. If the viewer of such materials becomes merely a spectator, nothing of educational value can result. The formation of a critical attitude, the development of proper habits of thinking and action, an increased vocabulary and better understanding of words, and other enriching educational results can accrue from the proper use of any or all of the following supplementary teaching aids.

Feltboards and Chalkboards

Feltboards and chalkboards should be used mainly to show symbols, words, numbers, and charts. All materials displayed should be neat and legible. Script writing should be used in the upper grades, and manuscript writing for the primary children. The pegboard, a variation of the feltboard, is best for showing three-dimensional materials; these can be obtained from educational supply houses at a nominal cost. Like the feltboard, it should be used during class discussions or in simplified "lectures" to illustrate important facts or points. The best flannelboards or feltboards are portable and lightweight. Such boards can be easily made by stretching and nailing flannel or felt over a large square of heavy cardboard or plywood. A piece of similar material or a rough grade of sandpaper should be placed on the back of pictures which are to be put on the board as the speaker tells the class a story involving illustrated objects or pictures. Children will delight in making up their own stories about animated characters such as a tooth, brush, or types of food, and making their own feltboard illustrations to use as they share various kinds of health education information with their classmates. Games involving choosing a balanced lunch or snack, word games, sentence completion, and

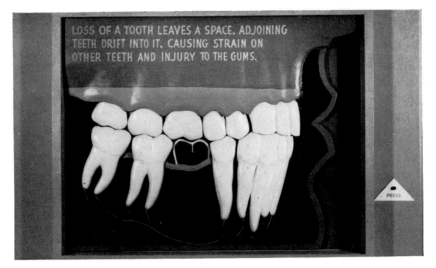

Figure 11-2. Visual aids can help children learn quickly and effectively. This exhibit shows teeth slowly move into the gap left by a missing tooth when the button is pressed. (Courtesy of Dallas Health and Science Museum)

word drills can all be used by a creative leader in all areas of health teaching. A whole "library" of feltboard dental educational materials can be made by the pupils, used, and then stored away for later use.

Models and Specimens

Models and specimens, available from local dentists, the American Dental Association, and toothpaste companies, can help enrich dental health education. These are ideal for showing the parts of the tooth, how the teeth fit into the gums, and the kinds of teeth, for such visual materials can help children gain in increased understanding of what they are studying about teeth. A class, through assigned committee projects, can also make their own models out of clay, papier-mâché, or other materials. Such created objects can range from a set of teeth, a single tooth, and the parts of a tooth, to a giant toothbrush and tube of toothpaste. Since these materials often exaggerate size, care must be taken in using them with primary pupils, so that the children know that the large things they are seeing and touching are like the "little" things in their own mouths or environment.

Bulletin Boards and Posters

Although many health agencies and commercial firms have an abundance of free posters which are available for educational purposes, those which children make themselves become more meaningful to them. The best posters and bulletin-board materials are those which concentrate upon a positive idea, thought, or message, are colorful, and motivate the viewer to do or reflect upon something. Suggested posters which the children might make in connection with a unit on dental health are:

1. Pictures of various teeth, or tooth decay germs.
2. How to have an attractive smile.
3. How to brush the teeth properly.
4. Why we should see our dentist regularly.
5. The different teeth and their functions.
6. Name and parts of a tooth.
7. The role that chewing plays in digestion.
8. How decay spreads from the enamel to the pulp of a tooth.
9. The best kind of toothbrush to buy and how to care for it properly.
10. The value of an x-ray examination.
11. Safety in play as a means of avoiding broken teeth.
12. Safety at the drinking fountain.
13. The relationship of good teeth to good health.
14. How to avoid malocclusion; how it can be corrected.
15. Snack foods which are good for teeth.
16. What sweets do to the teeth; those which cause the most damage.
17. The dentist as a friend.

Although bulletin boards can be one of the most effective means of visual education, they too should be used with care. They can be an excellent way, however, of informing pupils about proper tooth care, increasing interest in this activity, as well as the latest news in the field of oral hygiene. Here again, the best boards are those which are planned and arranged by the pupils themselves. This can be done by committees, or by several interested individuals guided by the teacher. The boards can also be used to advise pupils when the school dental examination will be given, remind them of the necessity of regular dental care given by their own family dentist, or even contain the name of an honor roll of pupils who had seen their dentist twice a year, or of those in a class or grade who have not had a single cavity. Such techniques often serve as strong motivational forces.

Radio and Television

Programs used in relationship with dental health are of two types: (1) those which are purely informative, and (2) those which have been prepared and presented by the learners themselves. The former is a one-way type of communication, and the latter, two-way, and therefore of richer educational value. Increasingly schools are installing public-address systems. These can be used for spot announcements and brief presentations on a wide variety of health topics including dental health, or for a solid week of concentrated effort in any one area. Dental Health Week in February would be an ideal time for such brief daily programs.

In the upper elementary grades stress can be placed upon consumer education, and children taught to purchase dentifrices wisely. Each child could be assigned to listen to and report on toothpaste advertising claims, and the class as a whole determine the differences between true and false advertising. Such projects might well be a part of a larger unit based upon the problem of self-medication and health protective measures, or they can be used in a single unit on dental health.

Mock or real radio and television broadcasts, whether these be pupil-created plays or panel discussions, might well cover informative program materials which all enable the listeners and viewers to learn how to maintain and retain their own teeth throughout life.

Photographs and Cartoons

Effective as a means of motivating interest and action for good dental health, photographs are especially well suited for educational use with older children. These can be photographs of the pupils themselves, showing each child at various stages of his development in each grade in the elementary school. Pictures showing malocclusion, taken from books and shown on the opaque projector, and the stages and measures used for its correction are especially helpful in teaching youngsters about the damages which can be done to the formation of teeth, mouth, and face by bad habits.

Cartoons appeal more to younger pupils. Those which show animated figures such as "Mr. Germ" or a talking carrot, however, should be used with caution, for often the children will merely be entertained by the antics of these characters, and learn little from watching such films unless the teacher draws "meaning" out of the pictures and helps them understand it. Commercially sponsored cartoon programs which appear regularly on television can also be utilized for dental health education. These may be watched by the class at school, in their own homes, or at a neighborhood recreation center after school, and discussed by the group later. Needless to say, the best use of cartoons can be made in the classroom, for the discussion which follows the showing can then best be guided and summarized by the class and teacher.

DESIRABLE OUTCOMES

If the materials presented in dental health education have been effective, the following desirable outcomes should result in the areas of knowledge, attitudes, and practices:

In the primary grades, the pupils will:

1. Know that there are different kinds of teeth.
2. Become alerted to what happens when they have unhealthy teeth.
3. Realize the importance of having and keeping sound teeth.
4. Develop a strong desire to maintain mouth cleanliness.
5. Understand the relationship between eating a balanced diet and having good teeth.
6. Be prepared for and get periodic dental examinations.
7. Take good care of their own teeth, have their own toothbrush, know how to use it properly, and to keep it hanging separately in a holder and dry.
8. Know that they have twenty baby teeth (ten above, like their ten fingers, and ten below, like their ten toes) and that the new teeth which appeared around the age of six are permanent and will last a lifetime, if cared for properly.
9. Know that "grown-up teeth" are behind baby ones and that if a baby tooth becomes loose it will not hurt much to pull it out.
10. Be aware that foods eaten when they have baby teeth and the good care taken of these will help make permanent teeth stronger and better.
11. Know that little, unfilled cavities will become bigger and cause pain.
12. Recognize that the dentist is a friend who can help make one's teeth last longer.
13. Avoid thumb sucking or other harmful habits which will cause the teeth to protrude or be crooked.
14. Know the danger of biting hard objects or cracking nuts with the teeth.
15. Become aware of the importance of brushing the teeth within five minutes after eating.

16. Eat apples, carrots, bread crusts, and other foods which require lots of chewing.
17. Guard against having or causing accidents which will break or injure the teeth, especially when drinking from a water fountain.
18. Make their own dental appointment or remind their parents to do so by the end of the third grade.

In the upper elementary grades, the pupils will:

1. Take good care of their teeth.
2. Know that human beings have two sets of teeth in a lifetime.
3. Know the names and functions of permanent teeth.
4. Be aware of the importance of and eat a balanced diet daily.
5. Know that major factors in causing dental decay are improper care of the teeth and the consumption of sugar or other sweets.
6. Be aware that dental decay is more prevalent in the preadolescent and adolescent years than during any other time in life.
7. Know the diseases of the mouth and gums and how to prevent them.
8. Be aware of the causes and treatmeut for malocclusion, and that one with malformed teeth should consult an orthodontist.
9. Carefully avoid accidents while playing active sports and games or when drinking from water fountains.
10. Understand the use of fluoridation in preventing tooth decay.
11. Know that by the age of 12 or 13 they should have 28 permanent teeth and will get 4 wisdom teeth between the ages of 16 and 25.
12. Know that teeth have different functions—that incisors cut, cuspids tear, and molars grind.
13. Be able to name the parts of a tooth.
14. Understand the role teeth and chewing play in digestion.
15. Be aware that a sound tooth is a well-fed tooth and know that gums can be kept healthy through diet.
16. Know that sweets produce tooth decay and that mouth bacteria turn sugar into acids which destroy enamel.
17. Be able to illustrate and describe how tooth decay spreads from the enamel to the pulp of a tooth.
18. Know the importance of and follow correct tooth-brushing practices and be aware that teeth should be brushed soon after eating.
19. Know the best kind of toothbrush and how to care for it properly.
20. Go to the dentist regularly.
21. Take pride in the appearance of their teeth and of themselves.
22. Be aware of the value of an x-ray examination given by a dentist in discovering between-the-teeth cavities and abscesses at the root of the tooth.

SUGGESTED TEACHING UNITS

Found below are suggested teaching units, lesson plans, and other instructional suggestions for teaching dental health to children grades K to 6:

Kindergarten

Approach

To increase the knowledge and understanding about:
1. The role of the dentist, and reduce any fears about visiting him.
2. The proper way to brush teeth.
3. Knowing that primary teeth will fall out and be replaced by permanent ones, and that everyone is different when losing his/her teeth.

Group Activities
1. Have a bunny party with fresh fruit or vegetables as refreshments and help children realize these are better for them than soft drinks or candy as refereshments.
2. Read *One Morning in Maine* (see student references).
3. Have children count their teeth.
4. Demonstrate and practice correct brushing techniques. Also demonstrate swish and swallow techniques to use if you cannot brush your teeth.
5. Play guessing games about teeth such as, "What is white, comes out of a tube, and you should use to brush your teeth?"

Individual Activities
1. Cut out smiling pictures, and paste them on paper.
2. Cut out pictures of animals whose teeth are showing.
3. Help each child make his own dental chart showing that he brushes his teeth three times daily.

Related Activities
1. Math
   a. Counting teeth, learning time concept of brushing three minutes by using hour glass or big clock.
2. Physical Education
   a. Tag games with "It" being tooth decay who is chasing healthy teeth. Home base is the dentist's office.
3. Drama
   a. Role play a child brushing teeth, going to dentist, eating correctly.
4. Art
   a. Draw teeth. Make Jack-O-Lanterns without some teeth around Halloween. Make papier-mâché teeth. Make "smile" pins with teeth showing.

Grade 1

Approach
1. Promote good dental health practices (including care and prevention by child and professionals).
2. Increase knowledge and understanding about:
   a. When and how to brush the teeth.
   b. Loss of primary teeth and appearance of first 6-year molars.
   c. Why people visit the dentist.
3. Help children learn that teeth are important for many reasons, such as eating, speech, and appearance.
4. Daily care of teeth is necessary even if you cannot brush.
5. Learn the fundamental rules of safety that pertain to teeth care.

Group Activities
1. Have the children learn the importance of teeth by trying to eat a piece of apple, celery, or carrot without chewing.
2. Read *Your Wonderful Teeth* (see student references) and discuss it in relationship to dental health.
3. Have class eat a cracker to feel the food coating, then eat raw fruit and feel cleaner teeth.
4. Show how primitive people used twigs to clean their teeth.
5. Discuss the importance of primary teeth, although they are eventually lost.
6. Give a lesson on proper brushing; use residue food detecting tablet to show food is still on teeth (available at most dentists).
7. Make a list of the improper objects in the mouth, such as hard objects, cracking nuts, etc.

8. Discuss how the cartoon character Bugs Bunny takes care of his teeth.
9. Have children look at and count their teeth as they look into small pocket mirrors.
10. Play riddle games such as, "You use this to clean your teeth," "You can buy it at a store," "It is a brush," "Can you show us how you would use it?"
11. Talk with the children about fears they may have going to a dentist.
12. Have a dentist or school nurse visit the classroom to discuss why a dentist is a good health helper.
13. Give out free toothbrushes and sample toothpaste and have the whole class brush their teeth proeprly.

Individual Activities
1. Have each child make his own dental chart to be kept at school so children can mark if they brushed or swished and swallowed after eating lunch at school.
2. Make dental chart for home use to record dental habits.
3. Encourage children to bring to class any animal teeth they may have in a collection or pictures of them.
4. Make a class mural notebook of cut-outs from magazines of toothpastes, brushes, and other aspects of dental care.

Related Activities
1. Music
   a. Make up songs about food, teeth, and smiling and put them to popular tunes.
   b. Sing together, "All I Want for Christmas Is My Two Front Teeth."
2. Drama
   a. Role play dentist and patient in the chair.

Grade 2

Approach
General Objective: To promote good dental health practices (including care and prevention by child and professionals).
1. To increase knowledge and understanding about:
   a. Proper brushing, time, technique
   b. Services dentists and others render to keep teeth healthy
2. To learn the different shapes of the teeth and understand what function they serve, some for biting, some for chewing, etc.
3. To understand that the food we eat affects our teeth.
4. To increase knowledge and practice of good safety habits which will preclude damage to teeth through accidents, such as being careful what you bite, standing far away from a batter, etc.
5. To learn that permanent teeth are already growing in jaw.
6. To understand that teeth are important for many reasons, such as appearances, speech, and eating.

Group Activities
1. Repeat proper brushing techniques, stress again the value of the swish-and-swallow routine.
2. Have each child demonstrate correct brushing techniques.
3. Have children bring pictures of smiling people to class. After discussion of how important teeth are for each person, have children black out some teeth in the smile to note the change. Use caution with this activity as some children may be sensitive about their own loss of teeth.
4. Assign students to read about animals, such as a dog, horse, etc., and for what purpose their teeth were designed.

Individual Activities
1. Have all draw all teeth in their mouths and have each child cross out the ones that are missing.

2. Continue to add smiling people to notebook started in Grade 1.
3. Let children report on snacks they bring to school that are good for their teeth.
4. Set up classroom display of toothbrushes, toothpaste, etc.
5. Discuss why babies have no teeth, and about old people who do not have teeth. Talk about false teeth.

Related Activities
1. Art
   a. Make class mural on foods or a visit to the dentist's office.
2. Drama
   a. Role playing about experiences.
   b. Have drama of sugar or candy attacking a tooth.
   c. Make puppets and perform play on dental health.
   d. Use words like dentist, cavity, decay, primary, etc., in story about yourself.
3. Social Science
   a. Make class project of discouraging candy and drink machines in school and consult with school dietitian to see that good foods are served for dessert.
   b. Study mouth and tooth shapes of animals (such as a tiger or squirrel) to show how they are different.
4. Science
   a. Have an experiment to show the effects of acid on calcium, using an eggshell.
   b. Show the effects of soft drinks on teeth by leaving a coin overnight in a glass of cola.
   c. Show effects of bacteria on an apple with broken skin, note discoloration.
   d. Make toothpaste out of soda, salt, water, and oil of peppermint. Discuss the cost of this in relationship to toothpaste.

Grade 3

Objectives
At the third-grade level the children need to learn the proper care of their primary teeth, the approximate timetable for these teeth to be shed, and the numbers, purpose, and kinds of teeth in their mouths. Methods of cavity prevention should be discussed. Stress the importance of tooth brushing and going to the dentist regularly.

Basic Concepts
1. What are the names of your teeth?
   a. Central incisor
   b. Lateral incisor
   c. Cuspid
   d. First molar
   e. Second molar
2. Why are our primary teeth important?
   a. For talking
   b. For chewing
   c. As guides for permanent teeth
3. What can be done if the primary teeth are lost too early? The dentist many times can replace the tooth successfully if the child comes in directly after the accident.
4. The parts of the teeth and their purposes are important.
   a. Crown, gums, roots, etc.
   b. The incisors and cuspids cut and tear food. They each have only one root.
   c. The molars grind food. They have two roots.
   d. Roots of primary teeth dissolve and in this way they are shed easily.

5. Preventing cavities is important in the maintenance of healthy teeth.
   a. Brush after each meal, or swish water around in your mouth.
   b. Visit your dentist regularly.
   c. Cut down on sweet foods.
   d. Have fluoride treatments regularly.
6. Discuss having teeth filled and cared for by the dentist.
7. Discuss foods for building teeth.

Correlation With Other Studies
1. Math
   a. Add and subtract, using teeth as an example.
   b. Count the number of teeth in your mouth.
   c. Add the number of your teeth or that of the person's on your left and right.
2. English
   a. Vocabulary, spelling bee, simple stories.
   b. Newspaper clippings on dentistry or accidents which result in tooth loss.
3. Drama and Art
   a. Pretend you are a tooth. Tell a story of what you do and how your owner treats you.
   b. Paint or draw pictures of smiles and what each child thinks his teeth look like.
   c. Posters made with paper cut-outs or crayons.
   d. Finger paint smiles and frowns to learn the difference in relationship to being friendly.

Group Activities
1. Discuss how it would be to have no teeth at all.
2. Look at and discuss the teeth mold on the science table.
3. Write a letter to the American Dental Association asking for the name of a good dentist in St. Louis, where you are moving to with your family.
4. Review the parts of the tooth and what the parts do.
5. Look at the side view of the primary teeth with the permanent teeth shown partly formed in the jaw bone under the primary teeth.
6. Why do some teeth grow straight and some crooked? Discuss.
7. What are space maintainers or other devices? Why do only some children have them?
8. What do dentists do? In what ways do they help us?
9. Show some x-rays of teeth to show relationship of primary to secondary teeth.

Individual Activities
1. Get complimentary toothbrushes for the whole class; give personal instruction to each child on tooth brushing.
2. What size food is easiest to swallow? Try different types of foods, carrots, crackers, etc.
3. Notice the importance of teeth in our daily lives. Write or tell about experiences with your teeth.
4. Draw pictures of your teeth without using a model to copy.

Audio-Visual Aids
"Dentist in the Classroom." American Dental Association.
"Dental Health; How and Why." Coronet Films.
"Healthy Teeth." Aims Instructional Media Services.
"Learning to Brush." American Dental Association.
Model: The Giant Tooth. Ideal School Supply.

Pupil References

Burchheimer, Naomi: *Let's Go To a Dentist.* New York: G. P. Putnam's Sons.

Greene, Carla: *I Want To Be a Dentist.* Children's Press.

Schloat, B. Warren, Jr.: *Your Wonderful Teeth.*

Teacher's References

Sandell, Perry: *Teaching Dental Health to Elementary Children.* Washington, D.C.: AAHPER & NEA.

Richmond, Julius: *Health and Growth.* Glenview, Ill.: Scott, Foresman & Co., 1971.

Health in the Elementary School. Los Angeles: Los Angeles School District Pub. Sec-201, 1959.

Grade 4

Objectives

The fourth grader should be given a more detailed view of the permanent teeth; their shapes, tissues, and purposes. The importance and purpose of dental visits should be discussed with the class in a relaxed but informative atmosphere. Help the child be at ease with his new knowledge of his teeth. Discuss further methods of tooth decay prevention.

Basic Concepts

1. Review the parts of the teeth.
2. The teeth are made of four kinds of tissue:
   a. Enamel
   b. Dentin
   c. Pulp
   d. Cementum periodontal membrane
3. Review the permanent teeth, including the second and third molars.
4. From where did the names of our teeth come?
5. When do our permanent molars come in?
   a. First molars at 6 or 7 years.
   b. Second molars at 12 or 13 years.
   c. Third molars at 17 to 21 years.
6. Our teeth are important in many ways:
   a. Talking
   b. Chewing
   c. Looking healthy and happy
7. Discuss bacteria, tooth decay, and its resultant drilling and filling the teeth.
   a. Bacteria breaks down enamel.
   b. Decay can spread from the enamel to lower layers of the teeth.
   c. When this happens the tartar and bacteria must be removed from the tooth and a filling is put in to take its place.
8. New discoveries in dental health:
   a. Fluoride
   b. The fluorometer, which detects cavities in their earliest stage.

Correlation With Other Subjects

1. Math
   a. Count the number of teeth of each kind for the entire class.
   b. Count the number of times you chew each bite of food. Which foods do you chew more than others?
   c. Count your teeth, remembering that filled teeth do count. How many are missing?
   d. Make a study of your class to find out how many have missing teeth, where they are located, and how many have cavities. Show your results in a graph and also in a pie graph.

2. English and Reading
   a. Read books from the list of pupil references.
   b. Build vocabulary by adding new words and having spelling bees.
   c. Make up stories about missing teeth, a gold tooth, or false teeth.
3. Drama and Art
   a. Imitate the tooth decay commercials.
   b. Role play being teeth, some foods that attract germs, and a dentist coming to the rescue.
   c. Make posters, pictures, and murals on dental health.
4. Science
   a. Discuss how milk helps teeth and bones.
   b. Have a dentist discuss braces and show how they can help a person.
   c. Use large models of teeth for learning experiences.
   d. Bring to class an animal's teeth, and have your classmates guess from which animal they came.

Group Activities
1. Show pictures of a dentist filling cavities and discuss it.
2. Have tooth test. Chew tablets containing sodium fluoride which turns food particles left on the teeth red.
3. Discuss orthodontia.
4. Talk about the dentist and his work, his tools and how he helps you.
5. Show the chart showing tooth decay and where the filling goes.
6. Discuss the astronauts; do they use toothpaste as we do? (They use powdered paste.)
7. Which food feels best when eating? Discuss.
8. Can tooth problems cause us to speak less clearly? If so, why?
9. Have a debate on whether fluoride should be put in the city water.

Individual Activities
1. Let the children explore and compare their teeth with the model.
2. Draw posters for the Dental Health Week contest.
3. Brush teeth after lunch on your own. Mark the chart.
4. Make a creative daily brushing chart. If no toothbrush, swishing will do.
5. Discuss the reasons for fluoride in the water.

Pupil References for Grades 5 and 6
Lapp, Carolyn: *Dentists' Tools.* Lerner, 1966
Project Teeth: Dental Health and Classroom Science (Film). American Dental Association.
Healthy Teeth, Happy Smile. Wexler, Distributed by Henk Newenhouse.
Showers, Paula: *How Many Teeth.* Crowell, 1969.

Materials for the Teacher
Giant Tooth. A plastic model made to show the inside structure of a molar tooth. Model Number S 230 is available from The Ideal School Supply Company, 11000 S. Lavergne Avenue, Oak Lawn, Illinois 60453. Cost is about $12.00
Also write to The American Dental Association for lists of available posters, charts, etc. Address: 211 E. Chicago, Illinois 60611.

Teacher's References
Health in the Elementary School. Los Angeles: Los Angeles Schools, Division of Instructional Services, Pub. #201, 1959.
Cornacchia, H. J. and Staton, W. M.: *Health and Growth 4.* Glenview, Ill.: Scott, Foresman & Co., 1971.
Richmond, Julius: *Health in the Elementary School.* St. Louis: C. V. Mosby Co., 1970.
Willgoose, Carl: *Health in the Elementary School.* 4th ed., Philadelphia: W. B. Saunders Co., 1974.

CHAPTER 12

body growth, structure, and function

A functional health education program aids each pupil to gain a clear understanding of and real appreciation for his own body, as well as to assist him to develop the knowledge and desire for taking good care of it throughout life. All materials included in this area should be directed toward learning the best ways to protect oneself and others from hazards and disease. In the primary grades a minimum amount of time should be spent in studying the names of various parts of human anatomy, for such facts as the parts of the teeth or names of bones mean little, if anything, to a child. Rather, emphasis should be placed upon developing good health habits which will ensure the protection of eyes, ears, and all other body parts as well as ways to increase their functional use. In the upper elementary grades, pupils should see their body as a whole, and know the relationship that exists between what they do and how they look, act, or feel. It is essential that each youngster, regardless of which school grade he is in, gain a lasting appreciation for the wonder, beauty, and miracle of his own life and the body in which it is housed. A visit to a health museum to see a transparent man or woman, or the use of models, or pictures of the entire human body in the classroom will be of great value in helping children see the unity of man—a masterpiece created by God. As the child progresses in school, he should be taught simple facts of the physiology and anatomy of the many organs and structure of the body. However, learning the scientific name of any body part is an educational waste if the child cannot or does not apply what he has learned. Teachers working in this area should primarily be concerned with helping children live healthfully.

SUGGESTED GRADED TOPICS

Units of study in this area might well include noncommunicable and contagious diseases, good grooming, and the care of the senses, as well as the structure and function of the various parts of the body. Suggested graded topics include the following:

GRADE 1

1. Keeping clean.
2. How to avoid colds and sickness.
3. Having good teeth.
4. How to have good posture.
5. Suitable clothing.
6. Play, rest, and sleep.
7. How we grow.
8. Why we should, and how we can, avoid accidents.

GRADE 2

1. Reasons for using personal toilet articles.
2. How to drink from the fountain without touching it; how not to spread germs at home and school.
3. Staying home when we are sick.
4. The body as a machine.
5. Protecting ourselves from accidents.
6. Common contagious diseases of children.
7. Exercise, nutrition, and sleep in relationship to growth.

GRADE 3

1. The framework of the body.
2. Care of the eyes, ears, and nose.
3. The skin and its care.
4. The systems of the body.
5. How disease germs get into the body.
6. Periodic health examinations.
7. Heart and circulation.
8. Dental health.

GRADE 4

1. Mechanics of movement.
2. Body care and grooming.
3. The value and need for good health habits in relationship to growth.
4. Effects of bacteria and viruses.
5. Diseases of the respiratory and digestive systems.
6. How the body protects and heals itself.
7. The effect of accidents and illness.
8. Structure and care of teeth.
9. The skeletal system.

GRADE 5

1. Our senses and how they work.
2. The brain and mental hygiene.
3. Skin, hair, nails, and good grooming.
4. Bones and muscles.
5. How the stomach works; the digestion of food.
6. Safeguarding the body at work and play.
7. Immunization.
8. Disease carriers and communicable diseases.

GRADE 6

1. The heart and lungs, their structure, function, and care.
2. The effects of alcohol, smoking, and drugs upon the body.
3. How we use food.

4. Problems of growing up.
5. The glands and growth.
6. Feet and their care.
7. How the body protects and heals itself.
8. The noncommunicable diseases of diabetes, heart disease, cancer, rheumatic fever.

CURRICULUM PLACEMENT

Instruction in the structure, care, and function of the human body should be included in the curriculum for every grade level from the first through high school. There are numerous ways which this may be done, and often these are through the means of a separate health and safety program, or integrating and correlating this subject with science, home economics, or physical education. However, there are other subject areas which can be used most successfully for correlating and integrating these health education foundational materials.

Social Sciences

The social sciences provide opportunities for children to see the relationship between good health and good living throughout the entire history of mankind. Older pupils will profit from finding out about a number of health devices, such as how eyeglasses have changed from those first bifocals invented by Benjamin Franklin to modern contact lenses or from learning of the serious health problems among primitive peoples in contrast to our own. Special reports can be given when the class is studying about wars and determining whether or not the advancement of scientific knowledge is a positive result of such struggles, or on how seeing-eye dogs are trained and how dogs are used in warfare or in apprehending criminals. They can also profit from learning how blind people read Braille and by listening to talking books in order to increase their understanding of the many problems sightless people have. Units on good grooming and boy-and-girl relationships will help older children gain needed social and physical skills which may have lasting effects upon them as high school and college students and adult members of society. The older pupils will also profit from learning about some of the famous historical medical experiments, such as that conducted by Dr. William Beaumont, who was the first person to look into the stomach of a living person, as well as becoming acquainted with medicine, nursing, or related fields as a profession. Heart disease and cancer might well be discussed from both social and economic aspects, and children be taught ways to protect themselves from these dreaded illnesses. Actually, the possibilities for intermeshing this phase of health education with the social sciences are as abundant as an alert and skilled teacher can make them.

Science

Children can become fascinated by learning more about themselves and what makes them the way they are. The class group on every grade level need not be kept together with all pupils required to study the same things, for some will be naturally more eager and interested to learn more scientific details than others. This is especially true of those even in the elementary grades who have decided that they want to become nurses, doctors, or scientists. Many dreaming of becoming spacemen can develop great interest in the physical hazards and effects of outer space upon the body, or the physical training program of the astronauts. In this scientific age, children tend to be more science-minded than their parents were and often, consequently, are all the more eager to learn many of the more scientific facts about human beings.

Conducting simple experiments and learning how to use such equipment as a microscope, stethoscope, dental mirror, height and weight scales, etc., are exciting experiences for growing children and should be a part of the skills taught in this area. Simple scientific experiments which can also help the pupils learn many new fascinating things about the body and how it works are:

1. Blindfolded, taste pieces of raw onion, apple, and potato in order to learn how the senses of taste and sight work together.
2. Blow through two sheets of thin paper to discover how quickly the ears pick up vibrating sounds.
3. Use an ordinary fork or a tuning fork. Observe how sound travels.
4. Strike a spoon against several glasses filled with various amounts of water. Note that sound has musical qualities.
5. Taste a fresh lemon, a piece of candy, and sugar in that order, then taste the lemon again. Note how the sense of taste is deceiving, for on the second taste the lemon seems sourer than before.
6. Blindfolded, touch a wide variety of objects such as a ball, bowl, etc. Note the connection between the sense of touch and that of sight.
7. Experiment blindfolded with hot and cold objects. Note the quickness with which the hands respond to these two temperatures.
8. Observe a small bird closely. Do birds have ears? If so, where are they?
9. Rub a piece of cleansing tissue over your face. Note that the skin has its own natural oil.
10. Look at a hair pulled out of your own head under a magnifying glass. Find the root and discuss how hair grows and if cutting or shaving it makes it grow faster.
11. Show how perspiration cools the skin as it evaporates by placing a bit of cotton which has been dipped in warm water on your forehead.
12. Examine an uncooked meat bone under a magnifying glass. See its spongy tissue, outer covering, and marrow.
13. Make a stethoscope out of a cardboard mailing tube. Listen to the heartbeat of a classmate through it.
14. Locate and feel the pulse of a classmate at his wrist, in front of the ear, along the jawbone line. Record your finding. Have your partner do vigorous exercise for one minute, such as run in place. Count his pulse again. Have him rest for one minute. Count his pulse rate and compare it to the first reading. Know that if the first and last rates correspond within five counts, your partner is physically fit.
15. Examine blood cells under a microscope.
16. Compare the skin on your hands and face, using a magnifying glass.
17. Make your own fingerprints, using ink and paper. Compare yours with anyone else's in class.
18. Observe a healing cut on your hand under a magnifying glass. Note how the body heals itself.
19. Place milk and four spoonsful of vinegar in a quart jar. Shake it up. Observe what happens to the milk. Discuss how the stomach, enzymes, and digestive juices churn and change food into liquid.
20. Examine unclean food and eating and drinking utensils under a microscope. Experiment with various ways to destroy germs. Review state and local laws for food handlers and restaurant inspection standards which must be met in public dining places.
21. Invite a local druggist to talk to the class about his work and show how pills are made. Have him list things which should be in every first-aid cabinet.

8

The Communicative Arts

Reading, writing, and speaking can be used in this area in the following suggested ways:

1. Read stories, talk about good nutritional habits, and supervise school lunchroom experiences; conduct play activities in the class at regular intervals.
2. Teach new vocabulary words and play quiz games built around them.
3. Divide the class into groups and assign each tasks, including room responsibilities. Discuss the value of work in life, stressing that it is a privilege, not a drudgery, and that everyone must share responsibility for the benefit of the group as well as himself.
4. Bring a book written in Braille to class. Demonstrate how blind people read. Discuss how blindness is caused, how seeing-eye dogs are used, etc. Stress why the eyes must be protected and well cared for at all times.
5. Have the class make a survey and report their findings of sanitary conditions found in the school toilets and public restrooms throughout their city. Discuss in detail local sanitation laws and how they could be better enforced.
6. Have the class bring pictures or tell about handicapped victims. Stress that in one way or another, all human beings are "handicapped." Discuss ways an exceptional person should be treated; how such a person can learn to help himself; great leaders or artistic geniuses who were handicapped, such as Franklin D. Roosevelt or Lord Byron.
7. Study the big muscles of the body by looking closely at charts or book illustrations. Discuss sprains, muscle soreness, and the recommended first-aid treatment for both.
8. Have each pupil keep a record of his activities for each 24-hour period in a week. Look at this report carefully as an adult friend and educator who desires to help each child become an increasingly independent citizen who is "health" educated.
9. Have a committee give a report and demonstrate safety measures taken in sports by showing many kinds of recommended equipment, such as a catcher's mask, float board for a nonswimmer, archery finger tab, football shoulder pads, etc.
10. Have each pupil write a summary of the findings of his yearly physical and dental checkup. Discuss the report with each individually.
11. Listen to several class panel discussions on "Why I Know I Am Growing Up."
12. Play a game "Guess How I Feel" in charade form, with one child having only his back toward the group. Have that child act out being angry, etc., and the class guess which emotion is being acted out according to the position of the spine, head, body. Discuss how posture reveals emotions.
13. Write letters to the American Medical Association asking for free health literature on any subject included in this unit. Use this in an oral or written report given in class.
14. Tell your own version of the life and work of any of the health heroes, such as Dr. Harvey, Dr. Salk, or others. Look into such books as *The Story behind Great Medical Discoveries* by Elizabeth Montgomery (Dodd, Mead) or *How Man Discovered His Body* by Sarah Reidman (International).
15. Write in your own words the story of how food is digested.
16. Make up and write health slogans and rhymes, such as "See Your Dentist Twice a Year" or "When Riding a Bicycle to School/Ride Safely, Don't Be a Fool."
17. Have a speaking contest, choose the best oral talk given on "The Human Body, the Greatest Wonder of Them All."

18. Consult the encyclopedia to gather material for a written report on any topic covered in this unit such as "How the Eyes See," or "A Bone Bank."
19. Invite an admired older boy and girl to talk to the class about the importance of having good health and grooming habits.

Mathematics

Many kinds of learning experiences can be devised which will help pupils gather and apply increased knowledge. Topics might include discovering the costs of medical, accident, and hospital insurance policies; life-expectancy predictions in relationship to obesity or lung cancer; height and weight tables for a variety of ages; advertising costs in relationship to increased sales in food and grooming products; hidden costs in drugs; yearly expenditures for patent medicines; costs for rehabilitating drug addicts or mental patients, etc.; or making graphs of temperature and barometer changes; reading and recording outdoor temperature; learning how to forecast the weather; making weather flags. Care must be taken that the pupils see the relationship of such mathematical problems to themselves and their own well-being. Knowing how much it costs to rehabilitate a mentally ill person is just another fact unless this knowledge motivates the learner to practice good mental hygiene in order to prevent him from becoming emotionally and mentally ill.

Drama and Art

Dramatic and art activities can be used successfully with each age group. Suggested ways for doing so are:

1. Have the group divide up into couples and have each give a demonstration of the many aspects of good grooming, care of the feet, etc.
2. Have the class draw pictures showing the effects of measles, scarlet fever, mumps, and other diseases of the body. Discuss the signs and symptoms of each of these.
3. Study anatomical charts or view models of all parts of the human body. Reproduce models of any body part or system for the class health museum made out of clay, papier-mâché, or plaster of Paris.
4. Make models or other types of visual aids to show how blood circulates; digestion; how the respiratory system functions; parts of the skin, or any other information gained from the library or other assignments. Pool gleaned information with the class.
5. See a film on the harmful effects of tobacco, alcohol, or narcotics upon the body. Assign the class a library reference project on this topic, and have each write a paper or make an illustrated poster or cartoon on his findings.
6. Bring a camera to class. Make a poster to show its similarity to the human eye.
7. Discuss the reasons the school requires immunizations before entrance, and what vaccinations each has had.
8. Make posters illustrating why wet clothing should be changed, how colds are spread through sneezing, etc.
9. Bring pictures of animals to school. Discuss how animals protect themselves; what is rabies; the importance of avoiding strange animals or reporting an animal bite immediately.
10. Visit the zoo and learn how animals are protected from illness. Illustrate by labeled drawings things learned from this experience.
11. Discuss cleanliness in public places. Write a letter to city officials suggesting ways these places can be made more attractive and sanitary.
12. Paint pictures of the activities of city employees who protect community health, such as the trash collector, dog catcher, etc.

13. Visit the city water department or the waste disposal plant. Write a short report or tape record a class discussion on important things learned from this experience. Make a poster on such topics as "Keep Our City Clean."
14. Give a puppet show to show health practices such as getting ready for bed, coming home from school, getting ready to go sledding, etc.
15. Paint or draw and color an illustrated panel showing ways food is handled from its source to the consumer. Explain each step in this process to the group.
16. Plan and make a window display on what the community is doing to protect the health of its citizens.
17. Give a puppet show, playlet, or make a cartoon motion picture on the life of any health hero or a large scale epidemic, such as the Black Plague.
18. Make a water color, oil, or illustrated poster the Red Cross might use for one of its financial drives. Select the five made best and display them in the school lobby.
19. Make a skeletal model of the human body, using cardboard, paste, and string.
20. Carve a human figure out of any kind of wood or soap. Have the class select the best one.

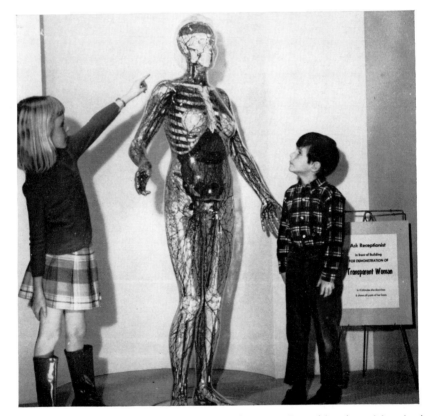

Figure 12-1.   Visi-Belle is a star performer and an experienced hand at giving simple yet complete talks about the wonders of the human body. Various parts of the transparent woman light up as she discusses how her organs and systems function. Field trips to museums are an ideal way for youngsters to learn about health. (Courtesy of Dallas Science and Health Museum)

Physical Education

There are many opportunities for correlating and integrating health instruction and physical education, through both direct and incidental teaching. The conscientious physical educator and athletic coach will capitalize upon moments for health education from situations which arise naturally out of class activity, on the playground, or athletic field. The following are suggested opportunities for relating this area of health education with that of physical education:

1. Emphasizing the relationship between exercise and physical activities to organic vigor and physical fitness.
2. Discussing the opportunities provided by taking part in play for widened social contacts and improved mental health.
3. Showing the carry-over value of activities and stressing the need for some kind of physical activities throughout life.
4. Stress that physical activities provide chances to work out feelings of hostility and aggression in positive ways.
5. Discussing the values of physical activity in modern, sedentary life.
6. Showing how the body recovers from fatigue.
7. Emphasizing the necessity of well-balanced diets for energy and growth.
8. Showing how bones, muscles, and joints work, and helping pupils learn the joy of well-coordinated body movements.
9. Discussing what causes muscle cramps, strains, and tears, and how these should be cared for and can be prevented.
10. Explaining the values of conditioning the body before strenuous activity and teaching basic exercises for doing so.

Safety Education

Pupils can put in practice knowledge gained and shape favorable attitudes toward the value of safety as a means of protecting themselves from injury and avoiding needless and costly accidents. Ways in which the importance of teaching safety can be stressed in this area include:

1. Teaching the proper use of equipment, showing how misuse can bring about injury.
2. Emphasizing common-sense rules and good techniques in and around swimming pools and other bodies of water.
3. Pointing out the reasons for matching competitors for weight, size, and maturity in some activities.
4. Emphasizing safe conduct in shower and locker rooms.
5. Teaching first aid and the recognition of emergency situations.[1]

Guidance and Counseling

Guidance, whether in groups or through individual conferences, can do much to help children find ways to solve their own health problems and answers to questions concerning their ever-changing and fast-developing bodies. Some will need to be referred to the school doctor or specialists within the community because of their own unique problems, such as a too rapid increase in weight or the onset of acute nervousness. Others will need special encouragement and parental help to have remedial defects corrected, such as a crossed eye or protruding teeth.

---

[1] *Health Education*, 5th ed. Washington, D. C., National Education Association and American Medical Association. 1961, p. 256.

Every teacher in the school, through the help of specially trained guidance personnel, should capitalize upon opportunities for integrating health with counseling and guidance, for this is essential if pupils are to be helped and reached as individuals in a large group to solve their own unique health problems. In the elementary school it is imperative that such health guidance and counseling include the parents.

USE OF TEACHING METHODS

Problem Solving

Group problem solving in this area can be done informally by day-by-day activities or by extensive problem units. Grout has reported that in one school there was too much fighting on the playground and too many children were being hurt. These problem incidents were discussed, and the children figured out ways of having just as much fun with less risk.[2]

Problem areas suitable for study in this area can be any aspect of physical, mental, or emotional health, In general these pertain to:

Nutrition and diet	Chronic diseases
Exercise and diet	Growth and development
Rest, relaxation, and sleep	Mental and emotional problems
Physical defects	

Older pupils will be interested in studying not only the problems which occur in their own school in this area, but also in their community and in the world. One group of sixth-graders in a school in Indiana recently became concerned about the fact that, although polio vaccine is available and is a known preventive, relatively few of the school-age children in their state had been inoculated. They determined to discover why this was true and what could be done about the problem. The group began by studying the cause, types, and effects of polio. Next they learned about the development of the Salk vaccine and how it works. One committee studied the polio problem on a worldwide scale, still another made a class-by-class survey first of the pupils in their own school and then in all of their city's schools in order to learn just how many had been protected, another committee interviewed one hundred adults from all walks of life in an attempt to discover how they felt about requiring by law that all school-age children be inoculated as a requirement for entrance and re-entrance to public schools. The class invited a leading pediatrician to talk to them about this subject. They saw three films, *The Magic Touch* (Avis Films), *What Is Disease?* (Institute of Inter-American Affairs), and *The Control of Communicable Disease in Man* (American Public Health Association). After spending two weeks on this problem, the class drew up a list of specific things which could be done in their community to eradicate polio. Through the efforts of their school principal, the class planned and gave a 30-minute televised program on this subject over a local station. The newspaper publicity received from this endeavor, the amount of education each pupil obtained, and pride among the parents for what the children had done did much to increase the appreciation of the citizens in that community for the teacher who had skillfully guided the whole project, as well as for their own school system.

---

[2] Grout, Ruth: *Health Teaching in Schools.* 5th ed. Philadelphia: W. B. Saunders Co., 1968, p. 103.

Every daily newspaper and many periodicals such as *Time, Reader's Digest, Today's Health,* and *National Geographic* contain materials which can be used to motivate pupil interest in any area of health education, including those which revolve around the human body, its structure, care, and protection.

Class Discussions

Discussions which will help the pupils gain better understanding of their bodies might include the following topics and activities:

1. Play several types of quiet games in the classroom often; talk about the value of doing tapering-off activities before bedtime.
2. Teach relaxation exercises to the class, such as playing at being a rag doll, floating like a big log lazily down a quiet stream, etc. Play soft music to the children as they stretch out on the floor and listen to it with their eyes closed. Discuss with them how the heart and other body parts rest.
3. Teach the group a wide variety of large-muscle activities, exercises, and games which require twisting, hanging, crawling, skipping, running, etc. Discuss with the group why they need vigorous exercise every day in order to grow and develop good posture.
4. Conduct vision and hearing tests and encourage the pupils to adjust their own seating arrangements according to the test results. Discuss the value of good sitting posture.
5. Elect or appoint a class health committee or inspector to check washing hands properly, drinking from fountains, or keeping objects out of the mouth. Change membership in these often enough to give each child an opportunity to serve. Discuss how children can prevent illness by being clean.
6. Have an outdoor and indoor clothing fashion show. Talk about the value of dressing properly for all kinds of weather.
7. Discuss why tissues may be safer to use than a handkerchief.
8. Teach and play more advanced quiet games such as "Human Checkers" or "Who Am I?"[3] Discuss the relationship between rest and fatigue and health.
9. View and discuss films about all phases of this unit; see filmstrips about health heroes.[4]
10. Have a playground clean-up period, dividing the group in teams. Discuss the reason for keeping the playground free from trash.
11. Read aloud or listen to Basil Rathbone's recording of Poe's famous short story, "The Masque of the Red Death." Discuss the significance of this story. Make up and tell a similar one about any epidemic which might happen in your local community.
12. Appoint certain pupils each week to change the room thermostat or adjust room temperature and lighting. Discuss how the body adjusts to change.
13. Discuss the future professional plans of each student. Tell the group about the training needed to be a nurse, doctor, or dentist. Help the group see the relationship which exists between success as an elementary pupil and as a professional worker in the medical field in the future.
14. Go on a hike during school time, or as a class group on Saturday. Report on birds, animals, plants, and other things seen. Discuss how animals and birds spread seeds, or destroy insects or pests. Talk about the creatures that spread diseases.

---

[3] For suggestions, see Maryhelen Vannier, *Techniques in Recreation Leadership.* 3rd ed. Philadelphia, Lea & Febiger. (In preparation.)
[4] These are obtainable free of charge from the Education Department of the Metropolitan Life Insurance Company.

15. Divide into groups and discuss ways that sanitation in your school could be improved. Plan and conduct a campaign for doing so. Evaluate the results.
16. Assign each pupil to teach a game to a group of first-graders or any younger children in the neighborhood. Have each give a brief oral report on this experience. Lead a class discussion on the value of older children setting a good example for younger ones by having good health, work, and play habits.

Demonstrations

Useful and beneficial demonstrations to pupils in this area are:

1. Demonstrate good sitting, walking, and moving posture. Use three blocks piled on top of each other to demonstrate body balance; have each child check a partner for good posture as well as look at his own in a large mirror during the day.
2. Demonstrate methods for sterilizing water, eating utensils, surgical instruments, etc.
3. Bring a dog to class and demonstrate the keenness of his hearing ability. Experiment with soundless whistles and other kinds of noises. Have the group observe birds and other creatures after school and report to the group how they hear. Stimulate interest by asking: if a tree crashed in the forest and no one saw it or was within ten miles of it, would there be a noise when it hit the ground? Why or why not?
4. Demonstrate ear, eye, and nose safety and the first aid which could be used to remove a foreign body from each.
5. Demonstrate how fast bacteria multiply in darkness, warmth, and moisture. Write a short summary of your findings.
6. Have pupils bring samples of improperly fitting shoes and socks to class. Demonstrate good foot care; the damage done to the feet by wearing shoes which are too small or large or have run-down heels, or wearing socks with many big holes or darns in them.
7. Conduct a Junior Red Cross First Aid course in class or as an after-school club activity. Demonstrate the latest methods of artificial respiration.
8. Have a handwashing demonstration; teach the necessity of keeping nails clean.
9. Demonstrate how milk is pasteurized; visit a dairy or ice cream plant. Have each child write a brief report on the value of drinking or eating pasteurized dairy products.
10. Demonstrate how the ear hears; play hearing guessing games by having the children close their eyes and identify certain objects dropped or sounds made in the room. Discuss how a hearing aid works. Show an actual hearing aid or pictures of people wearing one.
11. Measure and weigh the pupils periodically. Discuss ways to stimulate growth. Show each child his own growth chart.

Field Trips

Field trips can be especially valuable in helping pupils gain a better understanding of their community as well as themselves. Suggested places to visit include:[5]

1. A visit to an aquarium to observe how fish breathe. Use bellows to demonstrate how the lungs work. Discuss diseases of the lungs; value of fresh air.
2. A tour of the school cafeteria—learn how the dishes are washed, food stored, and waste disposed of.

_____

[5] See also suggested field trips in the chapters on nutrition, dental care, and safety.

3. A visit to a pet shop or an animal hospital. Discuss the value of protective rabies shots or those given for hepatitis or other diseases common to pets.
4. A visit to interview a local physician, public health official, or nurse. Summarize the important things learned from this experience.
5. A visit to a pharmacy to learn how prescriptions are filled, records are kept, etc.
6. A visit to a blood or bone bank to learn how these are stored and used in emergencies.
7. A trip to see the village dump or waste disposal plant. Discuss how diseases are spread.
8. A visit to a housing project and a slum district. Discuss how good housing affects health.

Storytelling

Stories can provide younger children with increased avenues for self-expression, as well as provide the teacher with added insight into their health habits, attitudes, and feelings. Almost any topic can be used for this purpose. The story can be told by the teacher, who should be well aware that children like stories best about real things they do and those characters which express feelings similar to their own. Some of the most revealing ones can be created and told by the children themselves about any of these suggested headings:

Birthdays	A farm
Why I like to play games	My favortie food
My house	How puppies grow
My parents	A broken front tooth
Any fruit or vegetable	Babies
What I want to be	

Role Playing

Also revealing and of high educational value is role playing. Although teachers should not try to be amateur psychiatrists, they can become skilled in understanding what the child is trying to communicate through this type of dramatic activity. This understanding is essential if adults are to have insight into what children say and do and why they are as they are. It is known that children in role playing assign to themselves parts which are an extension or expression of their own problems, and what they do is an indication of what they think and feel. Imitating adults, such as playing at being a nurse, doctor, mother, father, teacher, etc., creates not only better understanding of what these people do but also helps promote a feeling of identification with these adults. Sex differences in role playing are striking, for girls often select roles to play which revolve around being the mother of the house, cooking, and feeding a family, while boys play variations on the one theme of riding or guiding vehicles, whether as a steamboat captain or an outer-space pilot, and rarely choose roles in which they identify with their own father. Although "cops and robbers" is played by most children, such roles are the favorites of children who are most aggressive. The axious and withdrawn child rarely shows aggression in role choice or actions.

The teacher can set up problem situations, and have the children act out their own selected roles in the following suggested ways:

1. Jane made a surprise present for her mother, who was in the hospital.
   The doctor said she was too sick to have visitors.
2. George's mother took him to the store to buy new shoes. The salesman
   helped him get a pair that were just right for a growing boy.
3. Tommy has a cold. He couldn't come to school, but he had a happy,
   restful day in bed.
4. Mary wouldn't eat vegetables for dinner. Her daddy told her why she
   should do so and helped her learn to like them.
5. Jesse never took part in the games the other children played. His teacher
   found out why.
6. Our family has a new baby brother. I can help him be happy and grow.
   My parents told me how.

USE OF INSTRUCTIONAL MATERIALS

Free graphic materials are available in an abundance in the form of posters,
charts, comic strips, and graphs, which can be powerful forces for shaping attitudes
and motivating action among pupils so that they will learn to understand and have
increased respect for their own bodies and know how to take better care of them.
The types and suggested use of these materials include:

Models and Specimens

Models which show the entire systems of the body or any specific part of it, such
as a cutaway model of the eye, can enable pupils to gain a clearer understanding of

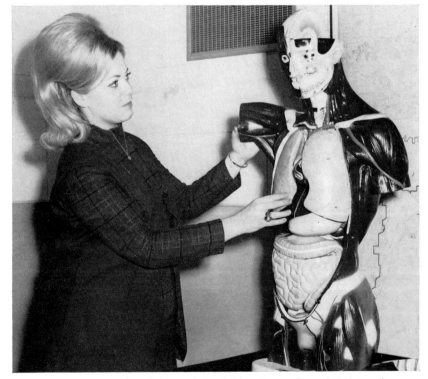

Figure 12-2. The use of models can help children learn about their internal organs.
(Courtesy of Dallas Health and Science Museum)

where each body part is and its function in relationship to other parts, senses, or systems of a human being. Many of these models can be obtained commercially and are relatively inexpensive. Pupils in some schools have made their own successfully from clay, carved soap or wood, papier-mâché, and other materials. Such models can be made of the entire body or almost any part of it including teeth, ears, bones, hands, feet, stomach, heart, etc. Such experiences help create increased pupil interest in and better understanding of materials covered.

Posters

Posters made by the children in this area might cover the following topics:

1. Any communicable disease, its symptoms, cause, and contagious period.
2. Outdoor play and exercise.
3. Cancer, diabetes, hepatitis, and other diseases.
4. The care and function of skin, muscles, teeth, etc.
5. How the body repairs itself.
6. Co-workers in health.
7. How to help yourself grow.
8. Kinds of germs, bacteria, and molds.
9. Harmful effects of tea, coffee, and alcohol.
10. How to protect your heart.

Cartoons

The daily comic strip and other cartoons are especially well suited for helping children realize the difference between positive and negative use of leisure time, how some people face problems concerning their health in a dentist's or doctor's office, hospital, at home, and elsewhere. Younger children will enjoy bringing in their favorite comics to illustrate material studied in this area, such as "Dondi" or "Little Orphan Annie" facing a health problem. The comic strip "Peanuts" is especially well suited for this purpose and can supplement study about how to avoid accidents, staying in bed when you have a cold, and other topics.

Books

Supplementary reading materials can also be used to a good advantage in this area. Older pupils will profit from looking at illustrated materials on the human body found in many kinds of reference works in the school or local public library. They would especially be fascinated by looking closely at the wonderful drawings of the human body in the book, *Man in Structure and Function* by Fritz Kahn (Knopf). This beautiful, two-volume work was written and illustrated by a physician in Germany and should be in every school library. Few other books can come close to it in helping the layman understand how each organ, part, and system of the human body looks and functions. Those who fear that these materials are too advanced for those in upper elementary school should remember that the unchallenged pupil will remain that way, and that our most gifted scholars, who are ready for and can digest a "banquet" of learning, are too often fed a steady diet of pre-digested Pablum.

Suggested books, as well as films, that each class will enjoy and profit from reading or seeing in all grades of the elementary school are listed at the end of this chapter.

Audio-Visual Aids

Films, television, and radio should also be used as supplementary teaching aids in this area.

DESIRABLE OUTCOMES

A well-conducted instructional program on the human body, its structure, function, and care should produce the following desirable outcomes.

In the primary grades, the pupils will:

1. After vision and hearing tests, understand why they should move their chairs closer in order to see or hear better and then do so by themselves.
2. Engage in quiet activities in their own homes before bedtime; rest well at school and know the value of, as well as take part in, several kinds of relaxing activities.
3. Engage in vigorous play with their peers and be aware of the value of doing so, both at home, during leisure, and at school.
4. Be aware of the existing relationship between balanced diets, growth, and good health; eat nutritious meals; be concerned with growing up healthy and strong.
5. Protect others as well as themselves from accidents during spontaneous, unsupervised play.
6. Be well aware of the importance of the uniqueness of their own bodies and desire to take good care of them; realize increasingly that this is their own responsibility.
7. Know the value of and enjoy cleanliness and neatness; wear appropriate clothing.
8. Have good toilet habits; wash hands after play, after going to the bathroom, and before eating.
9. Know the relationship of lighting and seating to posture and good health, and act accordingly.
10. Remove heavy clothing such as snowsuits and boots by themselves and put them in their proper places at home, as well as at school.
11. Go to bed at the proper time according to their age; know the reason one needs lots of sleep; get up eagerly in the morning; use good health habits before retiring and coming to school every morning.
12. Know the value of having good posture and being physically clean and attractive and act accordingly; enjoy being clean and neat and be popular among their peers.
13. Know correct terms related to elimination, perspiration, and the names of some of the parts of their own body.
14. Make effective use of their own leisure; know how to relax and rest when tired.
15. Perform work duties and understand the need for being a worker in society.

In the upper elementary grades, the pupils will:

1. Understand the scientific reasons why they should have good health habits and keep themselves clean.
2. Keep good care of their own bodies, including teeth, nails, hair, and skin.
3. Be aware that many diseases can be spread through the unclean handling of food and eating utensils.
4. Use toilet and other facilities at home, school, and in public places correctly and be aware of good sanitary practices; avoid spitting on floors or sidewalks.

5. Adjust to any physical defect they may have and learn to compensate for it.
6. Be aware that good foot health contributes to good posture; practice good foot health habits.
7. Know the structure, function, and care of their own bodies.
8. Know the relationship which exists among all parts and systems of the body.
9. Be aware how blood circulates, food is digested, fresh air is used, skin and bones protect the body, and other such information which will help them desire to have and maintain good health.
10. Know how the human brain works; the role emotions play in health; what causes fatigue and how it can be eliminated.
11. Have good posture; know the relationship of body posture to body function.
12. Assume responsibility for their own sleep and rest and the room conditions under which they sleep.
13. Know the relationship of adequate sleep and rest to a happy state of mind, being safe, using good behavior, and having the ability to do good school work.
14. Know how to rest and relax frequently during the day.
15. Take part in vigorous physical education and leisure-time play activities.
16. Cooperate with parents and the teacher in planning and carrying out a healthful daily program of work, rest, and play.
17. Be aware of the relationship which exists between bacteria and viruses and health, and know how to protect themselves from such dangers.
18. Avoid handling or tasting unfamiliar medicines, cleaning agents, and insecticides.
19. Show individual evidence of growth, and adjust to body change.
20. Contribute to happy mealtimes at home and school; know the value to good digestion of eating in a pleasant environment.
21. Have periodic dental and physical examinations; know the value of such check-ups in the prevention and control of disease.
22. Increasingly become more self-disciplined and independent; know the value of setting a good example for younger children.
23. Engage in many wholesome boy-and-girl relationships.

Kindergarten

Objectives
1. To introduce an awareness of the foods essential for growth.
2. To introduce an awareness of bodily growth.

Suggested Approaches
1. Use the snack time to reinforce good eating habits that aid the body's digestion (i.e., take small bites, eat slowly, chew thoroughly).

Basic Concepts To Teach
1. Body Growth
   a. Good food for body growth; milk and milk products, eggs, bread and cereals, vegetables and fruits.
   b. Body development: compare the size of babies to the pupils; compare pupil sizes; keep track of the pupil's growth during the year.
2. Body Structure
   a. Identification of external parts (i.e., shoulder, elbow, head, hand).
   b. Observation of different body builds in the classroom.
   c. Identification of the senses (sight, hearing, touch, taste, smell).
3. Body Functions
   a. Digestion—how to eat to aid digestion (chew thoroughly, take small bites, eat slowly).
   b. Elimination—stress the importance of regularity, cleanliness.

Group Activities
1. Make a bulletin board of hens, eggs, and the association of the two.
2. Have a party using vegetables and fruits for refreshments.
3. Show pictures to the class and ask the students which sense detects or identifies the picture in actuality.

Individual Activities
1. Have each of the students tell what would be a good breakfast.
2. Have students bring pictures of themselves or others as babies.
3. Keep a record of how much they grow over the school year.
4. Make a list of safety measures for the senses (i.e., keep scissors away from the eyes).

Correlation With Other Subjects
1. Science
   a. Blindfold the students and have them identify objects by smell and touch.
2. Drama and Art
   a. Make collages of food that they like to eat.
3. Physical Education
   a. Play hide the button.
   b. Show pictures to the class; have them close their eyes; take some of the pictures away; when they open their eyes see how many of the missing objects can be identified.
   c. Any kind of rhythm work.

Pupil References
Borten, Helen: *Do You Hear What I Hear?* New York: Abelard-Schuman, 1960. (Also *Do You See What I See?; Do You Move As I Do?; Do You Know What I Know?*)
Krauss, Ruth: *Eyes, Nose, Fingers, Toes.* New York: Harper & Row, 1964. (Also *The Growing Story.*)

Teacher References
Teacher editions of health texts (*Health and Growth.* Glenview, Ill.: Scott Foresman & Company, and others).

Audio-Visual Aids
This Is You. (Filmstrip series) Walt Disney Productions.
You the Human Being; You and Your Ears; You and Your Eyes; You and Your Five Senses; Your Sense of Touch; Your Sense of Smell and Taste.
Living and Growing. Churchill Films.
Skimpy and a Good Breakfast. (Filmstrip) Cereal Learning Corp.

Other Teaching Aids
Let's Sing with Ella Jenkins. Glenview, Ill.: Scott, Foresman & Co., 1971. Long-playing record of 8 health and safety songs. It is included in the kit *Health and Safety Highlights: Pictures and Songs for Young Children.*
Posters from the National Dairy Council: *Let's Make Butter; Milk Made the Difference; Every Day, Eat the 1-2-3 Way.*

Grade 1

Objectives
1. To reinforce the knowledge of foods essential for growth.
2. To reinforce the awareness of bodily growth.

Suggested Approaches
1. Talk about what the students are eating while you share lunch with them.
2. Bring a snack of fruits and vegetables to the class and talk about why this kind of snack was chosen.

Basic Concepts To Teach
1. Body Growth
   a. Individual growth over the year.
   b. Body builds of students in the class.
   c. Foods essential for good growth (the four basic food groups).
   d. Need for rest and exercise.
   e. Need for sunshine.
   f. Need for enough sleep.
2. Body Structure
   a. Identification of external parts (nose, neck, hand).
   b. Senses: identification and usage; care; associated diseases and germs (colds, sore throats).
   c. Care of the body: bathing and washing, exercise, rest, and nourishment.
3. Body Functions
   a. Digestion: major organs (i.e., mouth, throat, stomach); aids (proper chewing, eating slowly, resting after eating).
   b. Elimination: necessity of regularity, cleanliness.

Group Activities
1. Visit a dairy farm.
2. Make a bulletin board of good snack foods.
3. Churn butter to show the process.
4. Visit a bakery.
5. Identify objects by feel and smell.

Individual Activities
1. Write a story about what you think a good meal should include.
2. List favorite foods and tell why they are your favorite.
3. Make a chart determining differences between fruits and vegetables.
4. Make a book of the uses of eggs and/or milk.
5. Make a list of safety measures for the senses.
6. Make a list of foods and label each sweet, salty, sour, or bitter.

Correlation With Other Subjects
1. Math
   a. To reinforce the usage of money, have the students buy foods at the class store.
2. Language Arts
   a. Write a story about what they ate for lunch.
3. Science
   a. Plant two seeds in individual pots, let one grow in the sunlight and one in the dark. Stresses the need for sunshine for good growth.
4. Drama and Art
   a. Make up and act a vegetable and fruit play.
   b. Play act a visit to the doctor for weight and measurement check.
5. Physical Education
   a. How many ways can you move your body, and other types of movement exploration.
   b. Arrange the students in two rows; one row hides their eyes, the other switches places; when the opposite group opens their eyes, they must arrange the mixed-up line into their original places. Pupils line up by height.
   c. Rhythm work—Games where the person who is "It" must identify the voice of another.

Pupil References
Aliki, Diogenes: *My Five Senses*. New York: Thomas Y. Crowell Co., 1962.
Brown, Myra: *Ice Cream for Breakfast*. New York: Franklin Watts, 1972.
National Dairy Council: *Milk for You and Me*. Chicago: The Council, 1972.

Showers, Paul: *Find Out by Touching.* New York: Thomas Y. Crowell Co., 1961.

Wolff, Janet: *Let's Imagine Sounds.* New York: E. P. Dutton & Co., 1961.

Teacher References
Teacher editions of health texts.

Audio-Visual Aids
Food for the City: Wheat and Flour. Bailey-Film Associates.
Eyes Bright. Avis Films.
The Five Senses. (Filmstrip series.) The Jam Handy Corp.: *Look How You See; Your Tasting Tongue; Here's Your Ear; How Your Nose Knows; The Feel of Your Skin.*

Other Teaching Aids
Floor Puzzle: Breakfast. Glenview, Ill.: Scott, Foresman & Co. Full-color picture floor puzzle 3′ × 2′ of a breakfast scene that provides leads for nutrition discussions. Teacher's leaflet included.
We All Like Milk. Chicago: National Dairy Council. Series of 21 photographs of animal babies and their mothers.
A set of food models in color together with a display chart can be obtained from the National Dairy Council also.
Muffin in the City. (Record) Creative Playthings. Sounds from *The Noisy Book* by Margaret Wise Brown.
Let's Sing with Ella Jenkins. Glenview, Ill.: Scott, Foresman & Co. Long-playing record of 8 health and safety songs.

Grade 2

Objectives
1. To teach how the heart and lungs work.
2. To help pupils learn how blood, the food of the body, feeds all the cells of the body.

Basic Concepts To Teach
1. How and by whom was blood circulation discovered.
2. What the circulatory system actually is.
3. What happens when the heart beats.
4. How blood is circulated through the body.
5. How our lungs work and how we can keep them healthy.

Group Activities
1. Have the class examine a beef heart cut in half to see the auricles, ventricles, valves, and muscle wall dividing the two sides of the heart.
2. Bring new clippings or make posters of the effects of smoking upon the lungs for a bulletin board.
3. Listen to each other's heartbeats through a mailing tube before and after running in place for two minutes.
4. With a partner learn the latest first aid methods of artificial respiration.

Individual Activities
1. Write a research paper of your special interest in this area such as heart transplants or the link of lung cancer to excessive smoking.
2. Bring to class magazine clippings of various kinds of cigarette ads and discuss the pros and cons of the truthfulness presented.
3. Interview five persons who are on an extensive physical fitness program to strengthen their hearts and health. Present your findings to the class.

Correlation with Other Subjects
Math: Make charts and diagrams on heart and cancer deaths.
Art: Make a plastic or papier mâché model of the human heart.

Language Arts: Read Edgar Allen Poe's story "The Telltale Heart" aloud in class.

Physical Education: Keep a weekly record of how far you can increase the distance you run.   Write a short paper on the effects of doing this and your health.

Social Science: Study the air pollution problem at your school and in your community.

Pupil References

Chester, Michael: "Let's Go To Stop Air Pollution." New York, Putnam Publishing Company, 1970.

Kavaler, Luch: *Dangerous Air.* New York, The John Day Company, 1969.

Lauber, P.: *Your Body and How it Works.* New York, Random House, 1971.

Teacher References

Diehl, Harold: *Tobacco and Your Health.* New York, McGraw-Hill, 1967.

Willgoose, Carl: *Teaching Health in Elementary Schools*, Philadelphia, W. B. Saunders, 1974.

Grade 3

Objectives

1. To help pupils know how their body works as a complete unit.
2. To learn the function of each body part.

Basic Concepts To Teach

1. How the brain controls body action.
2. How each body part works to keep you healthy.
3. How emotions, sleep, and food affect the body.
4. The vital organs of the body and their duties.
5. The machines your doctor uses to check brain waves, heartbeats, bone injuries, etc.

Group Activities

1. Make up riddles about body parts for the class to guess such as, "It produces juices to help your small intestine work.   What is it?"
2. Experiment using each body part to find out how many ways you can bend each part of your hands, feet, whole body. Why can you move in so many ways?
3. Role play the different emotions and discuss how each can help or hurt you and your body.
4. With a partner, make a model of the brain and label the parts that control movement, speech, etc.

Individual Activities

1. Draw a human body and label where the endocrine glands are. Know the function of each.
2. Prepare a 5-minute oral report on why we need to exercise every day to keep our muscles in good shape.
3. Write a paper on the x-ray and its use.
4. Bring an animal bone to class and tell why it is like and also different from one in our own body.

Correlation with Other Subjects

Math: Make a chart of the number of hours you sleep and play outside for a week.   List three things you learned from doing this.

Art: Make a soap or wood carving of any body part.

Language Arts: Read any magazine article, such as "I Am Joe's Heart" in the Reader's Digest, and give an oral report on it.

Physical Education: Experiment to learn how fast or slow you can use any part of your body.

Pupil References
    Coy, Harold: *Doctors And What They Do.* Englewood Cliffs, New Jersey,
       Prentice-Hall, 1971.
    Krumgold, Joseph: *And Now, Miguel.* New York, Crowell, 1969.

Teacher References
    Kogan, Benjamin: *Health.* New York, Harcourt, Brace and World, Inc., 1970.
    Read, Donald, and Greene, Walter: *Health and Modern Man.* New York,
       The Macmillan Company, 1973.

Grade 4

Objectives
    1. To help the student become acquainted with the ways the body has of
       protecting itself.
    2. To help the student realize the five main senses and the body's outpost
       that warns it of danger and thus helps protect it.
    3. Help student learn how to get adequate sleep and rest (10 to 11 hours).

Basic Concepts To Teach
    1. How does body help itself?
        a. Body keeps itself at safe temperature.
        b. Your body can store food and water.
        c. You sleep to get the rest you need.
        d. Other special protective actions.
    2. Help students answer questions about the body.
        a. How does a cut heal?
        b. How does a broken bone mend?
        c. How does body fight diseased gums?
    3. To help students understand more clearly.
        a. Heart: How exercise increases heart beats (simple terms).
        b. Pulse.
        c. Lungs.
        d. Intestines.

Group Activities
    1. Class makes a booklet called "My Body and How It Works." Make
       this as simple or complex as you think class can handle.
    2. Visit a health museum. Have the class start its own health museum.
    3. Have nurse or doctor visit and talk about the body and how to take
       care of it.
    4. If possible, let students visit a health clinic or first aid station.
    5. Have class discussion on how your senses help protect you today.

Individual Activities
    1. Let each pupil feel his pulse at the wrist. Count the heartbeats before
       and after three minutes of vigorous exercise.
    2. Show how body works as unit using hands and arms.
    3. Take pictures or movies of students at the start of school and at the
       end, showing how they have improved.
    4. Test food for starch and fats and discuss how both affect growth.

Correlation With Other Subjects
    1. Math
        a. Have students count number of bones in the body and the number
           of teeth.
    2. Language
        a. Write a story about using one of the five senses.
    3. Art
        a. Make pictures to illustrate stories written about ways to solve health
           problems.
    4. Social Studies
        a. Make report on health problems of early pioneers.

Pupil References
Lewis, Alfred: *The New World of Food.* New York: Dodd, Mead & Co., 1968.
Aglesworth, Thomas G.: *This Vital Air and Water.* Chicago, Rand McNally, 1968.

Teacher References
Teacher's edition, *Health and Growth 5.* Glenview, Ill.: Scott, Foresman, & Co., 1971.

Models
Major organs of body. Reserval, Mineola, New York, 11501.

Films
Eat To Your Heart's Content. McGraw-Hill Co.
Digestive System. (Filmstrip) Rand McNally.
The Five Senses. (Filmstrip) Jam Handy Corp.
—*The Feel of Your Skin; Look How You See.*

Grade 5

Objectives
1. To help students understand how bones and muscles work.
2. Learn how the body digests food.
3. To help students know how senses help and what they do.

Basic Concepts To Teach
1. How many senses there are and what each does to help the body.
2. How bones fit together and stay in place.
3. How bones grow.
4. What are voluntary and involuntary muscles.
5. How does the body digest foods and get rid of waste.
6. How food is used by the body.

Group Activities
1. Have a variety of objects—eraser, chalk, key, bobby pin, etc. Let pupil be blindfolded and identify objects. This shows how many things can be identified by touch.
2. Let pupils talk about things they like to taste and smell. This is a good time to make a point of things that can be harmful by smelling and tasting.
3. Demonstration. Put a lump of sugar in a glass; put crushed sugar in another glass. See which dissolves first. This can be done to show how teeth aid in digestion.

Individual Activities
1. Ask pupils to find some key words relating to hearing, other than the word ear. Have them tell what volumes of the encyclopedia in which they can be found. Example: Sound—S, Deafness—D, Hearing aids—H.
2. Make a listing showing the importance of bones. Example: Bones give body support, etc.
3. Ask a butcher for some bones. Make a chart or exhibit showing sugar and salt forming crystals. Use microscope for hair, skin.
4. Assign each student an organ or sense to research. Help them find books and material for an oral report to the class.

Correlation With Other Subjects
1. Math
   a. Make a schedule for a 24-hour period. Note the balance of active and inactive periods. Determine what time to get up if you retire at 8:00 P.M. and get 8 hours of sleep.
2. Language
   a. Discuss bedtime procedures, and write a story on "What I do before Bed."

Pupil References

Goldsmith, Ilse: *Anatomy for Children.* New York: Thomas Y. Crowell Co., 1965.

McGovern, Ann: *The Question and Answer Book about the Human Body.* New York: Franklin Watts, 1964.

Raveilli, Anthony: *Wonders of the Human Skeleton.* New York: E. P. Dutton & Co., 1961.

Teacher References

Health and Growth. 4th ed. Glenview, Ill.: Scott Foresman & Co., 1971.

Other Teaching Aids

  Models

Sensory Models—Eye, Ear, Skin, Nose, and Tongue. Ideal School Supply.

Human Skeleton—Model No. 5228. Ideal School Supply.

Grade 6

Objectives

1. Age where questions about the body are important and essential to their all-around development.
2. Help them to understand the changes taking place in their physical makeup (voice, hair, etc.).

Suggested Approaches

1. Designate a study period to the aspects of the body and good body care.
2. Good film strips are sometimes beneficial in this area.
3. Guest speakers.
4. Field trips which are carefully planned.

Major Points To Stress

1. Body Growth.
   a. Physiological growth.
   b. Different approaches to weight control.
   c. Good food, nourishment.
2. Body Structure.
   a. External and internal parts of body (not in depth).
   b. Conditions which cause bad structure (posture).
3. Body Function
   a. Drugs, alcohol, etc. which affect body function.
   b. Major body systems, ways they function.

Group Activities

1. Open class discussions concerning body changes.
2. Lab experiences with major posters.
3. Give students an animal and let them explain how it differs from man in muscle development, and how it is similar.

Individual Activities

1. Have each one do some research in the area of his personal growth over the past few years.
2. Let them decide what they would like to talk about in area of body growth and function.

Correlation With Other Subjects

1. Physical Education
   a. Correlate body types with different sports. How we walk, run, why the swimmer has long muscles, the weight lifter has big bunchy muscles.
2. Art
   a. Body structure seen in paintings and pictures.
3. Science
   a. Study all aspects of body.

Pupil References
Check school library and public library for recent editions dealing with all types of body development.
Do some research around the area on what material other schools are using.

Audio-Visual Aids
Check with the junior high school and other schools to see what films they are watching, then after seeing and screening films choose some appropriate for your class.

Teacher References
Many good books available, but it is essential for one to use up-to-date material. Thus check with others and do some research on your own on recent editions.

CHAPTER 13

safety

The chief cause of death among children is accidents. The leading types of accidents of school children are those caused by motor vehicles, drowning, fires and explosions, firearms, and falls. Based on the National Health Survey, the time lost from school annually because of accidents serious enough to call for medical attention is 39.2 days per 100 boys, and 23.3 days per 100 girls.[1] Forty-three per cent of accidental deaths among school-age children are connected with school: 20% occur in school buildings, 17% on school grounds, and 6% on the way to and from school in pedestrian-motor vehicle and bicycle-motor vehicle accidents.[2] In the school plant, two out of every five accidents occur in organized athletics, principally football and basketball. Accidents which occur in auditoriums and classrooms are second most common, and those which happen while playing on playground apparatus rank third. Many pupils are seriously injured going to and from school and are involved in accidents caused by their own carelessness or that of drivers of motor vehicles. In addition, many children are injured, and some are killed, while riding in school buses. Although in 1959 29 children were killed in school-bus accidents, these vehicles were involved in some way in 7186 accidents, and 1580 children were injured while riding in them while on their way to or from school. Although safety education should begin at home and largely be parental responsibility, every school throughout the nation must also assume increased responsibility for conducting a well-planned and well-conducted safety education program. Likewise, pupils must be taught in a safer school environment by more well-rounded teachers who are alert to their needs for safety education and are able to help them gain emotional maturity and safety competence. Furthermore, the program of safety instruction must become a closer and more vital part of the school curriculum

---

[1] Oberteuffer, Delbert, et al.: *Health Education.* New York: Harper & Row, 1972, p. 264.
[2] Anderson, C. L.: *School Health Practice.* St. Louis: C. V. Mosby Co., 1970, p. 193.

and strive harder to develop understanding, shape the attitudes, values, apprecia-tions, habits, and skills which will enable children to assume responsibility for their own safety in the danger-filled world of today. Safety education experts believe that a vitalized safety education program can and should provide rich experiences through which many of the desirable traits of personality and character, which reflect the democratic ideal of concern for others, can be developed by the school.

The National Safety Council, which has an abundance of outstanding materials for teaching safety effectively, has made the following recommendations for those planning a program in school safety education.[3]

1. Safety education should be concerned with worthwhile activities rather than negative prescriptions and should thereby contribute to the enrich-ment rather than the impoverishment of living.
2. Since the field of safety education is as broad as life itself, it should be approached from every angle.
3. The curriculum should be closely related to community needs—"commu-nity" being defined as the area in which the pupil lives—but ability to meet the problems of a new environment should also be developed.
4. The curriculum should emphasize pupil growth in safety responsibility.
5. Although there are marked limitations in the use of personal first-hand experiences in safety education, this method should be used insofar as practical and possible.
6. The curriculum should be developed in the light of best practices of mental hygiene which place emphasis on the development of personal security.
7. The curriculum should be evaluated in light of each of its objectives, in-cluding the intangibles as well as the tangibles. The Standard Student Accident Reporting System[4] should be an essential part in the evaluation of the tangibles.
8. Safety instruction, to be effective, must be an integral part of the curricu-lum. Certain areas of the program, however, may best be provided for by special "courses" or "units."
9. Safety can well be used as a spearhead in the development of current curricular trends.
10. Safety education activities in the school should be properly integrated and correlated with worthwhile programs of safety education of all other appropriate agencies.

As Patty points out, the three major factors which should govern the allocation of subject matter in safety education to each grade are (1) the immediate needs of the child for this education, (2) the child's ability to comprehend materials, and (3) the interests of the child.[5]

Every city school should have a safety patrol. Since the youngest children, aged 5 to 9, have three times more pedestrian injuries than the 10- to 14-year-olds, school safety patrols, police, and teachers need to work together with parents in sharing responsibility for pedestrian safety education.[6] Careful supervision and planning are necessary if the safety-patrol system is to be an effective educational

[3] "Curriculum Planning for Safety." *Safety Education* (December 1961), 18–19.
[4] Available from the National Safety Council upon request.
[5] Patty, Willard: *Teaching Health and Safety in Elementary Grades.* Englewood Cliffs, N.J.: Prentice-Hall, 1951, p. 249.
[6] Ridgeway, William: "Protection without Education, A False Sense of Security." *Safety Education* (February 1960), 10–12.

and protective program. Most states have adopted standards and governing rules for such patrols, which can be obtained from state departments of education upon request. The National Safety Council also has such materials available and will gladly work closely with schools or other organizations on all matters pertaining to protection or safety education. The functions of the school safety patrol should be to (1) instruct, direct, and control traffic of the pupils in crossing the streets and highways at and near schools, and (2) assist teachers and other adults in teaching children safe practices in the use of streets and highways at all times and in all places. In addition to the traffic safety patrol, schools should have a fire patrol, building safety patrol, and playground safety patrol. Each of these groups should have clearly defined duties to perform, and it should be considered a school honor to be selected to serve on any of these patrols.

The safety education program should also be bolstered by an all-school safety council, as well as a class or homeroom safety committee. The former might well consist of selected teachers, including those from shop, laboratory, and physical education classes, the nurse, school physician, selected pupils, and the principal who would serve as an *ex-officio* member. The homeroom safety group should be made up of several pupils and their teacher. The purpose of such a committee should be to prevent accidents in the classroom or any place else at school. Membership changed periodically will help increase the effectiveness of the group as well as help sustain pupil interest in such a committee.

Children do not want to be hurt or killed, and yet many of them are involved in serious accidents at school, while traveling, or in their own homes every day. They must be made aware of existing dangers in their environment and know how to cope with them successfully. Rules, warnings, and threats mean little to most children. Consequently, teachers must somehow help youth develop safety habits, values, and the "know-how" which will enable them to survive and enjoy a long lifetime of happy living. In the primary grades, safety should be stressed informally daily. First aid should be taught in the intermediate grades so that pupils will learn how to take care of their own simple injuries, as well as know what to do in an emergency. Bicycle care and safety should also be included in the safety education programs at this level, for every 16 minutes some young cyclist is seriously injured, and every 18 hours a bicycle rider is killed by an automobile.[7] The majority of those maimed or killed in such accidents are children between the ages of 6 and 16. Every school should also have a training program in bicycle safety, and each community should enforce a program for the periodic inspection and licensing of all bicycles.

SUGGESTED GRADED TOPICS

Suggested graded topics in this area include the following:

GRADE 1
1. Safety in going and coming to school.
2. Safety in the classroom.
3. Safety in the entire school building.
4. Safety using scissors, sharp pointed articles, and other equipment.
5. Playground safety.
6. Safe places to play.
7. What causes accidents; how can they be prevented.

---

[7] *Accident Facts.* Chicago: National Safety Council, 1972, p. 15.

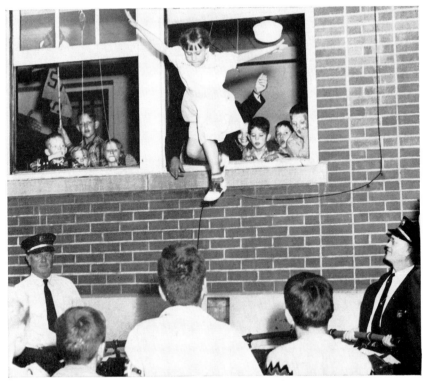

Figure 13-1. Fire drills should be held periodically. (Courtesy of Nashville Public Schools)

GRADE 2

1. Review of all the above-mentioned topics.
2. Safety at home.
3. Safety around pets and other animals.
4. Fire safety.
5. Extent and cause of accidents.
6. School bus safety.
7. Safety riding in automobiles and other vehicles.
8. Safety on hikes and cookouts.
9. Safety rules for summers and in boats.

GRADE 3

1. Bicycle safety.
2. Fire prevention and protection.
3. Safety using tools and equipment such as a knife, saw, plane, scissors, ice pick, nail file, etc.
4. Community protection of the health and safety of children.
5. Safety laws.
6. Safety at home.
7. Why we should report accidents.

GRADE 4

1. Safety problems of school-age pupils.
2. Hazards in the school, home, and the community.

3. Safety in physical education and recreation.
4. Weather hazards.
5. Community and governmental agencies of protection.
6. Safety for special events and happenings, including Halloween and Christmas, floods, and air attacks.
7. Gas and poisons.
8. Rabies and tetanus prevention.

GRADE 5

1. Junior first aid.
2. Home care and nursing.
3. Use of flammables.
4. Accidents in the home, including falls and burns.
5. Water safety.
6. Accident facts, cause and prevention.
7. Electricity and electric appliances.
8. Industrial safety.
9. Safety on the farm.

GRADE 6

1. First aid.
2. Safety problems in the community.
3. Predriver training.
4. The home medicine cabinet.
5. Self-medication; poisons.
6. Forest conservation and fire prevention.
7. Safe use of laboratory equipment.
8. Safety in sports.
9. Safety in aviation.
10. Travel safety.

CURRICULUM PLACEMENT

Many schools allocate safety education to the various areas already established in the curriculum. There are certain elements of safety education in every program area, for if pupils are learning to use laboratory equipment they should be taught to use it safely, or if they are learning to use a hammer or cut paper dolls with scissors in the first grade, they should learn to use this kind of equipment without danger to themselves. In some schools, the physical and safety education programs are combined, while in still others the physical education director or a teacher specialized in this field coordinates the entire safety program. In still others, it is taught as a separate subject. Ideally, safety education should be a major part of the course of study in health and safety and should be correlated and integrated with other subjects at every grade level. Throughout the elementary grades, safety education should be the classroom teacher's responsibility, and the educational program should consist largely of helping children develop desirable habits and attitudes toward healthful, safe living. The alert teacher will relate her instruction to such life experiences as the proper use of toilet and hand-washing, medical and dental examinations and tests, weighing and measuring, visits of the school health specialists, playground activities, and the lunch program. Thus, the amount of time needed for health and safety instruction cannot become set or predetermined. Fortunately, capable administrators and skilled teachers will always provide whatever time is needed to help boys and girls live healthfully and safely at school and elsewhere. Since health, its development and protection, is one of the primary objectives of education, the amount of time devoted to this area should be at least equal to, if not more than, that devoted to any other major area included in the school curriculum.

Suggested subject areas and ways in which safety education can skillfully be correlated and integrated include the following.

Social sciences can be used successfully for this purpose. As pupils study materials in history, civics, government, geography, economics, and sociology they can also learn about safety problems and their solutions in each of these subjects. Suggested topics which could be used for doing so at the elementary level are:

1. The westward movement and pioneer days.
2. The periods of colonization and settlement of early America.
3. Safety developments in transportation.
4. The development of the machine and resulting problems.
5. Types and causes of major accidents in America.
6. Accident prevention in the home, school, community, and nation.
7. The cost of accidents in comparison to safety education and safe practices.
8. The work of the state and federal government in local safety education and protection.
9. Fire prevention and control in the community, state, and nation.
10. City planning.
11. The rights, duties, and obligations of citizenship.
12. Protective safety laws and their enforcement.
13. Standards of living and the effects of poor housing and inadequate education upon accidents.
14. The growth and kinds of industrial safety programs.
15. Public utilities and community safety.
16. Community safeguards in time of flood or other catastrophes.

Science can become a splendid avenue for integrating and correlating certain materials in safety education. Suggested ways for doing so are through the use of the following broad topics:

1. Fire control and prevention.
2. Use and dangers of electricity.
3. Air, weather, and ventilation and their effects upon the health and welfare of people.
4. Sewage and waste disposal.
5. Food and drug laws.
6. Patent medicines.
7. Land, water, and air transportation safety devices.
8. Conservation of human and natural resources.
9. Hazards of smog and poisonous gas.
10. Germ warfare.
11. Cause and prevention of epidemics.
12. The relation of plants and animals to human life and welfare.
13. Survival procedures when lost in the woods, shipwrecked, or in a plane crash.
14. Effect of drugs and drinking and their relationship to rising accident and crime rates.
15. Handling of hot substances.
16. Proper use of radio and television aerials and grounds, dangers of power and electric lawn mowers, size of fuses, insulators, and electrical circuits.
17. Emotional causes of accidents and accident proneness.
18. First aid.
19. Safety engineering as a profession; the duties of a safety engineer.
20. Safety devices and programs used in industry.

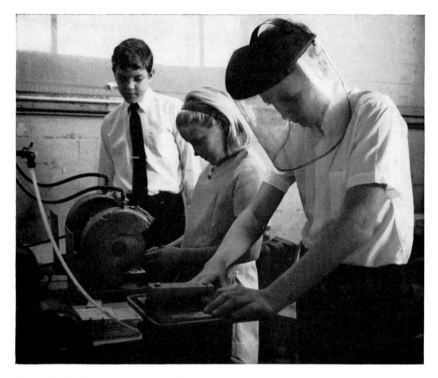

Figure 13-2. Youngsters in laboratories and carpentry and metal-working shops should
learn proper safety procedures. The boy wearing the clear mask
practices what he has learned about eye safety, but the other two lack
safety awareness. (Courtesy of Dallas Health and Science Museum)

Physical education includes many vigorous activities wherein children can have
adventurous, joyful experiences. Many activities are danger-filled, which is the
reason they are so appealing and challenging to youth. However, under skilled
leadership and proper instructions, physical education classes need not be any more
dangerous than those in other subjects. One way to safeguard against accidents is
to be sure that pupils engage in activities for which they have been prepared in age,
strength, and skill. Adults should help children see that if they are safety conscious
they can have fun over a longer period of time.

All teachers, whether or not they are trained physical education specialists, who
are assigned gymnasium or playground instructional or supervisory duties can
safeguard against accidents by:

1. Checking all apparatus and equipment periodically and keeping everything
   in good repair at all times.
2. Finding and marking all hazards with the pupils.
3. Directing all pupils in safety measures.
4. Using activities in a graded program which are best suited for the children
   at each grade level, and for those who are awkward and poorly skilled.
5. Insisting that all pupils wear suitable protective apparel for all activities.

6. Teaching children to swim, if possible, at school. Encourage parents to see to it that their child has lessons and learns during the summer or at other times, if the school does not have a pool. Teach basic water, boating, and fishing safety.
7. Supervising children during recess or other play periods. Know whether they are playing according to rules, and if not, insist that they do so. Discuss with the class the necessity of playing according to game rules, taking turns, and why one should be aware of his own safety and that of others, especially during play.

There are numerous ways in which the physical education teacher or classroom instructor teaching physical activities can integrate and correlate materials in this field with those in safety education. These include discussing with the pupils at teachable moments such topics as:

1. Cause and prevention of accidents in the playground, in the gymnasium, and elsewhere.
2. The effects of alcohol, drugs, and tobacco on health, safety, and efficiency.
3. The danger and proper use of all equipment, such as bat, archery bow, trampoline, swing, etc.
4. Prevention of water accidents.
5. Prevention of accidents and diseases such as athlete's foot, ringworm, itch, etc., through proper use of pool and locker-room facilities.
6. First-aid treatment for minor injuries.
7. Protective sports equipment and its proper use.
8. The causes of injuries in sports and games such as fatigue, lack of skill, and other factors.
9. Why and how game rules protect the safety of the players.
10. Kinds and use of accident reports and insurance plans for players.
11. Allocation of different sections of the playground for each grade for the safety and protection of the children, assigning to those in the primary grades a spot close to the building, those from the oldest group being farthest removed.
12. The proper location of all apparatus, equipment, and game space for courts, horseshoe pitching, and other activities along one side or at the end of the play area.
13. Common types of athletic injuries and how to avoid them.
14. Why all pupils should have a physical examination before participating in strenuous activities.
15. Why pupils are classified for competition.
16. Adequate supervision of all participants; safety procedures to follow when playing alone.
17. How and why the body should be warmed up before strenuous activity.
18. Why proper skill progression in sports and games is taught and how this is done.
19. How accidents are recorded and why.
20. Diets for competitors as a means of avoiding illness and accidents.
21. The results of a survey made *with* each class of the hazards in the gymnasium, playground, pool, locker room, and shower room.

Mathematics can also be correlated and integrated with safety education. Here again, however, the purpose for doing so should not primarily be to give pupils added experience in learning to apply mathematical concepts, but to teach them significant facts about safety, and the causes and preventions of accidents in order that they may better protect and prolong their own lives, as well as those of others.

Suggested areas of study and activities include those which will enable the pupils to:

1. Study the accident statistics of their own school, community, county and state. Classify these by types and within age groups.
2. Make graphs showing the accident problems of primary, intermediate, junior, and senior high school groups.
3. Make graphs showing accident trends among elementary and secondary school age groups from 1960 to the present.
4. Study the accident reports of a school system for one year. Classify reported accidents. Draw up an accident prevention plan for your own school from these data.
5. Evaluate the school's accident-prevention plan by tabulating accident causes for a 6-month period.
6. Make a study of the extent, types, and costs of accidents in your own family for one year. Combine your findings with those made by all other pupils. Draw up a preventive plan from this study which could be adopted in every home.
7. Interview the high school coach to find out which athletic benefit insurance plan is used. Learn the costs, benefits derived, and value of such a plan. Report your findings to the class.
8. Discover the total cost of school bus transportation in your county and state.
9. Inspect your own home and a farm. Make a comparative study of hazards found in each place.
10. Find out the number of school buildings in your state or the nation which were destroyed by fire last year. Determine the total cost of these fires.
11. Make a study of the costs of motor vehicle deaths in your community, state, and nation for one year. Determine in percentage the causes of those accidents reported.
12. Make a bar graph of the principal types of accidents which occur in your school.
13. Make a pie graph showing the location in which accidents of school-age children most frequently occur.
14. Make a line graph showing the increase of accidents as reported by the National Safety Council from 1970 to 1973.

As McGill has pointed out,

> Relating classroom lessons in safety to safe living at home is the most effective technique. Teaching activities which help children to identify the hazards to safe living in the home and school and to examine their activities for the potentially injurious consequences which may be present are basic to safety education. The safety rules which parents stress should be further emphasized through classroom study.[8]

If children are to learn to live safely, all teaching in this area must be conducted in a functional way. This means that besides direct safety instruction, all elementary teachers must be much more effective in correlating safety learning with all other subjects included in the curriculum. Likewise, they must increasingly relate safety lessons to all activities which enter into each pupil's daily life at home, at school, and in the community.

THE USE OF TEACHING METHODS

Almost every kind of teaching method can be used in safety education, providing they produce desired results. The following methods are especially adaptable for effective instruction in safety.

---

[8] McGill, John: "How to Teach Children to Do Things the Safe Way." *JOHPER*, *310*, 29, 1961.

Problem Solving

There are many problems which can be studied in safety education through the use of this method. Safety education itself is a gigantic problem which remains unsolved, for we still have to discover ways to prevent the tragic loss of human lives from accidents. Indeed, the problem is becoming increasingly greater, in spite of the fact that more Americans are now going to school and staying there for a longer time. Seemingly, then, education which consists of doing the same old thing in the same old way is *not* the answer.

Suggested problem areas which pupils would profit from exploring should be those which are meaningful to them at their own particular stage of development in each school grade. Primary youngsters should study safety problems which have a direct effect upon their behavior, whether this be when coming and going to school or while they are at school, home, or at play. Upper elementary pupils, who are increasingly becoming more civic-minded, might well study larger safety problems, such as traffic accidents in their own city and state. Regardless of the problem selected for study by each class through teacher-guided class discussion and planning, these problem areas must become real and vitally important ones to each learner.

Each school and each class in it has a safety problem of some kind which can be solved (either partially or completely) by pupils, guided by their teacher. Some of these problems are:

1. Pupil traffic in corridors, lunchrooms, etc., which may be solved by re-routing or channelization.
2. Horseplay in locker rooms, in the playground, toilets, and around drinking fountains.
3. Problems involving the transportation of pupils to the school in a school bus, private car, or public bus.
4. School ground and play area hazards.
5. Safety problems which center around the arrival and dismissal of school students every day, and before holiday periods.
6. Parking of vehicles, including bicycles.

Also, every school has its own unique safety problems due to its location, as when the school has been built near a railroad crossing or a jet airport. Still others have increased in-school traffic problems, due largely to the vast influx of children. Regardless of the cause and type of safety problem, it cannot be solved by the adults alone. Merely setting up conduct rules certainly will not do it, nor punishing children for disobeying rules. The pupils themselves can help solve it, but not by themselves, for the solution of all school safety problems lies only in the working together of both the children and adults involved. Safety work *must* be carried on by pupils if education in this subject is to be effective.

Class Discussions

In safety education, discussion can revolve around many kinds of topics. Here again, the role of the teacher is to draw the pupils out and to enter into the discussion at the best moment. Suggested topics for discussion and activities are:

1. Have each child report on exit signs he has seen in theaters, restaurants, stores, etc. Encourage each to tell how he would escape if his own house caught fire. Discuss protection from fires.

2. Show and discuss safety films or filmstrips.
3. Have each child report on an accident he saw and tell what caused it. Discuss what causes accidents.
4. As a class group, draw up safe passing rules to be observed when changing rooms at school or going from one place in the building to another. Talk about why people break rules and what should be done about this.
5. Bring newspaper clippings for the class bulletin board of accidents which happen in the local community. Discuss these as a class group.
6. Invite a local safety specialist to the class to describe the work he does. Have the class discuss what they learned from this experience.
7. Divide into groups of four to make an on-the-spot survey of pedestrian and motor traffic at several of the busiest city street intersections. Compare results, draw conclusions, and make recommendations from the information gathered from this experience.
8. Show pictures of accidents taken from magazines or newspapers. Select various students to discuss how such an accident might have been caused, how it could have been prevented, etc. Listen carefully to answers given in order to determine if pupils have gained workable knowledge concerning safety.
9. Discuss as a class or in panel groups why one should obey traffic rules and school safety rules.
10. Compare American life today with that of a century ago.
11. Discuss what evidence you have that man has failed so far to adjust to his changing environment.
12. Discuss, plan, and conduct a safety program in your school.
13. Discuss how accidents among adults can be prevented.
14. Discuss, plan, and give a P.T.A. program designed to secure parent cooperation in the prevention of child pedestrian injuries.
15. Discuss the values and problems of bicycle training programs.
16. Talk about ways in which you can help prevent accidents in your own home, at school, and on the playground.
17. Discuss seasonal play activities such as roller skating, kite flying, and sledding from the standpoint of safety.
18. Discuss water and boating safety.
19. Discuss the formation of a safety club in your class, define its purposes, activities, etc.
20. Secure and study free educational materials available from the National Safety Council in Chicago. Discuss these with the class.
21. Keep a class record of all accidents which happen in the classroom, while going to and from school, or in the playground. Discuss this record periodically.
22. Talk with parents, bus drivers, patrol boys, and others in order to learn if the pupils are becoming more safety conscious when away from their teachers. Discuss transportation safety.
23. Determine through observation if some children have become overcautious or afraid, or if any pupil seems to be accident-prone. Talk individually with such children, and help them recognize and overcome these handicaps.
24. Ask the class whether as a group they think that they generally practice good safety habits. Have them give suggestions of how they can still improve. Select one pupil to list these on the board. Refer to this list periodically and have the children again evaluate their progress.

Demonstrations

In many areas and activities demonstrations can add to the effectiveness of knowledge gained in safety education. It has been often said that one of the most effective ways to teach youth the importance of using equipment and facilities safely is the way the instructor herself uses her own tools and body skillfully. Well-conducted demonstrations on the safe use of equipment can and should set an example for the children to copy. Excellent opportunities to teach safety concepts by demonstrations are available in the areas of fire prevention and control; transportation via school bus, private car, or public bus; bicycle safety; common use of home electrical appliances; playground, laboratory, and other types of equipment safety. Pupils must not only see these demonstrations, but be taught through them. Other suggested demonstrations which can be used to teach safety concepts include the safe use of:

Scissors	Apparatus in the gymnasium, including ropes, the horizontal bar, traveling rings, and trampoline
Crayons, pencils, and pens	
Knives	
Playground apparatus	Outdoor cooking and camping equipment
Combustible materials	
Hard-surface areas	Apparatus on the playground, including the monkey bars, jungle gym, chinning and knee-hanging bars
Breakable materials	
Ways to use the body skillfully in sports and games	

As a cumulative activity, it is suggested that the group plan a school picnic and use this experience to learn about transportation safety, a first-aid kit and what it should contain, how to avoid sunburn, poison ivy, etc. Integrate previously learned materials in nutrition, and have pupils plan and cook a simple luncheon in foil.

Field Trips

Field trips interest pupils in the affairs and facilities of their own community, and in turn, stimulate interest among local citizens in what is happening at school. Visits to such places as a traffic court, a modern industrial plant, an airport, fire station, police station, emergency room in a hospital, railroad or bus station, or shipyard can help make safety education a vital and thrilling experience to youth.

Surveys

Surveys can best be used to teach pupils how to utilize the results of their findings and find ways to improve conditions. Those who come into contact with safety problems in their school or home environment and learn how to solve them correctly are ready to learn next about the larger safety problems which are found in their community, state, and nation. Often, the results of surveys made by just one class in the school can improve conditions as well as help other pupils in the entire school become more safety-conscious. Subjects suitable for school surveys include pedestrian problems in the building and in the playground, traffic problems in and around the school, fire-prevention methods and practices, bicycle safety, and field-trip safety. A survey of community agencies conducting safety education and accident-prevention programs will give pupils direct contact with these organizations, as well as acquaint both the pupils and teacher with speakers from these agencies who might be brought into the classroom as guests.

Many results can accrue from surveys made by pupils of conditions in their own school. These may include the establishment or enlargement of school safety patrols, the building of bicycle racks and a bicycle inspection program, the allocation of safer play areas, the building of a fenced-in playground, or even the resurfacing of outdoor play areas.

9

Guidance

To reach those pupils with unique safety problems, guidance can also be brought into the educational program. Those children who are accident-prone, too afraid to try new skills, always fearful of getting hurt, and those who play too recklessly without consideration of the well-being of others, all need special help. Often these can best be reached by individual counseling.

THE USE OF INSTRUCTIONAL MATERIALS

Many kinds of instructional materials can be utilized to help children develop good safety practices and safety consciousness. These include:

Equipment

The "real thing" should be brought into the classroom and used to its fullest educational extent. Such articles as the following can be used for teaching boys and girls how to use play and work equipment safely:

Football shoulder pads, helmets, mouth protectors	Jigsaw
	Stoves
Catcher's mask	Electric fans, lawn mowers
Scissors, knives	Can openers, razors
Sewing machines	Matches
Saws, hammers	Fishing rods and hooks
Bicycles, roller and ice skates	Band saw, power drill
Bows and arrows	Auto engine
Sander	Horseback-riding equipment
Oil and gasoline lamps and engines	Track and field equipment such as a
Cleaning equipment, including oily rags and mops	javelin, vaulting pole, shot, and others

Photographic and Related Materials

Many schools are increasingly utilizing the camera as an instructional device. Often pupils are assigned to photograph school-ground and play-area hazards, and then use these pictures in posters. Such photographs help children become cognizant of the location and type of hazards they are likely to encounter. The teacher can also make her own colored slides of a dangerous location, action, or situation to show to her class as she discusses safety problems with them. Still other schools are making their own movies of children at play or at work in the school, with the pupils planning, writing, and producing the film. Their finished product can be used for both classroom and community educational purposes.

The National Safety Council and the state departments of education have many splendid free films available for classroom use. Other visual aids suitable for presenting facts, shaping attitudes, and motivating behavior are cartoons, drawings, water colors, stencils, and linoleum blocks. Suggested activities using these creative materials are the following:

1. Explore the schoolroom, home, and school playground in order to discover existing hazards. Point these out and list those found in the classroom. Paint those found on the playground, such as rocks or tree trunks, with bright yellow paint. Mark off safety areas for waiting one's turn to swing or seesaw with a line of paint.

2. Walk in a class group to the nearest traffic light, and discover the safest way to walk to school. Learn the meaning of the various light signals, or those given by a policeman or patrol boy. Make a stop-and-go sign from a milk carton, colored paper, stick supported on a base, and a flashlight. Draw a traffic route in chalk on the floor. Have the class practice operating and responding to the changing signals.[9]

3. Bring or make pictures to show dangerous creatures found in their state, such as the coral snake, a bull, etc. Teach why the pupils should avoid these.

4. Have children bring newspaper or magazine articles for a scrapbook on any phase of the safety education program.

5. Take snapshots of existing school and playground hazards. Elect a committee to plan the removal of these hazards. Write a final report of the project, or have the committee present it orally in a school auditorium program, at a P.T.A. meeting, or over the local radio or television station.

6. Take "before" and "after" snapshots of a playground clean up campaign. Evaluate the success of this group endeavor, and plan another such campaign to be conducted later.

7. Study and make a chart of common poisons, giving suggestions for keeping these away from curious children or animals.

8. Appoint a bulletin-board or display committee to show the best pictures taken and posters made by class members.

9. Have each child make a poster on the safety practices to be carried out during any holiday. Display these in a department-store window.

10. Make an illustrative poster for a fire prevention unit.

Dramatic Activities

Role playing, skits, safety plays, puppet shows, and charades can all help pupils express what they have learned in safety education. They can also be used by a creative teacher as a means of having the children "teach" each other. Suggested activities in which dramatic activities can be used are:

1. Play "community" in the sandbox or by moving the chairs in the classroom. Using toy automobiles and trucks, have this traffic respond to hand traffic signals by a pupil "policeman."

2. Act out carrying, passing, and using scissors, knives, saws, hammers, and other tools correctly.

3. Show cans of lye, roach powder, shoe polish, or other products which are dangerous for human beings to swallow.

4. Dramatize the danger of toys left on the floor, medicines or poisons left where babies can get to them, food left cooking on a stove that a child can reach, or other causes of common home accidents.

5. Demonstrate safety at the drinking fountain.

6. Bring a pet cat or dog to class and demonstrate petting it correctly, and approaching animals with the hand held out, the back of it toward the floor as though the animal was about to be fed. Warn the class about approaching strange animals. Have the class make a poster on this subject.

7. Have periodic fire or other protective drills, and train each child so that he knows what he is to do in case of such an emergency. Have the class make posters on the cause of fires, and write a play about them.

8. Practice getting on and off a stationary school bus, and learn how to ride in it safely.

9. Using chairs for a two- or four-passenger automobile, dramatize the good and bad ways to be a passenger in the family car.

---

[9] Obtain a set of New Road Poster Signs from St. Regis, Consumer Products Division, 3300 Pinson Valley Parkway, Birmingham, Alabama 35217.

10. Dramatize what to do when injured at school.
11. Demonstrate blanket-wrapping in case clothing catches on fire; how to put out a small grass fire.
12. Have children move folding chairs or other room equipment, demonstrating first incorrectly in an exaggerated fashion, and then showing how to do it correctly. Give a skit on this topic.
13. Play "telephone and emergency," noting carefully if each pupil knows what to do in case of an emergency.
14. Make safety posters, miniature traffic signs. Act out being a policeman, patrol boy, pedestrian, auto driver, etc.
15. Demonstrate safe methods for riding a bicycle. Show the safety devices which should be on every bicycle, such as a horn, reflector light, etc.
16. Have a weekly clean-up contest between squads of playground area. Show dangerous articles found which could cause injury. Act out the wrong and right things to do.
17. Make up and act out walking safely in the rain or when snow or ice is on the ground.
18. Practice safe ways to climb, jump, hang upside down by the knees, or other movement skills.
19. Practice turning electric fans, television sets, irons, and other electrical equipment off and on. Demonstrate how to do these things safely.
20. Ask a safety patrol boy to talk to the class in order to acquaint the children with his job and how they can help him do it better. Give a skit showing the problems he has with some pupils.

Radio and Television

Many schools have real or mock radio and television safety education programs. Short radio dramas, skits, panel discussions, and other types of presentations can be given on a variety of safety topics such as "Safety at Play," "Swimming and Boating Safety," "Our School Safety Patrol," "Bicycle Safety," "Accidents in the Home," and others. Such experiences are often exciting ones in the lives of children, for they like to show adults what they can do, and they should be given many opportunities for them.

DESIRABLE OUTCOMES

A well-taught program in safety education will produce the following desirable outcomes in terms of knowledge, attitudes, and practices. In the primary grades, the pupils will

1. Become aware that their own home, school, travel route to school, and playground have hazards, know where these are, and how to cope with them successfully.
2. Know the meaning of traffic signals and the safest way to travel to and from school.
3. Be aware that policemen and firemen are protecting friends and that the school janitor, bus driver, nurse, doctor, and teacher are concerned about their safety too.
4. Know that scissors, knives, saws, or other articles can cause pain or serious injury, and know how to use these tools safely.
5. Know the danger of petting strange animals or picking up queer-looking insects or worms.
6. Be aware that medicine, insect powder, or other similar articles often found in the home can cause death or serious illness if consumed.
7. Know the meaning of school warning signals such as the fire alarm, the air-raid siren, and know what to do when these warnings are sounded.

8. Be safety-conscious while riding in the school bus or family automobile and act accordingly.
9. Be safety-conscious while using the playground apparatus or drinking at the water fountain, and act accordingly.
10. Wear tennis shoes while playing in the gymnasium, and rubbers when it is slick and icy outside.
11. Know what to do when they are hurt at school or at home.
12. Know their complete name, age, address, parent's names and where they can be reached by phone, their family doctor's name, and whom to call in case of an emergency.
13. Know what to do if their clothing catches fire or when a building is burning.
14. Become skilled in using all play equipment, such as the jungle gym, horizontal bars, swings, etc.
15. Know water safety rules and be able to swim.
16. Understand how weather affects safety and precautions which should be taken during adverse conditions.
17. Know how to handle correctly folding chairs or other movable school furniture.
18. Know how to use the telephone in case of an emergency and whom to call.

In the upper elementary grades, the pupils will

1. Review previously learned safety knowledge and skills.
2. Practice good housekeeping and safety in the playground, at school, in the classroom, and at home.
3. Know the danger of burns, poison ivy, poisonous snakes, and other things which can cause pain or serious injury.
4. Desire to prevent fires, and know what to do in case of a fire.
5. Practice traffic safety while riding a bicycle, in the school bus, or family car.
6. Have favorable attitudes and real concern for the rights and safety of others at work and play.
7. Know how to pass safely from room to room or floor to floor at school, and to use the drinking fountain, dressing-room shower, and other school equipment safely.
8. Play according to game rules, wear protective equipment such as shoulder pads, catcher's mask, or knee guards.
9. Know what to do in case of an emergency at school, home, on the playground, and while traveling.
10. Have earned the Junior Red Cross First Aid Certificate.
11. Use tools and experimental equipment carefully and skillfully in the classroom, manual training room, or science laboratory at school, and in home workshops during leisure time.
12. Recognize fire and accident hazards and remove them.
13. Obey safety patrol and other traffic signals.
14. Be a skilled bicycle rider.
15. Be a skilled swimmer; know how to fish and use a boat safely; be able to handle a gun for hunting safely.
16. Be skilled in body movements and be able to support their own weight while hanging; be able to jump over objects if necessary, swing across space by ropes, and have the strength, confidence, and courage necessary to do so.
17. Know how to care for and repair their own bicycles, skates, and other play equipment.
18. Ride licensed bicycles and have passed a bicycle rider's safety test.
19. Practice safety precautions while traveling on a bus, train, motor scooter, taxi, or airplane, or when using any other method of travel.

20. Understand the hazards of using matches improperly, firecrackers, guns, etc.
21. Practice safety while on a field trip, camping out, or picnicking.
22. Help members of their own family become more safety-conscious and develop good safety habits.

Found below are suggested teaching units, lesson plans, and other instructional aids for teaching children in grades K to 6 about safety education.

Kindergarten

Objectives
1. To establish the basic safety rules.
2. To establish an awareness of safety in basic activities.

Suggested Approaches
1. Show the movie *Primary Safety in the School Building.*
2. Read the book *Red Light, Green Light.*

Basic Concepts to Teach
1. Walking to and from school
   a. Safe routes
   b. Unsafe routes
2. Bus behavior
3. Playground safety
   a. Behavior
   b. The role of the school nurse

Group Activities
1. Have a safety-patrol member talk to the class
2. Play red light, green light
3. Sing traffic songs
4. Practice hall and drinking fountain safety
5. Use scissors safely in art activities
6. Practice fire drill safety
7. Talk about playing on the ice and in snow in winter and playing safely near the water in the summer

Individual Pupil Activities
1. Have each child learn his name, address, and phone number; play games with this information, such as baseball. You get a home run if you can say all three, first base if you know only your name, etc.
2. Have the students draw pictures of the safe way to school. Help them find the lights and crosswalks to do so.
3. Ask each student with whom he walks to school. Emphasize the importance of walking with a friend.

Correlation With Other Subjects
1. Language Arts
   a. Read stories about policemen, firemen, and doctors.
2. Drama and Art
   a. Make pictures of stoplights and explain their meaning.
   b. Make collages of the proper clothing for activities and time of participation.
   c. Wear white at night.
3. Physical Education
   a. Talk about dressing for activities.
   b. Talk about playground safety.
   c. Play games for inside only, and then those for outside only.

d. Have the children point out the hazards on the playground and have them paint each bright yellow.

e. Have children make up safety rules for the use of each piece of playground equipment.

Pupil References

Burton, Virginia: *Choo Choo.* Boston: Houghton Mifflin Co.

McDonald, Golden: *Red Light, Green Light.* Garden City, N. Y.: Doubleday, Doran & Co., 1969.

Tooze, Ruth: *Tim and the Brass Button.* New York, N. Y.: Julian Messner.

Teacher References

Bauer, W. W., et al.: *Just Like Me.* Glenview, Ill.: Scott, Foresman & Co.

Audio-Visual Aids

Live and Learn	SID
Playground Safety	CORF
Primary Safety: In the School Building	CORF
The Bus Driver	EBF
The Fireman	EBF
Safety to and from School	YAF
Safe Use of Tools	CORF

Evaluation

Can the students walk home without parents?

Do they know their name, address, and phone number when playing games?

Do they know what the different lights mean?

Grade 1

Objectives

1. To reenforce the basic safety rules.
2. To help the child gain an ability to use these rules.

Motivation

1. Show the movie *Safety Can Be Fun.*
2. Have a safety patrol student talk to the class.

Basic Concepts To Teach

1. Crossing Safety
   a. Crosswalks.
   b. Traffic signs and lights.
   c. Crossing between parked cars.
   d. Playing in the streets.
   e. Riding with strangers.
   f. Petting strange dogs.
   g. To hold palm up when approaching a dog, not palm down as if you were going to hit the dog.
2. Playground Safety
   a. Safety in games.
   b. Proper use of equipment (swings and slides, etc.).
3. Car and Bus Safety
   a. Use of seatbelts.
   b. Minimum amount of noise.
4. Home and Classroom Safety
   a. Spills on the floor.
   b. Temperature of tub water.
   c. Toys on the floor and stairs.

Group Activities
1. Visit a police station.
2. Talk about special occasion safety—Halloween, Christmas. Portray what they have discussed in role-playing.
3. Have the school nurse talk about bruises, bumps, scrapes, cuts and what to do in case of dog bite or other accident.

Individual Pupil Activities
1. Make a safety booklet with a story about each traffic sign on the child's way to and from school.
2. Make pictures about playground safety during the different seasons.
3. Make a list of safety hazards in the home.
   a. Playing with fire.
   b. Toys on floor and stairs.
   c. Playing with tools and knives.
   d. Electrical outlets.
   e. Getting up in the night; need of a night light or flashlight.

Correlation With Other Subjects
1. Arithmetic
   a. Count the number of each kind of traffic safety instrument between the students' home and school.
2. Language Arts
   a. Make up a story about policemen, firemen, safety rules, etc.
3. Science
   a. Discuss the care of cuts and bruises. What makes a fire?
4. Drama and Art
   a. Plan a puppet show demonstrating safety rules, role of safety helpers, etc.
5. Physical Education
   a. Play red light, green light. Demonstrate safe use of equipment.

Pupil References
Leaf, Munro: *Safety Can Be Fun.* Rev. ed. Philadelphia: J. B. Lippincott Co., 1962.
Lenski, Lois: *Policeman Small.* New York: Henry Z. Walck, 1968.
McDonald, Golden: *Red Light, Green Light.* Garden City, N. Y.: Doubleday and Co., 1969.

Teacher References
Safety Education Data Sheets: *Matches, Falls, Pedestrian Safety, Play Areas, Playground Apparatus, School Bus Safety, School Fires.* National Safety Council, 425 N. Michigan Ave., Chicago, Ill., 60611.
Yost, Charles P.: "Teaching Safety in the Elementary School." Washington, D. C.: AAHPER, 1969.

Audio-Visual Aids
Fire-Exit Drill at Our School. Coronet Films.
Safely Walk To School; Safety Rules For School; Stop, Look, And Think. Aims.
Safety in the Street. (Filmstrip.) National Film Board of Canada.

Evaluation
1. Can they carry on the fire drills properly?
2. Can they give their name, address, and phone number?
3. Do they fear or trust safety helpers?

Grade 2

Objectives
1. To increase the awareness of the need for safety in daily life.
2. To develop more self-reliance in using safety rules in daily life.

Motivation
1. Do the bicycle safety test presented by the police department.
2. Use fire prevention week activities.

Basic Concepts To Teach
1. Safe routes to school
   a. Walking.
   b. Bus.
   c. Bicycling.
2. Bicycle Safety
   a. Signals.
   b. Where to ride.
   c. Equipment needed for bike safety.
   d. When to ride safely.
3. Fire Safety
   a. Home hazards.
   b. Fire drills: school and home.
   c. Cookouts.
4. Home Safety
   a. Tub water.
   b. Animals and their handling.
   c. Toys and playing safety.
   d. Poisons.

Group Activities
1. Take a bus trip and talk about how to act safely.
   a. Hands and head inside.
   b. Proper boarding.
   c. How to sit safely.
   d. Safe level of noise.
2. Rules to obey in sports and games.
3. Take bicycle test.
4. Talk about the proper care of bikes.
5. Visit public helper departments.
   a. Have them tell the students how to get help when these helpers are needed.
   b. Have the helpers discuss their job.
   c. Include policemen, firemen, postmen, and lifeguards.

Individual Pupil Activities
1. Know the safest route to school.
2. Know your own name, address, and phone number.
3. Make a diagram of home fire drill route.
4. Make pictures of safety hazards in your own home.
5. Make a list of bicycle rules for proper care and safety.

Correlation With Other Subjects
1. Language Arts
   a. Make a story about jobs of the safety helpers after each visit.
2. Social Studies
   a. Study the evolution of the wheel and of bicycles.
   b. Study the different types of bikes.
3. Science
   a. Talk about what makes a fire live and what makes it die.
   b. Do experiments in fire extinction.
4. Drama and Art
   a. Make a booklet showing evolution of bicycles.
   b. Role-playing concerning safety helpers and a lost boy.
   c. Make a booklet of all the traffic signs and signals for bicycle safety.

Pupil References

Miner, Irene: *The True Book of Policemen and Firemen.* Chicago: Children's Press, 1970.

Rey, H. A. and Margaret: *Curious George Rides a Bike.* Boston: Houghton-Mifflin Co., 1971.

Smaridge, Norah: *Watch Out.* Nashville: Abingdon Press, 1969.

Teacher References
    Safety Education Data Sheets: *Matches, Falls, Pedestrian Safety, Play Areas,
    Playground Apparatus, School Bus Safety, School Fires.* National Safety
    Council, 425 N. Michigan Ave., Chicago, Ill. 60611.
    Yost, Charles P.: *Teaching Safety in the Elementary School.* Washington, D.C.:
    AAHPER, 1969.

Audio-Visual Aids
    Bicycle Rules of the Road. Aims Instructional Media Services.
    Playground Safety. Coronet Films.
    Strangers. Sid Davis Productions.

Evaluation
    1. Do they know their hand signals?
    2. Can they obey traffic signs?
    3. Do they know how to care for their cuts, scrapes, and bruises?
    4. Do they know how to handle fire safely?

Additional Films
    Safety With Animals. Garner-Jennings Productions.
    Donald's Fire Survival Plan. Walt Disney Productions.

Grade 3

Main Objectives
    1. Awareness; most accidents are caused by ignorance.
    2. Help students learn ways to help prevent the unnecessary accidents.
    3. A very elementary explanation of first aid, since wrong aid is worse
    than none.

Suggested Approaches
    1. Class explanation with students helping in demonstrations, using
    Show and Tell.
    2. Role playing.
    3. Take field trips.
    4. Show and tell (students relate own safety stories).
    5. Guest speakers (from school personnel, such as nurse or principal).

Major Points To Stress
    1. Playground safety.
    2. Transportation safety (walking, riding cars, bikes, bus).
    3. Keep things out of mouth, ears, and nose (drugs from medicine case,
    sharp objects, beans).
    4. Stay away from strangers going into houses, cars.
    5. Fire, matches, lighters.

Group Activities
    1. Show and tell, where students relate their own safety experiences with
    what the class is discussing, such as water safety.
    2. Draw pictures of different traffic signs; discuss what they mean.
    3. Practice fire, air raid, tornado, and other disaster drills.
    4. Do some simple role playing (especially with one child seeking help)
    of ways to get help in case of an accident.
    5. Have students make bulletin boards.

Individual Activities
    1. Have each student learn his full name, home address, and telephone
    number and the name of his doctor.
    2. Write down where to go in case of emergency (around school facilities)
    such as to the teacher, nurse, etc.
    3. Pass out simple matching test dealing with safety (pictures of a first-aid
    kit, titles such as a nurse, etc.).

Correlation With Other Studies
1. Art and Drama
   a. Pictures and role playing.
2. Reading
   a. Read safety stories, and have them read some.
   With a little imagination, one can improvise into his own daily exercises safety points.

Audio-Visual Aids
Use only films which you have carefully screened.

Teacher References
1. There are innumerable sources for teacher texts; the library is the starting point.
2. Ask other teachers at different schools their advice about books to read.
3. Write the National Safety Council, 425 No. Michigan Ave., Chicago, Illinois, for all kinds of free materials.

Pupil References
1. Bendick, Jeanne: *The Emergency Book.* Glenview, Ill.: Scott, Foresman & Co., 1967. Made to help prepare young people to meet unexpected emergencies.
2. Check school library and public library for recent materials dealing with all types of safety.

Evaluation
1. Be alert, concerned, and intelligent and you will be "aware" of your progress with your class by watching their behavior in situations which call for wise judgment making.

Grade 4

Main Objectives
1. Help students to learn major first-aid techniques.
2. Broaden "awareness" and stress prevention.
3. Make students aware that all injuries can end up as major ones if they do not take care of them, have first aid or medical treatment, if needed.

Suggested Approaches
1. Bulletin boards made by students.
2. Class walks off school grounds to observe safety hazards.
3. Group presentations of various facets of safety.
4. Demonstrations of first-aid techniques.
5. Guest speakers from the community.

Major Points To Stress
1. Bicycle safety.
2. Playground safety (playground leadership).
3. Water safety (use of the buddy system).
4. Drug abuse and dangers of self-medication.

Group Activities
1. Organize class into groups to give demonstrations dealing with some safety hazard and what to do in case of emergency.
2. Have the class arrange a safety board with all bringing in articles and pictures dealing with recent hazards and modern modes of preventing them.

Individual Activities
1. Have students list hazards around school or home.
2. Each student draw one picture displaying many safety signs, items, etc.

3. Have students discuss safety on minibikes and other motor-powered vehicles that children ride, such as go-carts.
4. Have pupils discuss vacation experiences and hazards they noticed at those spots.

Correlation With Other Subjects
1. Art and Drama
   a. Drawings and role playing dealing with safety aspects.
2. Reading
   a. Read and make oral and/or written reports on common and uncommon safety problems.
3. Spelling
   a. Tie spelling into safety education.

Audio-Visual Aids
Screen all films you use carefully.

Teacher References
Health Readers, Glenview, Ill.: Scott, Foresman and Co., 1971.
Contact local fire and police stations for pamphlets and sources of other safety information.
Write National Safety Council, Chicago, Illionis for materials for this grade level.

Pupil References
Bendick, Jeanne: *The Emergency Book.* Glenview, Ill.: Scott, Foresman & Co., 1967. Deals with children and their encounter with emergencies.
By keeping in touch with school librarian, find good recent material which ties in with your present teaching.

Evaluation
1. Be alert on playground, as this is where most students will make it apparent whether they are aware of safety rules.
2. Classroom activities will also reveal students' ability to deal with safety mishaps.
3. Let students demonstrate simple first-aid techniques they have learned in class.

Grade 5

Objectives
1. To help students identify and avoid the causes of minor accidents.
2. To help the student know what to do in case of minor accidents.
3. To teach the student simple first aid for the treatment of minor cuts, bruises, and burns.
4. To teach the students basic rules of safety while using bicycle and loading and unloading.

Suggested Approaches
1. Bulletin boards.
2. Demonstrations.
3. Guest speakers (fire marshal, police officer).
4. Role playing.
5. Field trips (how to cross streets while on a bicycle, motor bike, or in a car). If possible, visit the emergency room in a local hospital.

Points To Stress
1. All pointed objects should be handled with care.
2. Children should never start a fire without adult help.
3. To be safe, children should ask an adult to administer medicine to them.
4. Children should swim only in places where a lifeguard is on duty.

Group Activities
1. Have fire drills so students can react to the situation, if it arises.
2. Fix a bulletin board of things to look for at home for fire hazards, bad wiring, etc.
3. Have a group or committee prepare a bulletin board showing bicycle outline with main parts and safety rule outline.
4. As a group prepare a list of safety rules for getting on and off the school bus.
5. Let students look around school for fire hazards or places which might cause injury to someone.

Individual Activities
1. Each student prepares a written report on bicycle safety.
2. Pupils conduct a survey to note traffic violations of bicycles to and from school.
3. Have pupils make drawings of ways to prevent fires.
4. Make a card for home use listing telephone number of fire and police departments, family doctor, nearest relative to call in case of an accident, etc.
5. Report on causes and results of home accidents that involved relatives or close friends within the last year.
6. Prepare list of foods, clothing, medicine, and equipment needed for an emergency.

Correlation With Other Subjects
1. Art
   a. Have students draw up a plan of grounds and buildings, pointing out areas considered unsafe.
2. Drama
   a. Dramatize action in case of an emergency; have one student dramatize basic first aid and another the behavior of an observer.
   b. Prepare skit of things not to do while boating, riding a bicycle, or in a car.

Audio-Visual Aids
National Safety Council.
Let's Be Safe At Home. McGraw-Hill, Text Film Division.

Teacher References
"Let's Be At Home in the Water." (leaflet). Minneapolis: Minneapolis Imagination.
"Let's Talk About Fire." (booklet) Chicago: National Board of Fire Underwriters, 1970.
"Ten Little Swimmers." (leaflet) New York: McGraw-Hill Book Co., Text Division.
American Society of Safety Engineers, 5 North Wabash Avenue, Chicago, Illinois 60602.

Pupil References
Richmond, Julius, Pounds, Elenore, Fricke, Irma, and Sussforf, Dieter: *Health and Growth Today.* Grade 5. Glenview, Ill.: Scott, Foresman and Co., 1971.
"Ten Little Children." (leaflet) Chicago: National Safety Council, 1971.

Evaluation
1. Watch how children conduct themselves in fire drill.
2. Watch children coming to and leaving school to see that they conduct themselves according to safety rules.
3. Safety rules test and quiz.

Grade 6

Objectives
1. What to do in case of emergencies.

2. Type of first aid you would give under certain conditions for different types of injuries.
3. Teach the students ways to avoid accidents.
4. Teach guides for safety at play and home.

Suggested Approaches
1. Guest speakers.
2. Field trips.
3. Bulletin boards showing: bicycle safety; fire safety; disasters (how to react and prepare); bus safety while riding, loading, and unloading; different types of injuries (burns, cuts, scratches, bruises, etc.).
4. Demonstrations.

Basic Concepts
1. Know how to react under pressure when accidents occur by acting out accidents causing injuries.
2. Appropriate dress for safety in play activities at school and home.
3. Gain knowledge of how to choose an area to play in for safety.
4. How to treat small cuts or scratches, mild burns, blisters, small bruises, nosebleeds.
5. What to do in case of emergencies: severe bleeding, broken bone, fainting, swallowing of poison by child, choking.

Group Activities
1. Have a guest speaker from police or fire department.
2. Have class discussion of correct clothes to wear while playing games and doing certain things at home and school.
3. Have class check the playground area for glass, rocks, and other harmful things which might cause injury.
4. Discuss the responsibilities of pedestrians on highways.
5. Learn the meaning of the various civil defense signals.
6. Plan a first-aid kit for home, automobile, camping, or biking.

Individual Activities
1. Have students make a list of the things your school does to help prevent accidents in the gym and on playground.
2. Write a short paragraph about a sport accident you had and how it could have been avoided.
3. Have students get the telephone numbers of all places where they think help might be obtained in case of emergencies (police, fire station, doctor).
4. Have students pair off to show ways of doing artificial respiration.
5. Have students collect newspaper articles on accidents, then discuss first-aid procedures that might have been used in each situation.

Correlation With Other Subjects
1. Drama
   a. Give skits to show what to do in case of severe bleeding.
2. Physical Education
   a. Have students run full-speed and see how long it takes them to stop safely (without pulling muscles, etc.).
   b. Measure how far bases should be from walls and fences.
3. Art
   a. Have students draw and label bicycle with all safety measures on it.
4. Language
   a. Using letters of his first name, have each student write traffic safety ideas, sports safety guides or other safety rules. Example: Dave— Do not throw bat in softball. Students can be creative and on their own.

Pupil References
Health and Growth. Grade 6. Glenview, Ill.: Scott, Foresman and Co., 1971.

"Safety Education." (booklet) Chicago: National Safety Council. Textbook *Health 6*—Byrd, Nielson, Moon. 1969.

Teacher References
   Health and Growth. Grade 6. Glenview, Ill.: Scott, Foresman and Co., 1971.
   Elementary Education. Grades 4–6 (Curriculum Guide). Dallas, Texas: Dallas Independent School District, 1964.
   Textbook *Health 6*—Byrd, Nielson, Moore. 1969.
   "These Are Your Children." (booklet) National Advisory Council on Child Growth and Safety, 1971.

Evaluation
   1. Give a test to see how much students know about various aspects of safety (fill-in-blank type)
   2. Let pupils show how to bandage injuries and do artificial respiration before class.
   3. Watch the behavior of class to learn if they are being safe at play and in the classroom.

CHAPTER 14

mental health

About 400 out of every 100,000 children under 18 years of age require psychiatric care as out-patients yearly.[1] These shocking figures are due to many reasons including poverty, overcrowding, social upheaval, and school busing in which children are being forced to move from their familiar environment to an often hostile, emotionally harmful, and ego-disintegrating one.

Our schools are full of socially disadvantaged children who suffer from parental neglect whether they come from poor, middle-class, or rich economic backgrounds. All children who are emotionally disturbed and have serious behavior problems need to be helped early in their development if they are to receive the greatest benefits from assistance. The school is second to the family as the most important unit in society affecting the mental health and behavior of children. Therefore, it must provide both a greatly improved and increased preventive and corrective program in the area of mental health.

The mentally healthy person is one who enjoys life, is on good terms with himself and other people in his environment, and can work and play well with others. Children who receive love and acceptance, feel secure, can control their emotions, show consistency in behavior patterns, can be intellectually stimulated, adjust to failure, accept success as something earned rather than automatically received, are reasonably independent for their age, and have a sense of values and a faith in a Creator are not only mentally healthy but possess a strong foundation upon which a happy, productive adulthood can later be built. All children need to receive as

---

[1] Willgoose, Carl: *Health Education in the Elementary School*. 4th ed. Philadelphia, W. B. Saunders Co., 1974, p. 9.

well as give love. Every child has the right to receive from his teachers at least three "A's" throughout his entire educational experiences in schools—affection, acceptance, and achievement. Some, unfortunately, are neither wanted nor accepted by their own parents. These children especially need to be in the class of a friendly teacher who cares about them and their well-being. Recognition and praise both are tremendous motivators among youth, but if used too much will lose effectiveness and even cause children to gain an inflated concept of themselves. All children need to feel that they belong to a closely knit class group, even though some few seemingly never have that feeling. Since youngsters are brutally frank and often cruel to each other, they early discover weaker classmates who can easily be run over and become their victims. It is the teacher's duty to observe class behavior closely for signs of such treatment and put a stop to such practices at once. Such minor negative actions, if ignored, can snowball quickly and soon get out of hand; they may even cause permanent damage to the poor victim. Every child also needs to be controlled and guided by a firm, strict, consistent, but friendly teacher who sets behavior boundaries and sees to it that they are not crossed; inconsistency and too much freedom cause children to become fearful and feel insecure, and can retard progress in school.

The teacher who is aware of the facts concerning mental health can do much to recognize symptoms and eradicate causes of emotional maladjustment. The following behaviors *when occurring very frequently* may be symptoms of an emotional or physical health problem. Before conferring with the principal, the teacher would find it helpful to have a record of specific incidents, settings, and steps taken to correct the problem.

BEHAVIOR	WAYS TO HELP
Provocative Behavior	
The pupil	The teacher should
Tattles	Be alert to clues of causes.
Talks back	Remember . . .
Is snobbish	Don't take it personally. The pupil is
Is untidy	talking back to trouble, not to the
Shows destructive leadership	teacher.
Complains frequently of being "picked on"	Events, little and big, piling up in the pupil's past make it difficult for him
Resists authority	to grow with stability and order.
Insecure Behavior	
The pupil	The teacher should
Clings to teacher	Notice the pupil and show this recognition by a smile or remark.
Is timid	
Is seclusive	Praise the pupil or his work.
Is overly fearful	Choose the pupil for special tasks.
Cheats	Catch the pupil's eye.
Does not play fair	Work with the pupil.
Is unwilling to participate in activities in which he may lose	Call upon the pupil for specific work.
Boasts	
Has easily hurt feelings	
Shows extreme desire to please	

Motor Disturbances

The pupil
  Has tics
  Bites fingernails
  Sucks lips
  Grimaces
  Stutters
  Shows undue restlessness

The teacher should
  Watch for times of strain or stress and try to reduce them.
  "Stand by" the pupil until he feels more sure of himself.
  Correct the pupil less and praise him more.
  Guide the pupil into more quiet activities until he builds up reserves within himself

Withdrawn Behavior

The pupil
  Daydreams
  Is inattentive
  Uses illness as an escape
  Plays hooky
  Is apathetic
  Lacks interest
  Doodles
  Is nonparticipating

The teacher should
  Help the pupil feel at ease.
  Encourage the pupil.
  Give recognition to the pupil or to his work in the presence of other children.
  Interest the pupil in new avenues of expression.
  Teach the pupil a skill in which he may excel.
  Help the pupil feel better about himself, such as suggestions about improvements in his appearance and grooming.
  Recommend a health examination.
  Plan committee work and include the pupil in the group.
  Encourage friendship with another pupil.

Aggressive Behavior

The pupil
  Is overactive
  Is mischievous
  Has temper outbursts
  Fights
  Steals
  Is rivalrous and quarrelsome

The teacher should
  Show the pupil safe and acceptable ways to exert his energy.

Attention-getting Behavior

The pupil
  Is competitive in school work
  Shows off
  Clowns
  Interrupts

The teacher should
  Give the pupil a "place in the sun."
  Discover the pupil's interests.
  Speak about the pupil's possessions.
  Help the pupil attain a specific skill.
  Compliment the pupil for any improvements.[2]

---

[2] Reproduced by permission from *Health in the Elementary Schools—An Instructional Guide*, Los Angeles Public Schools, 1971, pp. 288–289.

Every experience a child has affects him to some degree, and serves to make him inwardly stronger or weaker, confident in his ability to solve his own problems or a "scaredy cat" who withdraws from social contacts. His experiences, like blocks piled on top of each other, can make him upright, wobbly, or can finally push him over. Seldom, it is claimed by psychiatrists, can one incident have a lasting damaging effect upon the emotions of a child, unless it be a traumatic one, such as the death of his parents. Yet constant tension, pressure, fear, anger, and hatred have a strong lasting influence not only upon a child's present behavior but also upon his future well-being. Some experiences which may prevent normal growth and might contribute to mental illness are:

Lack of parental affection.
Overprotection of parents.
Failure of adults to accept normal childish behavior.
The frustration of being constantly faced with expectations, standards, or
    ideals which cannot be achieved.
Few opportunities in childhood to associate freely with other children.
Unrealistic viewpoint of many adults toward normal sexuality in life.
Frequent experiences of hostility from adults, particularly parents.
Insecurity, because of economic factors and attitudes of others to economic
    background.
Attitudes of others toward uniqueness in appearance, intelligence, dress, etc.
Poor nutritional status.
Glandular disorders.
Prolonged or frequent illness of the child or his parents.
Separations, including divorce.
Death of a parent.
Membership in a minority group.
Placement away from home.
Membership in a migratory family

Although a child's basic behavior patterns have been largely set by the time that he enters the first grade, this does not mean that his personality cannot change. Certainly, the school can and should guide, direct, and mold youth into developing socially accepted actions and values, as well as provide boys and girls with many opportunities to rid themselves of their feelings of guilt, hostility, fear, and aggression in legitimate ways. Although behavior cannot be changed overnight, the daily contributions made by a teacher who really cares about any particular pupil can in the long run be of major importance and serve to steady an emotionally wobbly child.

Psychologists say that learning to live with other people is a major life task. Those who best fit into and contribute to worthwhile group endeavor are those who are independent, sure of themselves, dependable, and capable of producing something of value for the benefit of all. Such people are mature and have a clear, realistic view of themselves. They are the balanced ones who have their basic psychological needs satisfied as growing children to the degree that their physical-emotional growth becomes consistent and normal. All school experiences, whether they occur in the classroom, in the hall, or on the playground, can promote or retard growth toward maturity. Actually, positive experiences which take place at school can do much more to develop emotional well-being and mental health than any instructional unit can do. Likewise, the relationship, rapport, and interplay between the teacher and the pupil are vastly more important than many lessons which stress the importance of freedom from worry or other simliar topics. Every instructor should realize that her "actions, indeed, speak louder than words" and, in order to foster good mental health among her pupils, she must "practice what she preaches" about the worth of *every* human being. Likewise, each teacher must accept each child as he is, not as she would like him to be. She must also realize (1) that all behavior is *caused* and is *understandable* to any child-sensitized educator, and (2) that her attitudes and actions toward children and other adults must serve as a model.

Children do grow, in spite of our fearful concern that they never will get over what some oldsters refer to as "a child's fool's hill." Because of admired adults who love and believe in them, young people can be helped to become not just children who have grown older, taller, and heavier but wisely educated, happy, and mature people. Educators must remember that children are not miniature adults but children who must grow into adulthood.

Direct instruction in mental health should be coupled with numerous opportunities for children to explore, develop, and practice social skills. Freedom of movement, approval for expressing oneself, opportunities to be boisterous and let off steam, frequent changes of activities, and a wide variety of problem-solving experiences can all help children in their search for and struggles toward maturity. The difference between childhood and adulthood is that between becoming and being. To grow up or become a mature person is for many children a long, arduous, and often painful task, in which the right teacher at the right place in their development who does the right things can play a major role.

SUGGESTED GRADED TOPICS

Suggested graded topics for instruction in mental hygiene are:

GRADE 1
1. How to be a friend.
2. Our classmates as friends.
3. Helping each other and our parents.
4. Talking things over with adults.
5. Our feelings.
6. Rules and why we should obey them.
7. Good health practices.

GRADE 2
1. Our emotions and how to control them.
2. Working and playing together.
3. Learning to be a good sport.
4. How to accept sadness and disappointment.
5. How to have others like you.
6. How our bodies show how we feel.
7. What to do about angry feelings.
8. Good health practices.

GRADE 3
1. Our actions and how to control them.
2. How to cooperate with others.

3. How our emotions can help or hinder us.
4. Developing good physical and emotional health habits.
5. Using time wisely for our own good.
6. How our body works and rests.
7. How to be a good leader and follower.

GRADE 4

1. Self-discipline.
2. How to express and control our feelings.
3. The correct name and function of bodily organs.
4. The role of parents and children in the family.
5. Ways to acquire new friends.
6. How to be considerate of those who wear correctional aids such as glasses, braces, or crutches.
7. The effect of stress and tension on the body.
8. Mental health and how to achieve it.

GRADE 5

1. Basic needs of all people.
2. Importance of self-acceptance.
3. Respecting the beliefs and rights of others.
4. How to solve personal problems.
5. Importance of attending church.
6. The nervous system.
7. How our brain and emotions function.
8. Why we act as we do.
9. Self-reliance and courage.

GRADE 6

1. How to be attractive and popular.
2. Importance of good health practices and grooming.
3. How to grow up successfully.
4. Solving individual and group behavior problems.
5. How to recognize the strengths, weaknesses, and capabilities of ourself and others.
6. Social habits, courtesy, and good manners.
7. Boy-and-girl relationships.
8. How we learn and think.
9. Emotions and their regulators.
10. Individual differences.
11. Behavior disorders.
12. The effect of alcohol, tranquilizers and other drugs, tobacco, and narcotics upon the body and behavior.
13. Mental health habits.

CURRICULUM PLACEMENT

Regardless of where instruction in mental health occurs in the school curriculum, and whether it is a part of a core, broad-fields, or any other curricular plan, materials covered in this area and learning experiences conducted around them are of little value if the day-to-day relationships between teacher and child, pupil and classmates, are strained and full of tension and frustrating fear. The child is the total product of the home, school, and playground. Each boy and girl needs help in learning how to solve his own unique personal problems as well as assistance in developing steady qualities which will ensure his successful adoption to his own ever-changing self and environment.

Studies show that teachers who possess the best mental health themselves have the most stable pupils. Research also discloses that the actions, attitudes, and behavior of the teacher have a marked effect on the pupils' sense of security, freedom from tension, courtesy, resourcefulness, and methods used for obtaining social recognition.[3] It is imperative, then, that the teacher set the example in her relationship with others and that her own conduct be worthy of emulation. Since the classroom is where the child spends most of his time when away from home, this must be a place wherein he is accepted and assisted as an individual and as a group member.

There are many ways in which mental health education can be integrated and correlated with other subjects in the school curriculum. These include the following:

Social Science

Social science is especially well suited for integrating mental health with history, civics, geography, and in other included areas. Actually, almost every daily classroom experience provides pupils with opportunities for personality interaction, whether these be when pupils are discussing problems, engaged in group planning, or working on committees. Every teacher with insight and concern for the rights and well-being of each individual child, will utilize every moment which arises for promoting good mental health as the pupils work and play together.

The following topics can be used for correlating and integrating mental health with social science:

1. Living in an urban versus a rural community.
2. Housing problems.
3. Cause and prevention of juvenile delinquency and crime.
4. Unemployment and its effect upon morale.
5. The reactions of people in wartime and peacetime.
6. The prevention and treatment of mental illness.
7. The effect of economic conditions upon health.
8. The functions and programs of voluntary health agencies.
9. Relation of labor laws to health.
10. The recreational, educational, and work patterns of early Americans or other civilizations in contrast to those of today.
11. Changing patterns of the role of men, women, and children in society.
12. Proper use of recreational facilities.
13. Citizenship and civic responsibilities.
14. The influence of the space age upon health.
15. The conservation of human resources.
16. Local and state resources for mental health.
17. Understanding the problems of the aged.
18. Minority groups and their problems.
19. Youth in other lands.

The Communicative Arts

Reading, writing, and speaking should provide children with numerous opportunities to learn more about themselves and other people, places, and things. Each classroom activity, whether it be reading a book about a famous health hero, writing a short paper on such a topic as "My Happiest Experience," or taking part

---

[3] Oberteuffer, Delbert: *School Health Education.* 5th ed. New York: Harper & Row, 1972, p. 363.

on a panel and speaking on the subject, "Health Careers and Health Workers in Our Community," should have the purpose of helping each pupil develop as an emotionally healthy individual and group member. Likewise, each activity selected by the pupil or assigned to him by the teacher, who wishes to correlate instruction in mental health with that in the communicative arts, should aid in the emotional development of that child from:

Dependence toward independence.
Being a receiver toward becoming a giver.
Self-centeredness toward socialization.
Ignorance and fantasy toward recognition and acceptance of reality.
Aggressive hostile actions toward self-satisfying activities.
Feelings of inadequacy, fear, and timidity toward realistic self-confidence.

The following suggested activities can help youngsters grow closer to maturity:

1. Provide children with a wide variety of opportunities to share experiences and stories in daily "show-and-tell" sessions. Encourage all to speak freely and bring things to share with others. Talk less and listen more as a teacher, remembering that actions can speak louder than words and people "tell on themselves" by what they do, just as much as by what they say.
2. Encourage individuality and creativity, as well as needed group conformity for the benefit of all by providing a variety of individual, small group, as well as class projects.
3. Use teacher-pupil planning as much as possible in all learning activities.
4. Give children opportunities to show their work to teachers, parents, and other schoolmates through displays, demonstrations, shows, or other means. Be sure that every child takes part, not only the best ones.
5. Provide many opportunities for children to be leaders and helpers. Help them learn to recognize the characteristics and techniques of democratic leadership; teach them how to elect their own leaders wisely.
6. Use praise for work done well. Talk individually with those who seemingly are kinder and more sensitive than others, letting them know how valuable such qualities are and how glad you are that each has these qualities. Such praise helps children by bolstering their desire to continue being the type of person a respected teacher admires.
7. Have a "high degree of expectancy" in each child and help him select tasks which will bring success, challenge, and individual growth. Help children realize that mistakes are a vital part of learning.
8. Discuss the necessity of having rules or laws. Help the class select a class motto, such as "One for all, and all for one," etc. Keep this in plain view of the group. Refer to it often, so that the motto becomes part of a foundation on which other life values can be built. Draw out the group through discussion as to individual and class progress toward reaching this ideal.

Other ways in which mental hygiene can be integrated and correlated with materials covered in the communicative arts are:

1. Let children read widely stories of their own choosing which stress courage as found in the actions of heroes, heroines, or animals. Have each tell his favorite story to the class and make a tape recording of this class experience.
2. Write letters or visit ill classmates or friendless, hospitalized adults.
3. Provide numerous opportunities for small group projects; rotate group membership frequently and assist each pupil to widen his circle of friends.

4. Give an oral book report on any courageous person you have read about.
5. Give an oral or written book report on any hero or heroine story read or told by a family member. Give reasons why the main character is to be admired.
6. Give a situation test to evaluate each pupil's ability to face reality by telling the class a story about a boy or girl who worked hard and wanted to be chosen for the main part in a school play, but who was not. Have them write down the suggestions they would give to this person.
7. Write a poem about why we should be considerate of those who are in wheelchairs, wear a brace, walk with a crutch, etc.
8. Draw up a class-devised good grooming checklist. Have each child write a short paragraph periodically about the progress he has made in developing good grooming habits.
9. Have the class make a typical individual day schedule. Counsel with each pupil, discussing the need to be alone sometimes, time spent in self-care, etc.
10. Prepare questions for a question box on any aspect of health, going on to junior high school, or any life experience the children have or might have.
11. Choose any trait of character any adult has. Write a story or play about it. Have the class draw their conclusions and list desirable character traits to have.
12. Write a short story about the meaning of the phrase "a sense of values."
13. Have the pupils write a paper on how they would spend a thousand dollars won in a contest. Arrange a sample of budget items, saying that so much should go for gifts, a trip, college, or other future plans, etc. Read this report carefully in order to detect if the class is developing a good sense of values.

Mathematics

Suggested activities for closely integrating and correlating mathematics with mental health are as follows:

1. Making graphs to show the rising cost and incident of crime and delinquency.
2. Determining the cost of mental illness to the family, community, state, and nation.
3. Showing by graphs the reported income from the sale of alcohol, narcotics, and tranquilizers in contrast to that spent on public education.
4. Discovering the amount of money spent in America on passive types of recreation such as movie-going, watching television, or attending football games.
5. Making pie graphs to show how much of the community's budget is spent on health and medical care; how much on safety protection for its citizens.
6. Determining the amount of money spent yearly by the nation on cosmetics or medication.
7. Comparing advertising costs on sleeping pills or other such articles to net profits and benefits to the individual.

Physical Education

Like music and art activities, physical education can also be well correlated and integrated with mental health by providing pupils with opportunities to (1) learn recreative skills with high carry-over value into adult life, (2) belong to a group and obtain status, and (3) participate in free, joyous activities which help them express their inner feelings. The greatest values found in physical education are in developing physical fitness, increasing movement skills, socializing the pupil, creating improved mental and physical health, and increasing knowledge of and appreciation for one's own body, its care, protection, and development. Like the two sides of a coin, a sound mind and a sound body are inseparable, and the health of one, or lack of it, affects the health of the other. Total fitness, physical, mental, and emotional, cannot be stored away for future use, like money or food, but must be maintained when once acquired, and replaced when used.

One of the greatest values of sports and games is in socializing the individual who, as a group member engaged in team effort, contributes and cooperates by substituting the finer "we" drives for selfish "I" drives. Through winning and losing one learns the give and take of life, the necessity of obeying and behaving according to rules, and being a good sport. It is when playing on a team that many of the techniques for successful group life, both for now and for future, are best learned. It is here that good followers and leaders can be made. It is then also when a fuller understanding of our American way of life, our cultural values of "all for one and one for all," "where there is unity there is strength," or "unite or perish," is gained.

Games and modified sports for children also give them chances to work out feelings of hostility and aggression in legitimate ways, such as hitting a ball with a bat, or "destroying" an opponent by tagging him out. Such activities as learning to take turns and playing games without a referee help a child gain friends, self-respect, and develop habits of independence and truthfulness. Just as a good teacher, like a wise parent, becomes progressively unnecessary, children will not automatically become self-controlled or mature in their behavior unless they have chances to experiment and learn how to become so.

How a child learns to spend his leisure time is vastly important to himself as well as to his civilization, for leisure time offers rich opportunities which, when rightly used, can benefit us all. Leisure can be spent in positive or negative ways. The former are made up of those activities which benefit each person and society, the latter are detrimental to the individual and the group. Playing on a kickball team can be as highly beneficial as robbing a store is detrimental. Both activities contain the same basic elements of trying to get away without getting caught. Since children seek adventure, they will find it. Because of teachers, their parents, and some few other adults, what they seek and discover can be of the highest value according to society's preconceived social standards of what is "good" or "bad."

Science

Science with its many facts can assist children in learning much about the many mysteries and wonders of their own bodies, as well as help them gain insight into their own behavior and that of others. The pupils should learn about the basic life processes of circulation, respiration, digestion, excretion, metabolism, movement control, and human reproduction, so that they can increasingly make more intelligent choices regarding their own health. Likewise, they should become aware of the psychosocial basic needs of all people to belong, be loved, have self-respect, and obtain recognition.

USE OF TEACHING METHODS

Among the many kinds of teaching methods which can be used successfully in mental health education are:

Class Discussions

Elementary pupils often express themselves more frankly and honestly than older students, thus making it easier for their teachers to gain insight into their behavior, feelings, and emotional needs. Care must be taken not to "pry" into the personal lives of each family member, for these younger pupils often unknowingly reveal family secrets without realizing that they have done so.

Suggested topics for class discussions might well include the following:

1. Homesickness.
2. Fear of competitive games.
3. Wanting to play and being alone.
4. Dislike of the opposite sex.
5. Stealing, cheating, and lying.
6. Temper flare-ups.
7. Poor sportsmanship.
8. Cruelty to others and to animals.
9. Inability to make decisions.
10. Dependence upon others for praise and attention.
11. Daydreaming and absent-mindedness.
12. Fear.
13. Feelings of inferiority and inhibition.[4]

Problem Solving

This teaching method is especially well adapted to the field of mental health. Although primary children have seemingly small individual and group problems, these can become larger learning and developmental stumbling blocks if ignored or neglected. Numerous moments for instruction arise in every class situation, whether it be one of masturbation or of stealing. As children learn to share limited materials, organize a club, or work together making a survey, they are learning to solve their own basic problems of how to get along well with others, and the give and take of life.

Upper elementary pupils will profit from studying larger group problems and areas such as learning why human beings become mentally ill, are prejudiced, or fail in life. Often current events, such as reading about the United Nations or a summit meeting, can help motivate student interest in determining which of these many larger problems of life they should learn more about. Regardless of what problem areas are selected, however, the teacher should help each pupil, through these learning experiences, to gain more insight and a better understanding of himself.

Frequently, problems arise in the extracurricular school program which can be brought into the classroom for study, such as boys clustering together like scared rabbits at a school party and refusing to dance with girls. Even those events which occur outside of school but which cause children to be unhappy at school and frustrated in their learning attempts can become problems for a class to study and solve. The following incident was reported by an elementary education major preparing to become a teacher. When asked to record her most memorable learning experience in grade school, she wrote:

> When I was in the fifth grade, I unknowingly almost caused a riot in our school. I shared with a sixth-grader a "secret" told to me by one of my

---

4 Oberteuffer, *op. cit.*, p. 165.

classmates. A distorted version of it spread throughout the entire school. My friends deserted me. The kids took sides, and called certain people, including me, "a dirty liar." The boys and girls took sides, and even several serious fights occurred. Finally, the principal called us all down to the auditorium. He talked to us for a long time, trying to find out what was behind all of this trouble. He made me understand that I was wrong to have told a secret, and that the class had made a serious mistake by magnifying and distorting it. He then asked us to go back to our classroom and work out an answer to our big problem of how to get along and work together better and in harmony as a class. We all were frightened but determined not to fight among ourselves any more. Our teacher helped us work out the answer to our problem, but it took a long time. I was miserable all during that year at school; my grades were terrible, and the poorest I have ever made in school before or since then![5]

Guidance and Counseling

Every teacher has a responsibility not only to help children become healthy, happy, and successful learners, but also to provide them with wholesome and meaningful educational experiences. Emphasis should be placed upon helping children develop proper attitudes, values, conduct, and appreciation. The teacher should not only set the example children will want to copy, but she should help them develop a respect for the rights and opinions of others, develop skills in learning to control their own behavior, become good leaders and followers, and learn to use their leisure time constructively. Children do not change in behavior overnight, and no teacher, regardless of her skill and understanding, can make any pupil over in a few months, for each has been developing behavior patterns for several years which cannot easily be changed or eradicated. Since misbehavior is usually a question of degree, and is not serious unless it interferes with a child's social, emotional, and physical growth, the role of the teacher working within the area of guidance and counseling should be to help the child determine reasons for his misbehavior. Regardless of whether the problem may be one of showing off, bullying, stealing, disobedience, or using dirty words, the following principles should help those dealing with misbehavior:

1. All behavior is caused; atypical actions occur when basic human needs or drives clash.
2. Each human being is unique; therefore a method that works with one child may not necessarily be successful with another.
3. When children are engaged in activities they have selected to do and when they have a feeling of taking part in that activity, they are less likely to develop problems.
4. Behavior changes can only occur slowly; each child must be patiently aided to learn to help himself and to solve his own problems.

When teaching children in learning, working, and playing, the best results will be obtained if the following suggestions are kept in mind:

1. Always be fair, considerate, and show a genuine liking for all children.
2. Avoid showing favoritism, even though some children attract you more than others.

---

[5] Reported in the class, "Teaching Health and Physical Education in Elementary Schools," Southern Methodist University, June 1961.

3. Be sympathetic and understanding of children's problems, even though the difficulty may seem absurd, unimportant, and small from the adult viewpoint.
4. Avoid being shocked at a child's actions; seek the reason behind them.
5. Give each child a genuine feeling of belonging, security, and achievement.
6. Give each child increased opportunities to assume responsibilities of real worth.
7. Remember that every human being reacts favorably to praise.
8. Become more sensitized to children—their hopes, fears, and ambitions.

Ullman has identified children with serious problems which need the attention of a psychologist, personal counselor, physician, or all three.

1. Frequent absences, tardiness, and inattention in school.
2. Nervousness, irritability.
3. Lying, cheating, evasiveness, shiftiness.
4. Fearsome, withdrawing, overly shy behavior; lack of confidence.
5. Bullying, selfishness, overaggressiveness, quarreling.
6. Dawdling, time wasting, lack of purpose.
7. Unacceptable sexual conduct, "mashing," overinterest in the opposite sex.
8. Noncooperation and negativeness.[6]

Although most teachers are not prepared to deal with such problems or such children, help should be found for these individuals. Many large school systems now have the services of a school psychologist or psychiatrist, and most large cities have child guidance clinics. The teachers of pupils who are referred to such specialists should work closely with them. Every attempt should be made to keep the child in school, even though this may require the adjustment of his schedule, closer supervision, and additional, more personalized, and patient understanding. Many of the problem children who are "kicked out of school" are harmed greatly by this action, for many of them are already burdened by their inability to belong and be accepted by the group, and this final act of rejection only helps them to become more maladjusted, and often even more delinquent in their actions. The "kicked-out" youngster too often, then, becomes "kicked into" more serious trouble.

Demonstrations

The use of this teaching method can assist children to see, hear, and take part in many kinds of splendid educational experiences in the area of mental health. Suggested activities suitable for demonstration purposes are:

1. Demonstrate ways in which feelings of anger, hostility, etc., can quickly get out of hand; how to keep emotions well under control.
2. Demonstrate a wide variety of movements for relaxation, such as how to be as limp as a rag doll, float with your eyes closed while stretched out on the floor, stand on your toes and pick fireflies from the ceiling, etc.
3. Demonstrate the techniques of good grooming.
4. Demonstrate role playing in couples: ordering a meal in a restaurant; walking together to school; dancing together at a party; going to a movie.

[6] Ullman, Charles: "Identification of Maladjusted School Children," *Public Health Monograph* No. 7. Washington, D.C.: Public Health Services Publication No. 2111, 1952, p. 72.

5. Demonstrate childish and mature behavior in the classroom and in the playground. Discuss how pupils can act in mature ways.
6. Demonstrate by using a cutaway model how each part of the human brain functions.

Dramatic Activities

Role playing, puppet shows, one-act plays, charades, story telling, and shadow plays can be used in the following ways to help pupils learn much in the area of mental health:

1. Make a class sociogram, keep a running leadership list, and see that each child becomes a leader or helper periodically. Stress the importance of dependability and being a good follower. Act out the difference between being a good and "bossy" leader.
2. Give a talent show, using all pupils, to some outside group. Evaluate the results with the class, using the approach of "how could we have done this better."
3. Have each pupil give, in charade form or verbal description, ways in which he is learning how to make wiser decisions and choices.
4. Dramatize a happy family sharing several experiences in and away from their home.
5. Act out your most embarrassing moment, and describe how you got out of it.
6. Give puppet shows showing the difference between good humor or clean fun and harmful practical jokes.
7. Divide into subgroups and create a clown act or animated cartoon. Discuss the value of laughter and fun in life.
8. Use role playing of problems commonly found in everyday human relationships at home or school.

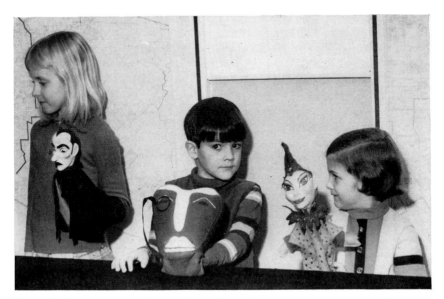

Figure 14-1. Puppets are fun to make and use. They can also correlate health education with the language arts if the children write and perform original puppet plays. (Courtesy of Dallas Health and Science Museum)

9. Have subgroups give puppet shows, playlets, or act out in pantomime how fear can be a means both of protection and of damage to a person; the harm that prejudice can do, etc.
10. Have children tell about their favorite adult neighborhood friends, and describe why they chose to tell about these adults. Make a list and discuss the qualities these respected adults possess.

Field Trips

There are many places the children can go on field trips within their community to learn from first-hand experiences more about mental health. Visits taken to such places as a kindergarten, day-care center, sheltered workshop for the handicapped and disabled, home for the aged, health museum, zoo, public library, traffic court, and baby clinic will broaden their understanding of other people, places, and problems in their own community. The maturity level, interest, and intellectual background of the class should be the determining factor in selecting which of these places can be profitably visited.

THE USE OF INSTRUCTIONAL MATERIALS

Throughout the school year, the teacher should observe the changes in behavior made by each pupil in his attitude toward himself, other pupils and adults, life in general, and his school work in particular. There are many ways in which the teacher can assist the children to be even-keeled, including listening carefully to what they say and watching closely what they do. It is wise occasionally to give pupils an assigned task, then leave the room briefly. If nothing has been accomplished, or the group has become rowdy during her absence, this is a warning sign that the relationship between the teacher and the class is not what it should be, nor is that among the children themselves.

There are many instructional materials which can be used to help teach the pupils needed material in the area of mental health. These include:

The Chalkboard

The pupils will learn new words for their ever-growing vocabulary more quickly when they see them written on the board, hear each pronounced and used correctly by the teacher, and then copy, pronounce, and use each correctly at frequent intervals throughout the class and week. Other suggested ways in which a chalkboard and bulletin board can be used for instructional purposes are:

1. Several times each semester, have the pupils write a paper and read it to the group on any new hobby developed. Keep a running chalkboard list or record in each child's folder of these new interests. Check this periodically for progress.
2. Have each child make a list of his New Year's resolutions or a list of bad habits he wishes to change. Post each list on the bulletin board. Check progress in this direction periodically.
3. Discuss ways of listening to and accepting criticism; have one pupil summarize the suggestions agreed upon by the class, and post these on the bulletin board.
4. Have a committee plan, make, and display a bulletin board expressing any idea stressed throughout this unit such as "Making Friends," or "Happy People Are Healthy People."

5. List on the chalkboard the ways pupils can protect themselves when playing active sports and games. Discuss permanent brain injuries, how they affect the body, and how they can be avoided.
6. Work in committees and draw up a list of reasons why laws should be obeyed. Have a person from each group write its list on the board. Have the class select the best one.
7. Make a list of those adults who might help children solve their problems. Write this on the board.

Cartoons and Comics

Every daily newspaper and many periodicals contain cartoons and comic strips which can be used to help children see humor in life, as well as problems faced by other people and how they solve them. The comic "Peanuts" is especially suitable for such classroom use. Many children who are afraid may not, like the character Linus in this comic strip, have to carry a blanket around with them to help bolster their courage, yet the teacher can use pictures of this little boy with his protective blanket clutched to his breast to stimulate a class discussion on fears. Another daily comic strip which could be used successfully is "Nancy," a most ingenious little girl who gets into and out of many of the problem situations faced by most children. For the older pupils, "Little Orphan Annie," "Mutt and Jeff," "Blondie," "Archie," and "Rex Morgan, M.D." are recommended. Some pupils will profit from and be interested in drawing their own cartoons, or making their own animated mental health films which they can show through improvised cardboard movie projectors.

Books and Supplementary Reading Materials

Children delight in being read to by their teacher. Those working on the primary level are well aware that most youngsters of this age are eager to come to school. Each soon finds out, however, that many other children are there competing with him for the teacher's attention and that many of them can do many things better than he can. These pupils need many opportunities to talk over the feelings they have, whether of fear, anger, shyness, or happiness. Knowing that everyone has these reactions, and that they are normal and can be handled, will often help these children gain increased self-understanding and control. Often a simple story read aloud by the teacher and discussed by the class can help each pupil gain needed insight into himself, increase his confidence in his own abilities and attitudes, learn how to face and solve his own problems, and give him courage to face challenging new situations, and an understanding of the correct place of emotion in life. Suggested materials to be used for this purpose are Joan Walsh Anglund's charming little books, *Look Out the Window* and *A Friend Is Someone Who Likes You* (Harcourt, Brace and Jovanovich), or *The Little Frightened Tiger* by Golden MacDonald and Leonard Weisgard (Doubleday).

Upper elementary pupils can profit greatly from reading books of their own choosing, as guided by the teacher and librarian. Boys will find the splendid book *Fear Strikes Out* by Jim Piersall (Little, Brown) especially interesting. Most girls will prefer books such as *The Diary of Anne Frank* (Houghton-Miffiin), *Desirée* by Annemarie Selenko (Morrow) or *The Yearling* by Marjorie K. Rawlings (Scribner). Reports given by each pupil on the book of his own choice will provide each with the opportunity to share with classmates and to express himself.

Radio and Television

Increasingly, large school systems are sponsoring their own television and radio educational programs. Teachers will profit from checking the weekly broadcast schedules found in most Sunday papers and requiring pupils to see certain well-selected programs. Class discussions should be planned so that the full educational values inherent in the programs are brought into proper focus. Serialized daily radio programs can also be used as a means of helping children learn how other people go about solving their problems. Another suggested activity is to have the class pick out the happiest looking faces they see on television programs, and tell what they think makes people happy.

The Phonograph

Most schools have a record player for classroom use. Children can gain a lifelong appreciation for good music from records played for them and explained to them by their teacher. They can be taught to pick out noisy, quiet, and happy sounds for a discussion of moods of people. Almost any type of light classical music can be used for this purpose, ranging all the way from Grofé's *Grand Canyon Suite* to Beethoven's *Pastoral Symphony*. Musical comedy tunes such as those from *Oklahoma!* or *My Fair Lady* can be played frequently to brighten a gloomy day at school or stimulate lagging interest in classroom work.

Since tension is one of the problems most Americans face, it is also recommended that children learn to relax through music, whether this be by doing mild exercises to records such as "Sentimental Journey" or "Sunrise Serenade," or pretending they are floating logs moving slowly down a lazy stream as they listen to a soothing melody. Children should learn why and how tensions build up as well as how pressures can be reduced by mild exercise, relaxing activities, and practicing good health habits.

Creative dance can be done in a classroom, gymnasium, or on the playground, and children can be given opportunities through this activity to express in body movements such feelings and emotions as joy, fear, hatred, anger, love, shyness, or bolstered courage. A child can lose his self-consciousness quickly in interpreting such things as a clock, bicycle, pony, or elephant. They can also express inner feelings by dancing out such colors as red, yellow, black, or green.[7] Imagination is innate in all children. It flowers richly in some but must be extracted with consummate skill from others. Whenever an exercise involves abstract feeling or a story or a theme, a picture should be painted by the teacher to fire the imagination.

DESIRABLE OUTCOMES

As a result of materials learned in mental hygiene, the following outcomes should accrue in terms of knowledge, attitudes, and practices:

In the primary grades, the pupils will:

1. Be able to get along well with others in their class, teachers, members of their family, and other adults.

---

[7] Vannier, Maryhelen, Foster, Mildred, and Gallahue, Daird: *Teaching Physical Education in Elementary Schools.* 5th ed. Philadelphia: W. B. Saunders Co., 1973, p. 161.

2. Understand and accept themselves.
3. Recognize that emotions of fear, anger, hate, jealousy, and love are universal, and be able to control these emotions well according to their present stage of development.
4. Feel accepted by a group and contribute to group welfare and projects.
5. Know their own weaknesses and abilities.
6. Understand that every group has rules which must be obeyed, and that such rules are for the happiness, protection, and well-being of all.
7. Welcome and enjoy new experiences.
8. Accept disappointment and adjust to things which do not always go according to previously set plans.
9. Be able to cooperate with other children and adults, realizing that their contribution will help make any group endeavor become successful.
10. Make friends easily.
11. Increasingly be able to evaluate their own actions and realistically analyze their contribution to group welfare or a group project.
12. Increasingly assume greater responsibility for their own actions, take the consequences for failure, and act according to rules.
13. Participate skillfully in solving individual and group problems.
14. Gain satisfaction from being alone sometimes and not always needing to be "doing something" or be entertained.
15. Accept those who have physical, social, or economic handicaps and be kind to more unfortunate people of all ages.
16. Receive pleasure from "doing the right thing" and taking turns.
17. Have a best friend and several close friends.
18. Take care of their own possessions and respect the rights and property of others.
19. Gain satisfaction from possessing acceptable work habits, and see an assumed task through to the end.
20. Be aware that to be a good leader one must use democratic methods, and practice this concept; good followers as well as leaders use increased understanding of the democratic method.
21. Know the difference between humor and harmful practical jokes which may hurt or embarrass others.
22. Gain real satisfaction from creative experiences, caring for a pet, and hobbies.
23. Play with others cooperatively and enjoy vigorous activities, be courageous, and sure of themselves.

In the upper elementary grades, the pupils will:

1. Possess deeper self-understanding and esteem for the rights of others.
2. Know how to express feelings of anger, hostility, aggression, love, joy, and fear in legitimate ways and can control these feelings.
3. Recognize their bodies are changing and ask frank, reasonable questions and know where to find information regarding their changing selves.
4. Understand their need for other people and yet know the value of independence.
5. Belong to a closely knit group of friends engaged in beneficial activities.
6. Recognize that home, church, and community approval for actions is a necessity.
7. Develop a higher sense of values; desire to have a good character.
8. Recognize and accept individual differences.
9. Develop greater appreciation for their families, home environment, and teachers as well as other adults.
10. Make increasingly wiser decisions and better choices.
11. Find that accepting and carrying out responsibility brings more satisfaction than negative behavior.

10

12. Be self-confident, loyal, trustworthy, dependable, honest, and sensitive to others.
13. Realize the importance of personal appearance, being popular, and respected among peers.
14. Participate, cooperate, and share in group activities.
15. Know practical ways to face failure.
16. Disagree with others without becoming angry or arousing anger.
17. Compete fairly and successfully against others; not always have to win in order to gain satisfaction from competition or cooperation.
18. Be a working member of any church or youth group.
19. Have a variety of skills for relaxation through creative experiences, clubs, and hobbies.
20. Appreciate the qualities of good leadership and select their own leaders wisely.
21. Accept the use of glasses, braces, or other correctional aids, if needed.
22. Have effective, independent study and work habits.
23. Become increasingly more skilled in solving their individual problems.
24. Recognize the value of strong emotional drive and possess favorable attitudes toward themselves, their school, and home.
25. Realize the importance of good manners and use them.
26. Use their individual talents for school and community services.
27. Increasingly practice self-discipline and feel responsible for their behavior when alone or away from adults.
28. Be well adjusted, happy, and eager for approaching junior high school experiences.
29. Have a high regard for the opposite sex and have both boy and girl friends.
30. Be courageous, independent, possess strong, skillful bodies, and take part in both vigorous physical activities and quiet recreational games.

Found below are suggested instructional materials for teaching mental health to children in grades K to 6:

Kindergarten

Objective
1. To aid the pupil to develop good mental health.

Suggested Approaches
1. Role playing.
2. Creative arts.
3. Bulletin board materials.
4. Use of the flannel board.

Group Activities
1. Discuss what it means to grow up.
2. Compare the differences between teachers, pupils, parents, brothers, and sisters.
3. Talk about the things you would like to be when you grow up.
4. Discuss the things you can do now that you could not do when younger.

Individual Activities
1. Draw a picture of your idea of "growing up" or a self-portrait.
2. Draw pictures of things you like to do.
3. Tell about things that disappoint you.

Correlations
1. Physical Education
   a. Have pupils draw pieces of paper with words describing emotional states (gloom, fear, etc.) and have pupils walk corresponding to the mood they drew.

2. Language Arts
   a. Write a story about a boy or girl with some negative behavior.
3. Drama
   a. Make up plays about disappointments which occur and how they can work for good.

Pupil References

McKean, Ellen: *Daird's Bad Day.* New York: Vanguard Press.
Leaf, Munro: *How To Behave and Why.* Philadelphia: J. B. Lippincott Co., 1970.
Leaf, Munro: *Play Fair.* Philadelphia: J. B. Lippincott Co., 1965.

Teacher References

Check periodicals which relate to this subject in schools, especially *The Journal of School Health* and *Today's Health.*

Evaluations

1. Can students explain what makes them sad, happy, etc.? Do they understand why?
2. Do they understand the importance of controlling such emotions?

Grade 1

Objective

1. To understand our emotions, how we can control them, and why we should.

Suggested Approaches

1. Role playing.
2. Bulletin boards.
3. Creative arts.

Basic Concepts

1. "You" as a person are very important.
2. Everyone is different and has different abilities.
3. Working and playing together are part of growing up.
4. Improving behavior tells others you are growing up.

Group Activities

1. Discuss how you can help at home.
2. Discuss the times you are happy and sad and what causes you to feel that way.
3. Talk about what you can do when you feel upset.
4. Discuss how you can help others when they feel upset.

Individual Activities

1. Tell a story about traits you like in others.
2. Role play how you get ready for bed and go to sleep.
3. Draw pictures showing joy and sorrow.

Correlations

1. Language Arts
   a. Write a story about how one person reacts to his mother's or father's discipline.
2. Drama
   a. Demonstrate how our voice and facial expressions can reflect our feelings although our words may not.
3. Social Studies
   a. Learn how children of different backgrounds do things differently.

Pupil References

Look up latest books in the libraries.

Teacher References

Look up information in latest periodicals and newest books.

Evaluation

1. Do students understand what good behavior is?
2. Do they show that good behavior is a sign of growing up?

Grade 2

Objective
1. To understand that as we grow we must improve our behavior and begin to consider others.

Suggested Approaches
1. Role playing.
2. Creative arts.
3. Bulletin boards.
4. Use of health readers.

Basic Concepts
1. We have many different feelings which are a part of life.
2. Consideration of others is important.
3. Our voice and actions reflect our feelings about ourselves.
4. We develop and change our behavior because of experiences we have.

Group Activities
1. Discuss the many ways in which you can show kindness to others.
2. Discuss relationships with brothers, sisters, parents, etc.
3. Discuss responsibilities of growing up.
4. Discuss differences between teasing and practical jokes.

Individual Activities
1. List traits of good follower and leader.
2. List the responsibilities you have now that you didn't have when younger.
3. Make a list of things about yourself you would like to improve.
4. Write a story about tolerating another's opinions.

Correlations
1. Drama and Arts
   a. Role play the different ways to settle an argument.*
2. Language Arts
   a. Write a story about how sad one can be when one is caught telling a lie.

Pupil References
Look up latest material in the library.

Teacher References
Look up latest materials in the library, including periodicals.

Evaluation
1. Do pupils understand the importance of controlling emotions, considering others, accepting responsibilities of growing up?

Grade 3

Objective
1. To help the student understand what makes him tick. Why do we become scared, angry or embarrassed?

Concepts
1. Individuality
   a. Similarities between each of us.
   b. Differences between each of us.

---

* Borrow a Teletrainer from the Bell Telephone Company. It consists of a box and two phones, and not only helps develop communicative skills but is especially good for role playing for shy children. Also available is a portable conference telephone. With it a whole class can talk to any person in the nation about a problem, such as a senator or a physicist. Its cost is between $10 and $15.00 monthly.

2. Mood and Personality
   a. Contributing factors: environment, experiences, heredity, physical health, relationships with peers and elders.
   b. Mood changes and their causes as natural occurrences.
3. Ways of expressing emotion and feelings
   a. Happiness: laughter and tears.
   b. Lacking of confidence; superiority (ego trip)
   c. Love: gentleness, hate, severe discipline.
   d. Fear.
   e. Anger.
4. Standing up for what you believe and being able to express your own concepts in the give and take of group relationships.
5. Making decisions
   a. Should I or shouldn't I?
6. Growing as a family member.

Group and Individual Activities
1. Class discussions are valuable in this area of education to help each individual become more aware of his inner self and his interaction with his classmates.
2. Have the class discuss the importance of making right decisions.
3. Role playing. Act out conflict scenes, such as being lonely, scared, or making right or wrong decisions when at home or at play with peers.
4. Keep a diary and record each day how you felt in relationship to conflicts, the weather, or adults.

Books to Read
Brenner, Anita: *A Hero by Mistake, The Story of a Frightened Indian.* New York: William R. Scott, 1953. This profound book is about fears and will help a child gain real understanding of bravery.
Buck, Pearl S.: *The Beech Tree.* New York: John Day Co., 1955. This beautifully written story tells how a family works things out when an ailing grandfather comes to live with them and how he became a real part of the family.
Bulla, Clyde Robert: *Indian Hill.* New York: Thomas Y. Crowell Co., 1963. This is about a young Indian and his family who move from the reservation to the city and have to adjust to new ways of living. Since many children move to new homes several times in their lives, this story will help them learn some of the problems they will face.
Burchardt, Nellie: *Project Cat.* New York: Franklin Watts, 1966. A homeless cat brings children living in a housing development into a closely knit group.
Dalgliesh, Alice: *The Courage of Sarah Noble.* New York: Charles Scribner's Sons, 1953. A modern classic set in 1707 with a neat message.
Vreeken, Elizabeth: *Kenny and Jane Make Friends.* Dobbs Ferry, N.Y.: Oceana Publications, 1963. Demonstrates the theme that it would be too bad if everyone looked alike, dressed alike etc.

Grade 4

Objective
1. To understand that different people have different needs. There are some things which we all need. As we grow older we express ourselves in different ways, and everyone must strive to be an individual.

Concepts
1. Growing Inwardly
   a. Developing curiosity; imagination.
   b. Developing skills; becoming independent.
2. Growing as a Family Member
   a. Age differences: ways in which age reflects duties which are assigned around the house.
   b. Cooperation
      Quarrels. Why do we quarrel? Advantages and disadvantages.

3. Feelings of Jealousy
   a. Ways in which we project jealous feelings onto others: teasing, bragging, bossing, being cruel to younger persons or animals.
   b. Why we have jealous feelings and what to do about them.
4. Getting Along With Others
   a. Our need for friends and self-understanding.

Individual and Group Activities
   1. Teacher acts out emotions and students guess what she is portraying. Reverse roles so the teacher guesses.
   2. Have a time for relaxing activities every school day for sharing fun and laughter.
   3. Use various types of music to help calm and relax children and to help create a beneficial atmosphere.
   4. Make stick, paper bag, or hand puppets, and tell stories or plays around such themes as fear, anger, and jealousy.
   5. Have each child tell a story about how he reacts to feelings of jealousy, anger, or sibling rivalry.
   6. Display work of each child as often as possible, and find ways in which each child can gain group recognition by being the best at something. Help each child to "shine."

Pupil References
   Estes, Eleanor: *The Moffats.* New York: Harcourt, Brace and Jovanovich, 1968.
   Heywood, Carolyn: *Annie, Pat and Eddie.* New York: William Morrow & Co., 1970.
   Friedman, Frieda: *The Janitor's Girl.* New York: William Morrow & Co., 1956.
   Stuart, Jesse: *The Beatinest Boy.* New York: McGraw-Hill Book Co., 1961.
   Bishop, Claire H.: *All Alone.* New York: The Viking Press, 1953.
   Nordstrom, Ursula: *The Secret Language.* New York: Harper & Row, 1972.

Teaching References
   Reading Ladders For Human Relation. 4th ed., American Council on Education. A source of books about human relations.
   Spolin, Viola: *Improvisation For The Theater.* Evanston, Ill.: Northwestern University Press, 1970.
   Read, Donald A., and Greene, Walter H.: *Creative Teaching in Health.* New York: The Macmillan Co., 1971.
   Health and Growth. Glenview, Ill.: Scott, Foresman & Co., 1971.
   Cornacchia, H. J., Staton, W., and Irwin, L.: *Health in Elementary Schools.* 3rd ed., St. Louis: C. V. Mosby Co., 1970.

Grade 5

Objectives
   1. Learn to respect yourself and others.
   2. Learn the importance of cooperation.
   3. Establish acceptable behavior patterns.
   4. Develop self-discipline at work and play.
   5. Realize your responsibilities as a member of the school, community, and the family.
   6. Learn to enjoy group activities.
   7. Learn that normal behavior incorporates mood changes.

Suggested Approaches
   Mental health is a wide area and is supplemented by the teacher setting a good example and by using her own creativity. Methods should include bulletin boards, crafts, role-playing, dramatizations, all contributed by the students. The teacher should have a mentally healthy attitude and aid

in creating an atmosphere conducive to good mental health. Have guest speakers from the community such as a grandparent, sports hero, etc. to help children build positive attitudes toward life.

Group Activities
1. Have pupils bring articles from newspapers and magazines concerning mental health problems and discuss how they could be solved or were solved.
2. Discuss traits an admired person has, as well as those who are disliked.
3. Discuss how to show appreciation, love, and respect to our friends, family, and adults.
4. Dramatize experiences that make a person happy, thoughtful, grateful, etc.
5. Have students report on handicapped persons who overcame their handicap to become productive and happy members of society, such as Beethoven, Keller, Edison, etc.
6. Have students make and contribute to a "worries box," and have the class discuss how each "worry" problem can be solved.
7. Dramatize how it feels to be different from others in terms of race, nationality, beliefs, and customs.

Individual Activities
1. Have each student draw a picture of how to be kind to each other.
2. Role play displaced anger projection.
3. Have the students listen to music and then let each write a poem or story about what the piece reminds him of.
4. Have each student write on unsigned papers their various experiences when they have felt angry, sad, fearful, etc. Read and discuss the different ways their emotions were handled.
5. Have a hobby show, and have each pupil tell how his hobby helps him relax and feel happy. Encourage each child to develop hobbies in many areas.
6. Have students write short reports for the school newspapers on jealousy, prejudice, anger, etc.

Correlations
1. Language Arts
   a. Write or tell a story that begins, "Once I felt very happy when."
   b. Write some stories in which the characters exhibit self-respect.
2. Drama
   a. Play "charades" using different emotions.
3. Art
   a. Make puppets and prepare plays with themes of different emotions such as fear, happiness, etc.
4. Social Studies
   a. Have students do research and report on the effect of mental health on certain leaders throughout history.

Pupil References
Goldenson, Robert M.: *All About The Human Mind: An Introduction to Psychology For Young People*. New York: Random House, 1963.
Alexander, Arthur: *The Hidden You, Psychology in Your Life*. Englewood Cliffs, N. J.: Prentice-Hall, 1962.
Limbacher, Walter J.: *Here I Am*. Dayton, Ohio: Pflaum, 1969.
Health and Growth. Glenview, Ill.: Scott, Foresman and Co., 1970.

Teacher References
Cornacchia, H. J., Staton, W., and Irwin, L.: *Health in Elementary Schools*. St. Louis: C. V. Mosby Co., 1970.
Greene, Walter H., and Read, Donald: *Creative Teaching in Health*. The Macmillan Co., 1971.

Health and Growth. Teacher's Edition. Glenview, Ill.: Scott, Foresman and Co., 1970.

Cameron, Norman A.: *Personality Development and Psychopathology.* Boston: Houghton Mifflin Co., 1963.

Audio-Visual Aids

"Evans' Corner." BFA Educational Media. Evans learns the value of helping others.

"Key of His Own." BFA. Explores the feelings of a child whose mother works and leaves him a key to the house and money for dinner and a show. Since many children come home to an empty house as both parents work, this film can help many of them.

Grade 6

Objectives—To help each child to
1. Be concerned about others and respect them as well as himself.
2. Experience leadership and the role of the follower in school situations.
3. Enjoy working and playing with others.
4. Learn to take in stride "routine changes and unexpected failures."
5. Understand that physical health is related to our emotional health and personal feelings.
6. Understand that as we grow more mature we generally become more effective, constructive, and self-directed.
7. Learn that a person has different responsibilities in society at different ages.

Suggested Approaches

Utilize student ideas by having them list areas in which they have real concern, such as racial prejudice or fear; how worry can make one ill; what the unconscious mind is and how it governs behavior.

Group Activities
1. Have students list the characteristics of a mentally healthy person.
2. Discuss constructive ways of handling mistakes or failures and give skits on how to handle and not handle mistakes, worries, or problem situations.
3. Have the class redecorate their classroom to make it more cheerful, and then talk about how one's environment and the weather affect moods.
4. Make a "sunshine package" for someone who is ill.
5. Have students do research on mental illness, suicide, and crime for oral reports.
6. Have each write a short paper on his worst habit or worst fault, showing how it can be eliminated.
7. Role play how fatigue or illness can make us "fussy" or "irritable."

Individual Activities
1. Report on how someone made you "feel better."
2. Give biographical reports on handicapped persons who overcame their setback to meet success, such as sports heroes, famous writers, etc.
3. Discuss the fact that everyone is good at something, and then have students write a paragraph on what they are most skilled in and like most to do.
4. Have each child relate how he finds relaxation and recreation, and tell how this relates to mental health by reducing tension and building confidence.

Correlations
1. Art
   a. Draw a picture of and discuss how you overcame worry.
2. Mathematics
   a. How mathematics can be "recreation" after vigorous physical activity and vice-versa.

3. Social Studies
   a. Discuss how individual differences make life richer. Discuss why it
   is important that we choose leaders and friends who are mentally
   healthy.

Pupil References
   Friedman, Frieda: *Ellen and The Gang.* New York: William Morrow and Co.,
   1963.
   Robinson, Veronica: *David in Silence.* Philadelphia: J. B. Lippincott Co.,
   1965.
   Health and Growth. Glenview, Ill.: Scott, Foresman and Co., 1970.

Teacher References
   Mead, Margaret: *A Creative Life for Your Children.* U.S. Dept. of HEW, 1966.
   Willgoose, Carl: Mental Health at an Early Age. *Instructor, 81*:58–59, 1971.
   Health and Growth. Teacher's Edition. Glenview, Ill.: Scott, Foresman and
   Co., 1970.
   Mental Health and School Health Services. Chicago: American Medical
   Association, 1965.
   Reading Ladders for Human Relations. 4th ed., Washington, D. C.: American
   Council on Education, 1970.

Audio-Visual Aids
   Shyness. (Film) McGraw-Hill.

CHAPTER 15

communicable diseases

Teaching children how to protect themselves and others from contagious diseases can make a significant difference in their health status throughout their entire lives. Each child should learn how he can and must cooperate with the community's efforts to control the spread of disease through personal care, sanitation, and law. It is of utmost importance that the total school environment serve as a model of cleanliness, for it is folly to give lip service to the need for cleanliness to check the spread of germs in a dirty classroom, or to have children eat in the school cafeteria where roaches and other vermin are also feeding.

In studying about diseases, all of the four principal ways to control communicable diseases should be stressed: (1) sanitation, (2) isolation and quarantine, (3) immunization, and (4) education. Since the common cold causes one-fourth of all school absences, children should be taught that fatigue, exposure, and malnutrition lower resistance to the germs causing this highly contagious disease. They also must learn to cough and sneeze into a tissue or handkerchief, to wash their hands thoroughly after handling anything used by someone with a cold, to wash all eating utensils of the ill person in very hot water and soap before they are used again, and to stay home when sick with a cold. Children as well as adults need to learn and practice good health habits and to know that one's personal health can lead to the prevention and control of disease not only within themselves but also in many others.

Children need to learn that personal cleanliness can help prevent disease and keep them well. Each should be taught to practice routinized health habits of bathing regularly, using his own toothbrush, towel, washcloth, etc. They should also learn as soon as possible that each has much responsibility as a citizen in the fight against disease, for disease control rests with each individual locally, as well as nationally and internationally.

Interest in this important area of health education can be aroused by thought-provoking questions such as the following:

If your little brother has a cold, how can you protect yourself so you won't get it?

How can we be sure that our drinking water is pure, or that the food we buy at the store is good for us to eat?

Why is air pollution a dangerous health hazard?

How and why is milk pasteurized?

What is a septic tank? Should every home have one, or only people who live on a farm?

How do our city, community, state, and national governments help us keep healthy?

How do germs, which make us sick, get inside our body? What can we do to keep them out?

What kind of immunization shots have you had? How long are they good for? What is a booster shot?

COMMUNICABLE DISEASE CONTROL
THROUGH DAILY OBSERVATION

Children are a hotbed for communicable diseases, for they are too young to have built up immunity for themselves. Since many contagious diseases are highly contagious *before* they start, all teachers should be alerted to watch for the appearance of

watery nasal discharge
headache or other body aches
fever (flushed face)
sore or scratchy throat
red, watery eyes

nausea or vomiting
a chill or chilliness
sneezing
tight, dry cough

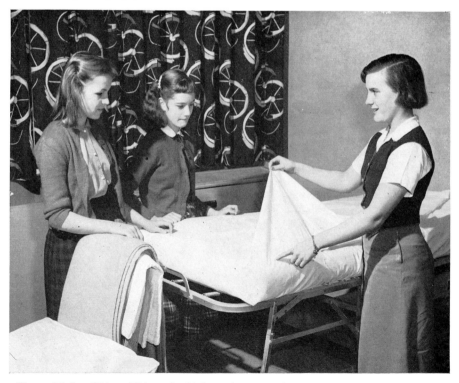

Figure 15-1. Older children should learn how to take care of someone who is ill. (Courtesy of U.S. Office of Education)

All of the above symptoms indicate the onset of an acute general infection and/or the onset of serious childhood diseases such as chickenpox, diphtheria, German measles, mumps, scarlet fever, polio, and whooping cough.

Found below are techniques of daily health observation of which every teacher should be cognizant. Children who are ill or are becoming so should be isolated. The school should have definite written policies concerning sending an ill child home, readmission procedures, and the alerting of parents of needed preventive injections for their own child should one of their classmates develop a highly contagious disease to which all others in his room have been exposed.

Daily Observations

I. *Day-by-day Association*
    A. Learn how each child normally looks and behaves when well.
    B. Observe the class as a whole and each child as an individual part of it.

II. *What Health Observation Embodies*

    A. Physical

        1. *Eyes*
            a. Sties or crusted lids
            b. Inflamed eyes
            c. Crossed eyes
            d. Frequent headaches
            e. Squinting, frowning, or scowling
            f. Protruding eyes
            g. Watery eyes
            h. Excessive blinking
            i. Twitching of the lids
            j. Holding head to one side

        2. *Ears*
            a. Discharge from ears
            b. Earache
            c. Failure to hear questions
            d. Picking at the ears
            e. Turning head to hear
            f. Talking in a monotone
            g. Inattention
            h. Anxious expression
            i. Excessive noisiness

        3. *Nose and Throat*
            a. Persistent mouth breathing
            b. Frequent sore throats
            c. Recurrent colds
            d. Chronic nose discharge
            e. Frequent nose bleeding
            f. Nasal speech
            g. Frequent tonsillitis

        4. *Skin and Scalp*
            a. Nits in the hair
            b. Unusual pallor of face
            c. Eruptions or rashes
            d. Habitual scratching of scalp or skin
            e. State of cleanliness
            f. Excessive redness of skin

        5. *Teeth and Mouth*
            a. State of cleanliness
            b. Gross visible caries
            c. Irregular teeth
            d. Stained teeth
            e. Offensive breath
            f. Mouth habits such as sucking

        6. *Growth*
            a. Failure to gain over a three-month period
            b. Unexplained loss in weight
            c. Unexplained gain in weight

        7. *General Appearance and Condition*
            a. Underweight—very thin
            b. Overweight—very obese
            c. Does not appear well
            d. Tires easily
            e. Chronic fatigue
            f. Nausea or vomiting
            g. Faintness or dizziness

        8. *Glands*
            a. Enlarged glands at one side on neck
            b. Enlarged thyroid

        9. *Heart*
            a. Excessive breathlessness
            b. Tires easily
            c. Any history of "growing pains"
            d. Bluish lips
            e. Excessive pallor

        10. *Posture and Musculature*
            a. Asymmetry of shoulders and hips

b. Peculiarity of gait
c. Obvious deformities of any type
d. Anomalies of muscular development

11. *Behavior Trends*
   a. Overstudious, docile, and withdrawing
   b. Bullying, overaggressive, and domineering
   c. Unhappy or depressed
   d. Overexcitable, uncontrollable emotions
   e. Stuttering or other forms of speech difficulties
   f. Lack of confidence, self-denial, self-censure
   g. Poor accomplishment in comparison with ability
   h. Lying (imaginative or defensive)
   i. Lack of appreciation of property rights
   j. Abnormal sex behavior
   k. Antagonistic, negativistic, continually quarreling

B. *Emotional*

1. Must change and adjust to conditions in environment
   a. Teacher must realize individual capability
   b. Find cause for deviation
   c. Remedy it with expert help

2. Teacher determines the atmosphere of classroom

3. In this atmosphere, child learns how to attack life's problems
   a. Make pupil's special abilities known to group
   b. Develop cooperative undertakings
   c. Provide opportunities for pupil to experience happiness and joy

4. Teacher *must* realize
   a. Social adjustment child is making
   b. Adjustment to authority
   c. Adjustment to own limitations
   d. Normal and abnormal methods of meeting these situations

5. Teacher must be objective about child's behavior.

a. Specific judgment of how child acts in concrete situations

6. Types of children needing help
   a. Different child
      1. May need help (so not permanently stigmatized as different)
   b. Suddenly changed child
      1. Physical cause
      2. Home relations
      3. Change (glasses) causing behavior problems
   c. Unhappy Child
   d. Solitary, friendless child
      1. Manifestations of pronounced withdrawal behavior
      2. Doesn't know how to break through
   e. Social rebel
      1. Gain in prestige
      2. Placate authority by tattling
      3. Chronic truant
   f. Accident-prone child
      1. Bad luck
      2. Physical defect
      3. Need to suffer felt
      4. Get attention

7. Behavior is always caused; find cause in order to eliminate it.

8. Use (for physical and emotional observation)
   a. Health histories
      1. Record past illness, present condition, and tendencies
   b. Height and weight records
   c. Accident records

9. Work with school nurse

10. Understand testing program
   a. Wetzel grid
   b. Snellen Visual test
   c. Audiometer

III. *Individual Differences Are an Important Factor*

A. Tommy as he appears to his mother as an individual.

B. Tommy as he appears to his teacher as one *among* individuals.

IV. *Types of Observation*

A. Formal inspection

  1. Done in a good light

  2. Points of observation

    a. Skin of forearm, hands, face, and neck

      1. Cleanliness

      2. Skin infection

      3. Rash

    b. Hair and fingernails

      1. Nits

      2. Neatness

      3. Cleanliness

    c. Teeth and gums

      1. Bleeding

      2. Inflammation

    d. Ears

      1. Discharge of ear canal

    e. Clothing

      1. Neatness and cleanliness

      2. Tissue or handkerchief

  3. Advantages

    a. Guarantees each child teacher's individual time

    b. Promotes a thorough check

  4. Disadvantages

    a. Embarrassing to individual child

    b. Psychological effect on child and teacher thinking that job is done

B. Informal inspection

  1. "Good morning" observation

    a. Hair and face

    b. Happy or sad

    c. Tired or rested

    d. Eyes—clear and bright or inflamed

  2. Closer observation of needy child

  3. Continuous observation

    a. Posture

    b. Contents of lunch box

    c. Adequate eating time

    d. Unduly quarrelsome

    e. Happy play

    f. "Hang back" from group

V. *Practice of Observation*

A. Look for *one* thing in the children you encounter each day.

B. Unobtrusive observation of individual children.

C. Practice observation for specific purpose of detecting departure from good health.

D. Teacher can act for nurse as mother of child does for the family physician.

E. To practice observation

  1. Must want to assume the responsibility for the health of her children.

  2. Must be able to recognize abnormalities.

  3. Must know what to do in a constructive manner.

VI. *Teacher—As Health Counselor*

A. Purposes to show the child

  1. Acceptance of self

  2. Ability to solve the problem at hand

  3. Ability to solve future problems

B. Teacher's qualities

  1. Interest in people

  2. Own personality

    a. Good listener

    b. Respects others' views

  3. Competency in counseling skills

  4. Her own health record

    a. Periodic health appraisal

    b. No fears and frustrations brought to class

    c. A feeling of adequacy in her work

    d. Interests outside her profession

    e. Not a depressed, sarcastic teacher, with an uncontrollable temper

    f. Teacher's health is a great factor in her ability to observe and to influence the health of her children

C. Results of conference

  1. Note sent to the parent a "must"

    a. State the problem to be discussed (not in full, though)

    b. The conference must be ended with a clear understanding of the steps to be taken

Summary

The teacher is the key to the school health program, both in the curriculum teaching and in a role of a member of the school health-service team. She must have abundant energy, a buoyancy, and the ability to think clearly and to plan carefully. She must have a wholesome personality, be healthy herself, be patient, and most of all, her outlook must be both promising and cheerful. The attitude of health and behavior of the teacher are of paramount importance. Our children's good health is one of our most valuable national resources now and for the nation's future.

COMMUNICABLE DISEASE SUMMARY FOR TEACHERS*

Chickenpox

Chickenpox is a very contagious but not a serious disease. There are rarely complications.

What to look for:

When cases are occurring in school or community, watch for symptoms of a "cold" or a rash. Many times chickenpox first appears with the rash, which resembles small blisters. Usually appear first on body, chest, or upper back 14 to 21 days after exposure. Child may have no sign of rash when he comes to school and by midmorning it may begin to appear.

How disease is spread:

By contact with case, often before symptoms appear in the case. Spread by droplets from nose and throat. Scabs are not infectious.

How to prevent:

No immunization. Child who has chickenpox should be kept away from others until no new "spots" appear (usually 6 or 7 days). Examine household contacts for symptoms before sending to school during incubation period.

Regulations:

Case: Exclude from school 6 days after first symptoms appear.
Contacts: None.

Common Cold

The common cold is easily spread from one person to another. Everyone is susceptible to common colds. Complications may occur, and parents should be urged to keep children at home at the first sign of a cold. Many times symptoms of colds are early signs of other childhood illnesses.

What to look for:

Common symptoms are runny nose, sneezing, general tired feeling. There is usually no fever unless complications have developed.

How disease is spread:

By contact with a person who has a cold. The discharges from the nose and mouth are infectious and are most dangerous through sneezing or coughing.

How to prevent:

No immunizing agent. Avoid people who have colds if possible. Urge parents to keep children with colds at home.

Regulations:

None.

Diphtheria

Diphtheria is a dangerous disease during the illness and because of complications. A child should be referred to his doctor immediately if symptoms suggestive of diphtheria occur.

* Materials condensed from *Communicable Disease Summary for Teachers*, published by the Colorado State Department of Public Health.

What to look for:

It begins with a sore throat and signs of fever. The symptoms rapidly become more severe. A person may develop diphtheria within a few hours to 4 to 5 days after being exposed.

How disease is spread:

By contact with a case or with a person who "carries" the germ in his throat but is not sick. The discharges from the nose and throat carry the germs.

How to prevent:

All children should be immunized against diphtheria. When cases occur in a community, school children should be given booster shots unless they have had a booster in the last year.

Regulations:

Case: Exclude until released by health department or private doctor.

Contacts: Household and other intimate contacts—same as case.

German Measles

German measles is a contagious but mild disease. Usually the only time there are any complications is when a pregnant woman develops it during the first 3 months of her pregnancy.

What to look for:

It may begin with mild symptoms of a cold, but usually the first symptom is a rash. The rash is fine and faint and appears on the face and chest. Glands are usually swollen along the hairline in the back of the neck and below the ear. These symptoms occur between 14 and 21 days after exposure.

How disease is spread:

By contact with a case. The droplets from the nose and throat are infectious, especially before the rash appears.

How to prevent:

A child should be kept home until the rash disappears, 2 or 3 days usually. A vaccine has recently been developed. Consult your physician.

Regulations:

Case: Exclude from school until symptoms are gone.

Contacts: None.

Head Lice (Pediculosis)

Pediculosis is infestation with head lice. It is common in areas where people live under crowded conditions or where children are in close contact as in school.

What to look for:

Itching is the main sign. One does not always see the lice; one sees the eggs which the louse lays on the hair—they look like tiny beads strung along the hair.

How disease is spread:

By close contact with infected persons or by using their caps, scarves, or combs.

How to prevent:

By the application of an effective insecticide promptly to the head of a case, to prevent spread. Children should not be in school so long as there are lice. They can be in school if they are under treatment.

Regulations:

None.

Impetigo

Impetigo is a highly contagious skin infection. It spreads easily if neglected. A child with impetigo must be excluded from school until all the sores are healed.

What to look for:
The first sign of impetigo is the appearance of crusty sores, often around the nose and mouth. The sores start as a small blister that soon breaks open and forms a brownish crust.
How disease is spread:
The discharge from the sores of impetigo is infectious. Articles used by a person who has the infection (towels, wash cloths, etc.) can also carry the germs.
How to prevent:
No immunizing agent. Prompt separation of cases from other children is important. When treated, impetigo clears up in 2 or 3 days.
Regulations:
Case: Exclude from school until sores are healed.
Contacts: None.

Infectious Hepatitis

Infectious hepatitis is a disease caused by a virus which produces inflammation of the liver. Often occurs in epidemics in schools and among members of households of cases.
What to look for:
Early signs of this disease are nausea, possibly vomiting, extreme fatigue, and often pain in the upper abdomen. Following these symptoms some cases develop jaundice—a yellow color in the skin and whites of the eyes. Many cases excrete dark (coffee-colored) urine and light (clay-colored) stools.
How disease is spread:
By person-to-person contact. The virus causing hepatitis is found in the human bowel and spread by dirty hands to the mouth. It can be spread by water if contaminated with human excretion.
How to prevent:
Gamma globulin may be given to the members of the family of a case. The supply of this serum is too limited to give in mass programs. Careful hand-washing, after using the toilet and before meals, will help control the spread.
Regulations:
Case: Exclude from school for one week or until symptoms are gone.
Contacts: None.

Measles

Measles is a contagious disease, especially the last few days of the incubabation period before the rash appears. This disease is dangerous for young children or children ill with some other condition. Complications can be severe.
What to look for:
This disease begins with cold symptoms: sneezing, inflamed eyes, a hard, dry cough. The fever is high and a rash develops after several days of fever—blotchy, dusky red in color. Symptoms develop 7 to 14 days after exposure.
How disease is spread:
By contact with a person who has it. Discharges from the nose and throat are infectious, especially early in the illness before symptoms appear.
How to prevent:
By vaccination with either killed or live measles vaccine or a combination of both, preferably in infancy.
Gamma globulin can be given to very young or to ill children after exposure. This serum will prevent a case or make it mild. Children in the family of a case, who have not had measles, should be observed closely for symptoms of illness during the second week after exposure.
Regulations:
Case: Exclude from school for 5 days following appearance of rash.
Contacts: None.

Mumps

Mumps is highly contagious, but so mild that one-third of all cases are un-recognized. Mumps is usually not dangerous except in teenagers or adults.
What to look for:
In a young child, the first sign is a swelling under the ear lobe. Symptoms appear 7 to 14 days after exposure.
How disease is spread:
By contact with a person who has it. Droplets from the nose and mouth are infectious from 2 days before the swelling appears until the end of it.
How to prevent:
A mumps vaccine is available but the period of immunization it provides is limited.
Regulations:
Case: Exclude from school until the swelling is gone.
Contacts: None.

Pink Eye (Conjunctivitis)

Conjunctivitis is not a single disease like mumps or measles. It is an eye infection and can be caused by a number of germs.
What to look for:
The whites of the eyes are reddened and drain matter. Sometimes the lids are swollen and stuck together. Usually develops 48 to 72 hours after exposure.
How disease is spread:
By contact with articles used by an infected person (towels, washcloths, etc.).
How to prevent:
No immunizing agent. A child should not be in school with an eye infection.
Regulations:
None.

Poliomyelitis

Poliomyelitis, like many other illnesses, causes headache and pain in the back. However, in polio, this pain is often followed by paralysis.
What to look for:
Headache or stiffness of the neck or back. If a child has these symptoms, he should see his family doctor.
How disease is spread:
This is not clearly understood. The virus is present in the throat secretions and stools of cases, unrecognized cases, and especially carriers. No way is known to prevent the virus from spreading.
How to prevent:
By immunization. Everyone should be immunized beginning at 6 weeks to 2 months of age. Schools should urge that all children be immunized before entry in school.
Regulations:
Case: Exclude case from school until released by health department or physician.
Contacts: None.

Ringworm

Ringworm is a skin infection that appears as a circular dry spot on the skin or as bald spots on the scalp that contain short, whiskery-like hairs.
What to look for:
Dry, circular patches on the skin and bare spots on the scalp.

How disease is spread:
By direct contact with children or animals who have it. By the use of caps, combs, towels of infected persons.

How to prevent:
Cases must be under treatment, including wearing a cap if the ringworm is on the scalp. When ringworm is present in a family or in school, children should be examined frequently for signs so that treatment can be started early.

Domestic animals, both large and small, affected with the fungus, should be separated and not handled until a cure has been effected.

Regulations:
Case: None if case is under treatment and wears protective cap.
Contacts: None.

Scabies

In scabies, the skin is infested by tiny mites.

What to look for:
Intense scratching. The mite burrows under the skin between the fingers, bend of elbow, or wherever skin touches skin. The small lesions resemble pinholes occurring along a line.

How disease is spread:
By direct contact with an infected person—hand shaking, contact with clothing or articles used by such a person.

How to prevent:
Cases must be treated. All infected members of the family of a case should be treated at the same time.

Regulations:
Case: Exclude from school until symptoms are gone.
Contacts: None.

Streptococcal Infections (Including Scarlet Fever)

Slight attacks of "strep" throat are just as contagious as severe ones. Scarlet fever and "strep" throat are the same disease except for the rash. Children should not be in school with a sore throat and should be treated.

What to look for:
Strep infections begin suddenly. Headache, fever, and sore throat are common. The glands of the neck are swollen. Scarlet fever rash appears within 24 hours—fine, "granular" to the touch. Symptoms develop 2 to 5 days after exposure.

How disease is spread:
By contact with case or carrier. Discharges from the nose and throat are infectious. Strep infections often spread through the mild, unrecognized case.

How to prevent:
Children should not be in school with a sore throat. Drugs can be given to other members of the family of a case with strep, and the spread of the disease may be limited in this way. Contacts of a case are no longer infectious after 24 hours if they are under treatment.

Regulations:
Case: Exclude from school 48 hours or until symptoms are gone if under treatment. If not under treatment exclude until symptoms are gone—not less than 7 days.
Contacts: None.

Tuberculosis

Tuberculosis is usually a long-term disease and usually is a disease of the lungs. It may involve bones or other organs. Primary tuberculosis, which is the kind most often found in children, usually shows no symptoms and is not infectious. When a child is found to have tuberculosis, it is rare that he has it in a stage where he could expose other children in school or his playmates.

What to look for:

There is no way to observe children for tuberculosis. Once in a while a child will show a low fever and be tired and listless because of tuberculosis, but these symptoms may be due to many things. Such a child should be examined by his physician for his own good, not because he may be a threat to others.

How disease is spread:

For all practical purposes, tuberculosis is an air-borne disease spread by inhalation of droplet nuclei resulting from coughing, sneezing, or talking by persons with active tuberculosis.

How to prevent:

There is no practical immunization. The best prevention is through locating infectious cases, usually adults, and keeping these away from others until released by physician or health department. General good health habits—adequate rest, good nutrition, and medical care for illness—keep up good resistance.

Regulations:

Case: Doctor determines whether child may attend school. When a child is kept out of school because of tuberculosis, it is usually for the good of his own health and not because of danger to others.

Contacts: None. May attend school.

Note: A positive tuberculin skin test alone does not indicate that a child is infectious. It does indicate that the child has been infected at some time in his life with tubercle bacilli and should be examined at regular one- to two-year intervals for evidence of active tuberculosis.

Whooping Cough (Pertussis)

Whooping cough is most dangerous in infancy. It is especially infectious during the first or second week, before the "whoop" occurs. Complications can be severe.

What to look for:

Usually not possible to recognize until characteristic whoop appears. Cough is only constant symptom and may be due to many diseases other than whooping cough.

How disease is spread:

By contact with a case. Discharges of the nose and throat probably most infectious before "whoop" appears.

How to prevent:

By immunization with whooping cough vaccine. Since these shots are not recommended after 5 years of age, all children should be immunized before starting school.

Regulations:

Case: Exclude from school 21 days after appearance of "whoop."

Contacts: None.

SUGGESTED TEACHING UNITS

Found below are suggested teaching units in the area of communicable disease control:

Grades 1-2

Objectives

1. To teach the child the difference between illness and well-being.
2. To help the child develop good health habits.
3. To teach how to prevent disease.
4. To help the child learn different types of diseases.

Concepts

1. Prevention of disease
   a. By keeping hands clean.

    b. By keeping hands out of mouth, nose, and eyes.
    c. By covering the mouth when coughing and sneezing.
2. Community health involves individual and group cooperation.
3. A common cold can lead to many serious diseases.
4. Draw cartoons to show that when we are ill we cannot do as well in school or be as happy.
5. Make posters to show that the respiratory system is vulnerable to germs.
6. Discuss the ways the human body has many natural defenses against disease.

Group Activities
1. Have pupils draw a picture of themselves when they are sick and when they are well.
2. Have school nurse visit class.
3. Draw a thermometer, mark your normal temperature; learn to read a thermometer (grade 3).
4. Make a list of childhood diseases they have had.
5. Let each describe how he looked with the mumps or some other disease they have experienced.
6. Make a rhyme about measles, mumps, or another disease.
7. Make a mural showing the kinds of clothes to wear in different weather; what a food inspector or a public health nurse does.
8. Play a game with a volleyball called "germ" or "flu," and have the children throw it to one another to show how germs spread.
9. Role play how to prevent disease spread; what to do if you get sick at school.
10. See germs and bread molds under the microscope.

Individual Activities
1. Practice the correct way to drink from water fountain.
2. Practice the correct health habits at home and away of washing hands, brushing teeth, keeping nails clean, etc.
3. Make their own survey on how many people wash their hands when they are through in a public rest room.
4. Have each child make a poster or write a story on any aspect of disease control.
5. Use dolls and puppets to dress to fit the weather.
6. Have each child tell how their animal pets groom themselves, sleep, and have good health habits.
7. Have each child tell how and what he does for fun in outdoor play.

Related Activities
1. Math
    a. Make a list of ten childhood diseases they have not had.
2. Physical Education
    a. Play tag game; the person who is "it" is the germ, and he tries to tag the healthy pupils.
3. Art
    a. Have the pupil draw himself when he is well and when he is ill.
4. Science
    a. Have the pupils look at germs in the microscope or on films.

Pupil References
Health and Growth Health Series. Grades 1, 2, 3. Glenview, Ill.: Scott, Foresman and Co., 1971.
Greene, Carla: *Doctors and Nurses, What Do They Do?* New York: Harper & Row, 1970.
Kohn, Bernice: *Our Tiny Servants: Molds and Yeast.* Englewood Cliffs, N. J.: Prentice-Hall, 1968.

Teacher References
   Barrett, Morris: *Health Education, Guide K–12.* Wynnewood, Pa., Health
      Education Associates, Ltd., 1971.
   Kansas City Public Schools: *Health Education in the Elementary Schools.*
      Kansas City, Mo., 1963.
   Texas Elementary School Health Education Guide. Bulletin 715. Austin: State
      Education Agency, 1971.

Grade 3

Objectives
   1. To acquaint the children with the concept of what microbes are and the
      role they play in their daily lives.
   2. To help them to understand how and why public agencies work to
      control diseases.

Concepts
   1. Microbes
      a. Are all around us, in the air, ground, and water.
      b. Are alive and eat, grow, get rid of wastes, reproduce, die.
      c. Size—they are so small that they can only be seen by a microscope.
      d. Helpful microbes: make changes in soil so that plants will grow
         well; used to make medicines; help to make food—bread, pickles,
         cheese.
      e. Harmful microbes: disease germs that make people sick; get into
         food and cause it to spoil.
   2. Bacteria
      a. Microbes that are likely to be in your house at all times: numerous
         —many thousands would fit on a pinhead; scientific names—rod-
         shaped, round, spiral.
      b. Bacterial growth: Divide and split in two when reaches certain size;
         each one doubles itself; some grow alone, pairs, chains, clumps,
         threads; grow best in wet places, dark places, warm places.
   3. What are Viruses?
      a. Classification: tiniest microbe of all; hard to determine if they are
         plants or animals.
      b. All viruses we know about are harmful—cause diseases such as
         chickenpox, flu, polio, mumps, measles colds.
   4. What are Molds
      a. How molds grow and under what conditions.
      b. Helpful molds: some make cheese taste good; scientists use them in
         making medicines.
   5. How You Keep Healthy
      a. Ways the body has of fighting off harmful microbes: juices in
         stomach; coughed up from lungs; role of white blood cells.
      b. Personal cleanliness: cover mouth during coughs and sneezes; wash
         hands before eating and after using toilet; use own towel and wash-
         cloth; keep pencils and other objects out of mouth.
      c. Things we cannot do ourselves to protect us from germs: public
         health nurse; dairy and meat inspectors; lab worker in air pollution
         department; street cleaner, engineer at incinerator; garbage col-
         lectors.
   6. Environmental Influences
      a. How water is made safe to drink and how it travels from plant to
         home
      b. Sewage
      c. Air pollution
      d. Garbage

Group Activities
1. Borrow a microscope from science room and show slides of bacteria.
2. To see how microbes from air settle on foods and grow, put a slice of banana, a slice of apple, and a slice of cooked potato on dish. Let food stand in open air for hour. Cover with aluminum foil and put in warm, dark place. Watch.
3. Watch bread mold grow—use moistened bread.
4. To show that microbes need moisture to grow, put some dry beans in one small glass. Put several spoonful of flour in another. Put dry beans and water to cover in third. Put flour and water to cover in fourth. Which ones begin to spoil?
5. Tell or write riddles about community health workers.
6. Visit a water treatment or a sewage treatment plant.
7. Make a mural of a doctor's day.
8. Role playing: a visit to the doctor, dentist.
9. Make a collage of our environmental helpers.

Individual Activities
1. Practice the use of a handkerchief.
2. Practice washing hands.
3. Look around kitchen for foods which are kept from spoiling by being dried.
4. Find out how the pioneers kept foods from spoiling.
5. Put one glass of milk on table, one in refrigerator, and one in warm place. Which one sours first?
6. Dress dolls in suitable clothing for the four seasons.
7. Learn the proper way to hold a phone in order to avoid contacting germs.

Pupil References
Frahm, Anne: *The True Book of Bacteria.* Chicago: Childrens Press, 1963.
Harrison, C. William: *The Microscope.* New York: Julia Messner, 1965.
Kohn, Bernice: *Our Tiny Servants: Molds and Yeast.* Englewood Cliffs, N. J.: Prentice-Hall, 1968.
Lewis, Lucia: *The First Book of Microbes.* New York: Franklin Watts, 1972.
Selsam, Millicent E.: *Greg's Microscope.* New York: Harper & Row, 1963.
Gilbert, Helen E.: *Dr. Trotter and His Big Gold Watch.* Nashville: Abington Press, 1948.
Bendick, Jeanne: *Have a Happy Measle.* New York: McGraw-Hill Book Co., 1958.
Sener, Josephine: *Johnny Goes to the Hospital.* Houghton Press, 1967.

Teacher References
Schneider, Leo: *Microbes in Your Life.* New York: Harcourt, Brace and Jovanovich, 1966.
Simon, Harold J.: *Microbes and Men.* New York: McGraw-Hill Book Co., 1963.
American Public Health Association: *Health Is a Community Affair.*
Blake, Peter: *God's Own Junkyard.* New York: Holt, Rinehart & Winston, 1964.
Health and Growth, 4. Teacher's Edition. Glenview, Ill.: Scott, Foresman and Co., 1971.

Films
Be Healthy! Be Happy! Newenhouse.
Cleanliness and Health. Coronet.
Health-Communicable. Aims.
Let's Keep Food Safe to Eat. Coronet.
Microbes and Their Control. Bailey.
Soapy, the Germ Fighter. Avis.
Community Helpers: The Sanitation Department. Aims.
A Community Keeps Healthy. Bailey.

Grade 4

Objectives
1. To understand what a communicable disease is.
2. To understand how one can prevent disease by immunization and vaccination.
3. To understand how our environment affects our health.

Concepts
1. Communicable disease as opposed to noncommunicable disease.
   a. Microbes (microorganisms) and germs.
   b. Ways of preventing the spread of a communicable disease: use of a handkerchief, etc.
2. Groups of disease germs: bacteria, protozoans, viruses.
3. Ways the body fights against germs
   a. Skin.
   b. Mucus.
   c. White blood cells.
   d. Antibodies—immunity.
   e. Vaccines.
   f. Booster shots.
4. World-wide efforts to fight diseases
   a. World Health Organization.
5. The Health Department
   a. Services.
   b. Advantages of periodic health checkups.
   c. Recognition of early symptoms of illness.
6. Ways our environment affects our health
   a. Water pollution as a source of disease; waste treatment plant, chlorine.
   b. Food pollution: dirty utensils, dirty hands, bugs.
   c. Air pollution: emphysema and bronchitis.
   d. Housing problems of the inner city.
   e. Noise: cause of nervousness; sleep disruption; causes one to tire more quickly than usual; development of hearing problems.

Group and Individual Activities
1. Appoint committee to assemble books about microbes.
2. Encourage pupils to bring in articles about communicable diseases. This could lead into direct involvement with community problems.
3. In Petri dishes grow germs from telephone mouthpiece, pencil, finger.
4. Place three pieces of sliced, cooked potato on three small, clean saucers. Rub a finger over first potato, cough on second one, sneeze on third. Put in plastic bags and watch germs grow.
5. Make maps showing location of community source of water, the water treatment plant, and the water storage towers.
6. Take class on trip to old buildings being reconstructed, to slums, garbage dumps, etc.
7. Make texture boxes—discuss the kind of environment you would be the healthiest in; where you would feel the most comfortable.
8. Build a space maze out of large pieces of cardboard bolted together. How do you feel in a small space as compared to a larger one? Are there some places you feel you should walk with your back turned to it?
9. Make a get well card for a fellow student or a sick friend. Use mixed media techniques.

Pupil References
Grant, Madeleine P.: *The Wonder World of Microbes.* 2nd ed. New York: McGraw-Hill Book Co., 1964.

Lietz, Gerald S.: *Junior Science Book of Bacteria.* Champaign, Ill.: Garrard Publishing Co., 1964.

Chester, Michael: *Let's Go to Stop Air Pollution.* New York: G. P. Putnam's Sons, 1968.

Knight, David: *The First Book of Sound.* New York: Franklin Watts, 1960.

Radlauer, Edward, and Shaw, Ruth: *Water For Your Community.* Encino, California: Elk Grove Press, 1960.

Schneider, Herman and Nina: *Let's Look Under the City.* Reading, Mass.: Addison-Wesley, 1962.

Teacher References

Dubois, Rene J.: *The Unseen World.* Rockefeller.

Saltman, Jules: *Immunization For All.* Public Affairs Committee.

Simon, Harold J.: *Microbes and Men.* New York: McGraw-Hill Book Co., 1963.

Farb, Peter: *Ecology.* Morristown, N. J.: Silver Burdette Co., 1963.

Lewis, Alfred: *This Thirsty World: Water Supply and Problems Ahead.* New York: McGraw-Hill Book Co., 1964.

Films

Bacteriology. Louis Pasteur and Robert Koch. Jam Handy. (From the Great Discoveries in Science Series.)

Cleanliness and Health. 2nd ed. Coronet.

Microbes and Their Control. BFA.

Problems of Our Cities. (Series of six filmstrips.) Urban Media.

Other Sources

Microbe-growing materials: Turtox Products.

CHAPTER 16

drugs, alcohol, and tobacco

Despite the efforts of teachers, parents, and other adults, the use of drugs, alcohol, and tobacco by children and older youth in our society is increasing. It is now imperative that educational programs be greatly revamped and be given to all children *starting in kindergarten* and extending through each school year thereafter. Even five-year-old children have already learned much about the use of illicit and licit drugs. They are well aware of the smoking and drinking habits of their parents, others in their own family, and the people they see on TV and movie screens. All children today in our affluent, temptation-filled society need much help in learning how to live wisely in the real world of which they are a part. Just as a child learns to brush his teeth long before he learns why he should do so, so must teachers in our schools and parents in their homes begin to shape his attitudes and behavior long before he begins to learn the factual information he must master in order to weigh wisely the making of his decision to turn to or away from the use of drugs, alcohol, and tobacco.

One approach that must be avoided above all else in this sensitive area is the "soap-box one," for nothing will turn student interest away from this program more quickly. As one authority has said:[1]

> Once the age of 11 has passed, we as teachers find ourselves in the position of having to compete with the closed-circuit peer group and with the full impact of the mass media aimed at our affluent young people. The extent of our effectiveness then becomes questionable—we have become 'The Establishment.'

TEACHING STRATEGIES

Studies show that youth begin using drugs, alcohol, and tobacco for three reasons: (1) they are curious and want to find out for themselves about them, (2) peer pressure

---

[1] Daniels, Rose: "Drug Education Begins Before Kindergarten." *The Journal of School Health* (May 1970), pp. 242–48.

and the need for peer acceptance, and (3) to escape an unpleasant situation. Those who do become involved seem to have a poor self-concept, lack respect for authority of any kind including law, and are unable to make responsible personal and social decisions alone or on their own. With these facts in mind, the teacher, through a well-planned preventive program can: (1) show actual drugs, not pictures of them, or do other things to satisfy curiosity except having students actually use these products, (2) help each individual gain in personal and social skills so that he is accepted by groups engaged in beneficial pursuits, rather than detrimental ones, and (3) aid each one to gain the courage to express his convictions by gradually building up his feelings of self-respect and individual worth.

All teaching methods used in this area should help students gain a clear understanding of the pros and cons of the use of these products. When medications are discussed, it should be stressed that the proper use should be fully explained by a doctor and that they should be obtained only from a physician. The teacher needs to read widely in order to know what is fact and what is myth in relationship to drugs and drug education especially. The use of scare tactics in teaching in this area is taboo. At all times the teacher should be able to answer children's questions with honesty and assurance. If the best deterrent to drug abuse is through each individual's value system and his knowledge of what great damage he can do to his body, personality, and self-concept, then these are the areas which must receive greater attention in any educational preventive program.

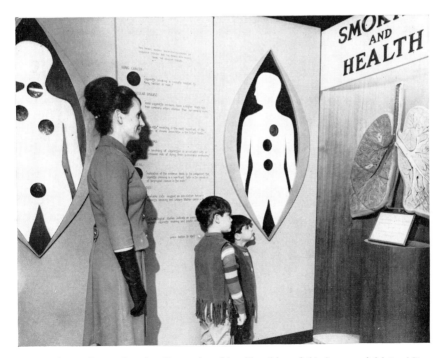

Figure 16-1. Comparing the diseased and healthy sides of this lung model lets visitors see for themselves the damage smoking can do. (Courtesy of Dallas Health and Science Museum)

Other suggestions are that teachers:

1. Take courses in a nearby school in drug education.
2. Read widely materials concerning the dangers of drug abuse and how to help children avoid them.
3. Develop improved communicative skills through workshops, taking part in "encounter" or "sensitivity-training" groups so that their students *do* feel free to seek their help with serious personal problems.

It is important for the teacher to remember that knowledge of facts alone cannot and does not change attitudes, beliefs, or behavior. How and in what context facts are presented, however, can do so especially with children. It is only when the learner puts in practice what he has studied in schools that learning actually takes place. Consequently, the *only* true test of any educational experience is what the learner *does* when *away* from the teacher. A real teacher, like a good parent, becomes progressively unnecessary, for her pupils will become self-motivated and self-directed.

Found below are suggestions for teaching about drugs to children in grades K to 6:

Kindergarten

Objectives
1. To realize that drugs have good and bad effects on the body.
2. To explain what adults and others mean when speaking of drugs.

Suggested Approaches
1. Have school nurse come in and discuss the purpose of a doctor. Show instruments he uses, such as a stethoscope.
2. Bulletin boards
3. Demonstrations

Major Points To Stress
1. Certain medicines are beneficial, if used properly.
2. Medicines can be dangerous as well as helpful.
3. Do not put things in mouth, ears, or nose unless parents or doctor advises them and gives it to them.

Group Activities
1. Have class tell about their experiences going to a doctor.
2. Discuss immunizations children have had.
3. Have class collect pictures showing effects of drugs on the individual.
4. Have class organize pictures showing how some drugs are made.
5. Show children the poison label on harmful products and understand what it means.
6. Discuss the danger of chewing on toys and sampling pills or other things just to learn what they are like.
7. Have the children tell about TV commericals they have seen.

Individual Activities
1. Have class use certain medicines to see effects of them (such as creams on skin).
2. Have them draw pictures of medicines they use.

Correlation with Other Subjects
1. Drama
   a. Role play visit to the doctor.
2. Science
   a. Discuss pollution, ecology tied in with effects of drugs.

Evaluation
1. Listen to what children say to each other about drugs.
2. Check with the parents if the children are becoming more concerned about carefulness of proper use of all kinds of drugs.

Audio-Visual Aids
Filmstrips and all kinds of other visual aids are available from The Tane Press, 6778 Greenville Ave., Dallas, Texas.

Teacher References
"Family Health Record." (Pamphlet) American Medical Association.
Check schools and public library for recent publications dealing with drugs, medicines, and alcohol.

Pupil References
Keep in touch with school librarian, find good recent material which ties in with your present area of teaching.

Grade 1

Objectives
1. To be aware of the constant presence and use of all kinds of drugs by everyone.
2. To teach children to be careful in taking all kinds of medicines or putting anything in their mouths.

Suggested Approaches
1. Guest speakers
2. Role playing
3. Show and tell
4. Demonstrations

Major Points To Stress
1. That drugs have to be used under the direction of a qualified adult. Discuss who is a qualified adult, and what makes him qualified.
2. The wide scope of drugs. Some products are detrimental to health, such as household cleansers and insect spray.

Group Activities
1. Role playing on areas safe for storing all medicines and household cleansers which are poisonous to pets and to children.
2. Read aloud the story of Snow White and discuss.
3. Role play what you should do if someone offers you something and if you know something might be dangerous, whom should you ask.
4. Role play what you would do if your little brother or sister puts something in your mouth.

Individual Activities
1. Have children make lists of where their mothers store medicines, and how they are kept out of reach of children and pets.
2. Have children make a chart of pictures of tablets, creams, mists, liquids, etc. Compare their pictures with things they have in home medicine cabinets.
3. Discuss how they can help keep drugs away from little brothers and sisters.

Correlation With Other Subjects
1. Art
a. Draw different dangerous drugs and good ones, too.

Evaluation
1. Note the carefulness with which children speak of medicines and see if you can notice any hints of carelessness around home. If you can, contact the parents to see if the problem can be alleviated.

Audio-Visual Aids
  Poison In The House. Associated Films.
  Children At Play With Poison. Creative Arts Studio.

Pupil References
  10 Little Tasters. St. Paul, Minn.: Imagination, Inc., 2651 University Ave.,
  St. Paul, Minnesota.
  Ask librarian where one can find good material for this age group of children.

Teacher References
  1. Contact local and national drug control councils for recent material on
     drug problems.
  2. Check with librarian.

Grade 2

Objectives
  1. To recognize that health can greatly be affected by drugs.
  2. To show how lives can be both lost and saved by the administration of
     drugs.

Suggested Approaches
  1. Demonstrations
  2. Show and tell
  3. Guest speakers
  4. Role playing

Major Points to Stress
  1. Safety in use of drugs must exist. Drugs must be used wisely and can
     help instead of hurt people.
  2. Begin to understand drug problem and why one must be careful when
     dealing with all types of drugs. Again explain the total area of drugs.

Group Activities
  1. Role play children finding candy or being given something by a
     stranger.
  2. Also do group activities dealing with the spoiling and safety precautions
     used for food.
  3. Have children tell about any hospital experiences they have had.

Individual Activities
  1. Have children list the medicines they think they need to be healthy.
  2. Have each draw pictures of people they think are qualified to recom-
     mend the use of drugs to them.
  3. Have children tell stories of vaccine and shots they have been given and
     tell why they were given these shots.

Correlation with Other Subjects
  1. The subject of drugs is important and should be tied in with all subjects,
     for this is such a wide term and can easily be discussed in all areas of
     study.
  2. Art and Drama
     a. Role playing with some students being patients and others being
        doctors and nurses.
  3. Math and Science
     a. How drugs were discovered. Why they were devised. How much
        do they cost?

Audio-Visual Aids
  Growing Up Day By Day. Encyclopedia Britannica.
  "Let's Talk About Drugs." Multimedia Productions.

Pupil References
  1. *Keeping Ourselves Healthy.* Chicago: Society For Visual Education. 1972.
  2. Check with librarian and other qualified teachers in area.

Teacher References
1. Check current magazines for good sources of information in this area.
2. Keep in contact with other personnel, and know where the nearest drug association or drug information center is located in your city. See the yellow pages in your phone book.

Evaluation
1. This is an important area of education and one must apply himself and be sure of giving the children knowledge of the need for staying away from hazardous drugs.

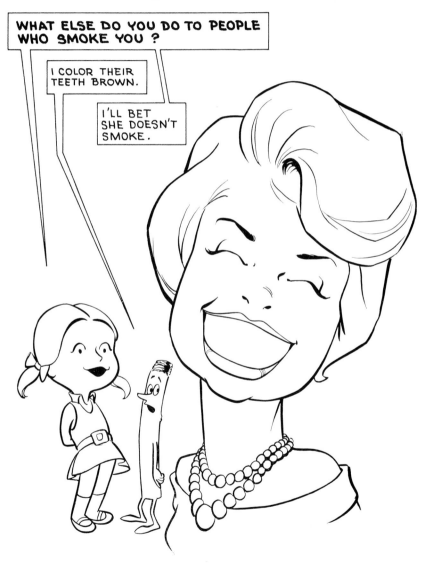

Figure 16-2. Excellent coloring books are available for children studying about drugs. (Courtesy of the Tane Press)

Grade 3

Concepts
1. Drugs can be both helpful and harmful.
   a. Helpful drugs can help a person recover from illness, prevent disease, and reduce pain.
   b. Harmful drugs can make a person ill and damage parts of the body.
2. To realize that too much of a good thing can be harmful.
   a. An overdose of helpful medicine.
   b. Too much food is harmful and can cause obesity, too much sun can cause damage to the skin and eyes.
3. Harmful agents are in common household cleaning products and should not be tasted.
4. To realize that anything that enters the body has some effect.
5. Sometimes nature can heal many problems without drugs, and that one should not be too quick to take medicines at the first sign of illness; e.g., scurvy and the story of the British limeys and other historical events which led to improved diets.

Approaches
1. Role playing
2. Discussion and demonstration
3. Bulletin boards and charts
4. Experiments

Group Activities
1. Discuss with students when they have had to take medicines during illness and point out importance of taking only the prescribed amount.
2. Have display of instruments used in medicine and the adminstration of certain kinds of drugs. Have nurse speak and demonstrate their uses.
3. Talk or role play about what you should do if you found a piece of candy or any kind of food, particularly around Halloween.
4. Demonstrate how oil and powder can change the texture of the skin. Sun, poison plants, or acid can cause rashes and skin eruption.
5. Have children learn the various poison labels.

Individual Activities
1. Collect pictures in scrapbook or notebook of the various instruments. Label and write a caption explaining their use. This could be a long-term project.
2. Have each child make a list of numbers used in case of an emergency. Check to be sure each child knows his phone number, street address, and doctor's number.

Correlation with Other Subjects
1. Drama
   a. Role play the discovery of an accidental poisoning. Instruct students on whom to call, what information to give.
   b. Teach rescue breathing.
2. Science
   a. Grow or buy an aloe plant. Discuss its use as an antiseptic by the Indians on open wounds. Use it in your class for first aid on minor scrapes.
3. Art
   a. Draw, collage, paint, papier-mâché bottles with poison labels.
4. Math
   a. Bring empty bottles of cleaning agents, old medicines, bottles, etc. Record price and amount inside and determine unit price per item.

Visual Aids — All available from The Tane Press.
   "Tell It Like It Is."
   "Alcohol Film Strip Set."

Books for The Pupils — All available from The Tane Press.
Cup of Fury; Let's Talk About Goofballs and Pep Pills; Gambling Is For Suckers.

Books for The Teacher
"Amphetamines," "Barbiturates," "Glue Sniffing," "LSD" and "Marihuana" available free from American Medical Association, Department of Health Education, 535 N. Dearborn St., Chicago 60610.

Public Health Service Publications #1827, 1828, 1829 and 1830. "Narcotics," "LSD," "Marihuana" and "The Up and Down Drugs: Amphetamines and Barbiturates." Available for 5¢ each from Superintendent of Documents, U.S. Government Printing Office, Washington, D.C. 20402.

Single copy of reprint from *Today's Education*, "Students and Drug Abuse," available free from National Institute of Mental Health, Box 1080, Washington, D. C. 20013.

Grade 4

Concepts
1. Learn difference between prescription and nonprescription medicines.
2. Realize the importance of taking only the prescribed amount of medicines.

Approaches
1. Role playing
2. Discussion and experiments
3. Demonstrations
4. Charts and bulletin boards
5. Individual research projects and book reports
6. Field trips

Group Activities
1. Have children bring the inside paper instructions which accompany nonprescription medicine. Read and discuss the instructions.
2. Discuss the role of the pharmacist, his training and duties. If possible, invite one to speak to the class. Visit behind the scenes in a drug store.
3. Have students trace drugs from their origin in plants, manufacturer, to drug store, to you, with your doctor's prescription, and present findings on bulletin board.

Individual Activities
1. Have each student write his own history, listing such things as when and what inoculations, etc.
2. Collect ads in newspaper, magazine, list those on TV about nonprescription drugs.
3. Have child think about how or why people might take the wrong dosage or the wrong medicine by accident or on purpose.
4. Have child make a survey of his own home for the proper storage of cleaning agents, medicines, etc. Point out the need for safe storage and proper disposal of old medicines and products, especially if there is a younger brother and sister.

Correlation with Other Subjects
1. Science
   a. Research history of drugs, what types of experiments researchers used, home remedies from various cultures, Indian cures, witchdoctors using herbs.
   b. Illustrate the growth of mold on a piece of bread or cheese to demonstrate discovery of some wonder drugs from such molds.
   c. List the drugs from plants and animals and those made in a laboratory.
2. Reading
   a. Book reports on such health heroes as Salk, Sabin, and Pasteur.

11

      b. Have students write a play on the life of one, bringing in informa-
         tion gained in reading the books.
   3. Math
      a. Research and make a statistical chart on how many people had polio
         in 1950, -55, -60, -65, -70. Make graph showing decline of other
         diseases as well (smallpox, tuberculosis, diphtheria, tetanus).
   4. Social Studies
      a. Study the effect of diseases upon history (Henry VIII, Alexander
         the Great, Beethoven, etc.).
      b. Trace the drug route of Marco Polo in the Orient.

Teacher References
   "Drug Education: Some Recent Resources." *Grade Teacher* 88 (April 1971):69.
   Bol. S.: "Philosophy and Objectives for a Drug Education Program." *Journal
      of School Health* 41 (January 1971):11–16.
   "Teaching About Drugs." Curriculum Guide K–12. *Consumer Information.*
      Pharmaceutical Association, 1155 15th St. N.W, Washington, D. C. 20025.
   Journal of Drug Education. Baywood Publishing Company, Inc. 1 Northwest
      Drive, Farmingdale, New York 11735.
   Escape To Nowhere, A Guide For Educators. Philadelphia: Smith, Kline and
      French Laboratories, 1967.
   Levy, Marvin P.: *Resource Book For Drug Abuse Information.* Washington,
      D. C.: AAHPER, 1972.

Student References
   Health and Growth, 4. Glenview, Ill.: Scott, Foresman and Co., 1971.
   Narcotic Education Bureau: National Women's Christian Temperance Union.
      1730 Chicago Avenue, Evanston, Illinois. 60201. Packets containing ma-
      terial on drugs, tobacco, and alcohol.
   Man, Sin and Drugs; The Drug Society; Decision. Internation Education and
      Training, 1776 New Highway, Farmingdale, N. Y., 11735.

Film and Filmstrips, Tapes
   Additional pamphlets and brochures available from:
   American Heart Association (or local offices).
   Texas Alcohol and Narcotic Education Bureau, 2814 Oak Lawn, Dallas, Texas
      75219.
   Blue Cross-Blue Shield, 222 North Dearborn, Chicago, Illinois, 60601 (or local
      offices).
   American Cancer Society (or local offices).
   Drugs and Our Lives. (Tape) International Education and Training.
   Don't Use It. (Filmstrip) Curriculum Studios.
   Drugs and the Nervous System. (Film) Churchill Films.

Grade 5

Objectives
   1. To know that drugs come from several sources.
   2. To appreciate their long history of use.
   3. To understand the difference betweeo prescription and nonprescription
      medicines.
   4. To recognize that drugs as medicines have many uses, along with a
      potential for producing both good and bad effects.
   5. To know that many widely used substances contain drugs.

Basic Concepts
   1. Drugs are defined as "articles intended for the use in the diagnosis,
      cure, mitigation, treatment or prevention of disease in man or other
      animals."
   2. There are four main sources of drugs:
      a. Plants

      b. Animals

      c. Minerals

      d. Laboratory (synthetic)

3. The history of drugs may be divided in three periods:

      a. Discovery

      b. Early use

      c. Modern use

4. Legally prescription medicine can be purchased only on the order of a doctor.

      a. Prescription of medicines by a physician or dentist for specific reasons and according to the needs of each individual patient; i.e., in terms of the severity of the disease, and of the age, weight, and individual characteristics of the patient.

      b. Need for purchasing prescription medicines from a registered pharmacist or doctor, or having them administered in a hospital.

      c. Necessity of carefully following directions for taking medicines.

      d. Desirability of destroying leftover prescription medicine upon relief of the condition, unless otherwise advised by a physician or dentist.

5. It is important to know how and when to use nonprescription medicines. Dangers associated with nonprescription medicines:

      a. Effects of excessive use

      b. Possible ineffectiveness, costliness, and harmfulness of self-directed medication

      c. Possible harmfulness of drugs which in combination may result in undesirable chemical interaction.

      d. Awareness that advertising claims for nonprescription medicines are designed to persuade the consumer to buy the product; dangers of failing to understand such claims.

      e. Danger that self-medication may seriously delay the proper diagnosis and care of illness in its incipient stages.

6. Medicinal drugs when properly administered

      a. Relieve pain

      b. Correct deficiencies

      c. Induce sleep

      d. Prevent diseases

7. The following substances that contain drugs are most commonly overused:

      a. Coffee, cola drinks (caffeine)

      b. Tobacco products (nicotine)

      c. Alcoholic beverages (alcohol)

8. Alcohol affects the user in the following areas of human activity:

      a. Judgment

      b. Muscular coordination

      c. Vision and hearing

      d. Memory

      e. Speech

      f. Breathing rate

      g. Heart action

      h. Social behavior (loud voice, desire to fight, etc.)

9. Alcohol can cause:

      a. Death

      b. Organic damage to digestive, urinary, nervous, and respiratory systems

10. Nicotine is a poisonous substance in tobacco smoke

      a. It causes increase of heart action

      b. Raising of blood pressure

      c. Irritation of digestive and respiratory tracts

      d. Stains the teeth.

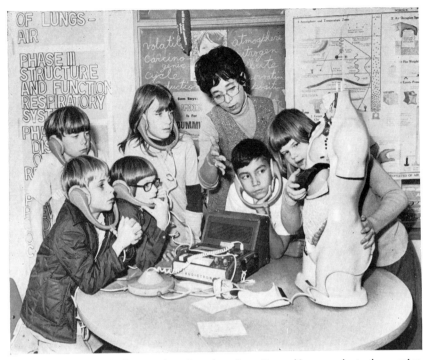

Figure 16-3. These children are learning what cigarette smoking can do to the respiratory system. (Courtesy of Dallas *Morning News*)

11. Caffeine is a mild stimulant found in tea, coffee, and cola drinks.
    a. May cause nervousness, sleeplessness (with excessive use)
    b. Is a source of undesirable stomach and intestinal reaction
    c. Increases heart rate

Suggested Approaches
    1. List examples of drugs which come from plants, animals, and which are synthesized in laboratories.
    2. Ask a physician to discuss how treatment with modern drugs affects illness.
    3. Write to Parke, Davis & Company for pictures of "Events of Medical History."
    4. Read and discuss stories about discoveries of important drugs, such as penicillin by Alexander Fleming.
    5. Describe to the class and discuss information included on a doctor's prescription; name and address of patient, name of medication, amount of dosage, form to be dispensed; directions to the patient; number of refills (if any); written signature of doctor, and date of prescription. Discuss why a second person, the pharmacist, is important in the use of prescription drugs.
    6. Have children make posters on how drugs as medicines contribute to healthful living.

Group Activities
    1. Role play the difficulties an intoxicated person would have in unlocking a door, tying his shoes, driving a car. Discuss what is incapacitating him and why.

2. Have children write a paper on why they or their friends do not smoke.
3. Describe positive ways of satisfying curiosity.
4. Act out positive ways of facing disappointment, stress, and grief.
5. Show children the warning label on a harmful substance and teach them its meaning.
6. Have children describe safety precautions that should be observed to prevent accidental poisoning.
7. Teach elementary first aid and have children practice on one another.
8. Discuss how easy is it to say "No" and on what occasions is it wise to say "No."
9. Present a panel on "What I can do to help prevent abuse of drugs."
10. Have students write to Food and Drug Administration and the Bureau of Narcotics and Dangerous Drugs for information.
11. Explore community resources that give help to people with drug problems.
12. Have children write a paper on how friends influence their choice of activities. Use a true experience.

Filmstrips

Let's Talk About Drugs. Multimedia Productions.
Who Are You? Society for Visual Education.
What Should I Do? Walt Disney.
The Mad Chemist. Professional Arts.
Rx Not For Kicks. Cathedral Films.

Pupil References

The Use and Misuse of Drugs. DCA Educational Products, Inc. 4865 Stenton Ave., Philadelphia, Pa., 19144.
How Safe Are Our Drugs? DCA Educational Products, Inc., 4865 Stenton Ave., Philadelphia, Pa., 19144.
Poison and You. Channing, Channing, L. Bete Co., Inc., Greenfield, Mass., 01301.
Irwin, Farnsworth, Fraumeni: *Finding Your Way; Understanding Your Needs; Choosing Your Goals.* Chicago: Lyons and Carnahan, 1970.
Byrd, Neilson, and Moore: *Health 5, 6.* River Forest, Ill.: Ludlow Bros., 60305.

Teacher Resources

Weitzman, Alice: "Guiding Children's Social Growth." Chicago: Science Research Associates, 1968.
Vogel, Victor H. and Virginia E.: "Facts About Narcotics and Other Dangerous Drugs." Chicago: Science Research Associates.

Books

Editors of Life: *Drugs.* New York: Time-Life Books, 1969.
Drug Abuse: Escape To Nowhere. Philadelphia: Smith, Kline and French Laboratories.
Stearn, Jess: *The Seekers.* Garden City, N. Y.: Doubleday & Co., 1972.

Grade 6

Objectives

1. To know that misused medicines, drugs, and other agents may have serious effects on the individual.
2. To identify common household products and to use them for their intended purposes.
3. To assume increasing responsibility for personal health.
4. To understand and appreciate the relationship of drugs to total health.

Basic Concepts

1. Medicine can be misused
    a. Through excessive or prolonged self-medication.
    b. By sharing medicine without consultation of a doctor.
    c. Through self-diagnosis and use of leftover prescription medicines.
    d. Through overdosage, accidental or intentional.
2. Various dangers are to be associated with misuse of prescription medicines.
    a. Tolerance to medication (so that larger dosages are required).
    b. Development of dependence, psychological and/or physical.
    c. Changes in personality, moods, goals, and outlook on life.
    d. Serious mental disorders.
    e. Possible organic damage.
    f. Death.
3. Various substances have an abuse potential that can be very harmful:
    a. Alcohol.
    b. Marijuana.
    c. LSD, mescaline, and other hallucinogens.
    d. Tranquilizers.
    e. Analgesics.
    f. Cough syrups.
    g. Certain foods.
    h. Tobacco.
4. Commonly abused drugs most frequently affect the brain and nervous system consequently altering body reactions.
    a. Stimulating or depressing the central nervous system.
    b. Inducing hallucinations, altering perception and subsequent performance.
    c. Altering mood and behavior.
5. People abuse drugs for a number of reasons.
    a. As a crutch.
    b. Desire for peer acceptance.
    c. Self-destruction that is deliberate.
    d. For "kicks."
    e. As an act of rebellion.
6. Manmade products, when properly used, provide essential benefits.
    a. Paint thinner.
    b. Antifreeze.
    c. Gasoline.
    d. Aerosols.
    e. Cleaning fluids.
    f. Glue.
    g. Foods.
    h. Plant foods.
    i. Insecticides.
7. Products are misused for various reasons.
    a. By accident.
    b. By experiment.
    c. By failure to read and follow directions.
    d. Through lack of knowledge.
    e. As a means of gaining peer acceptance or leadership.
8. The consequences of drug misuse are:
    a. Nausea, vomiting.
    b. Suffocation.
    c. Poisoning.
    d. Organic damage.
    e. Mental damage, temporary or permanent.
    f. Death.

9. Part of growing up is to become independent and responsible for personal health and the health of others.
   a. The need to help others in emergencies.
   b. Importance of a child's telling adults when he is ill.
   c. Importance of following the advice of a doctor.
10. Habits develop in several ways.
   a. Through motivation.
   b. Through conscious effort.
   c. Without conscious effort.
   d. Through influence of friends and their behavior.
11. Certain habits affect health.
   a. Personal health habits, eating, sleeping, exercising, cleanliness.
   b. Study habits.
   c. Safety habits.
   d. Recreational habits.
   e. Habits of using medicines and drugs.
12. Problems of drug abuse may be avoided
   a. By making wide choices based on accurate information.
   b. By having courage to say "no" to friends or others who insist on experimenting.
   c. By knowing and respecting the laws.
   d. By not experimenting with drugs or with any substance for other than its intended purpose.
   e. By recognizing that the normally healthy individual does not need regular medication.

Suggested Approaches
1. Role play how to cope with pressure from friends who insist that others use drugs.
2. Surveys. Ask children to survey their homes with either parent or another adult to learn where potentially harmful substances are stored. Report to the class on safe places to store substances (aerosols, glue, rubbing alcohol).
3. Speakers. Physician or nurse to discuss the consequences of product misuse. Have a past drug addict to speak on his experiences.
4. Bulletin boards. Cut out pictures of substances or products which are frequently misused. Discuss.

Group Activities
1. Learn the meaning of the following terms: stimulants; narcotics; depressants; hallucinogens; physical and psychological dependence; tolerance.
2. Have children describe or role play how their friends affect their behavior. Should one always follow advice? Are there disadvantages in following the leader?
3. Discuss the difficulties of breaking the habit of smoking.
4. Conduct a class debate on the question, "To smoke or not to smoke."

Correlation With Other Subjects
1. Spelling and Vocabulary
   a. Learn to use new terms in this unit on Drug Education.
2. Language Arts
   a. Bring interesting pictures related to drugs and use these for the children to create a story about them.
3. History
   a. Study the history of drug discoveries, people who used drugs such as Edgar Allen Poe.
4. Art
   a. Collages of the new terminology and pictures about drugs.

Filmstrips
"Drugs, Helpful and Harmful." Wexler Film Productions.
"To Save Your Life." Eli Lilly & Co.
"Bridge to Tomorrow." Modern Talking Picture Service.
"Alcohol and Your Health." Society for Visual Education.
"To Your Health." Mass Communications Center.

Pupil References
Irwin, Farnsworth, Fraumeni: *Finding Your Way.* Chicago: Lyons and Carnahan, 1970.
Pictures: *Events of Medical History.* Parke, Davis & Co.

Teacher References
"Drugs the Children Are Using." (Pamphlet) National Instructional Television Center, Box A, Bloomington, Ind., 47401.
"Drugs of Abuse." (Pamphlet) Journal of American Pharmaceutical Assn., 2215 Constitution Ave., N.W., Washington, D. C., 20037.
"The Medicine Your Doctor Prescribes." (Pamphlet) Washington, D. C.: Pharmaceutical Manufacturers Assn.
"Respect For Drugs." (Pamphlet) Washington, D. C.: U. S. Government Printing Office.
"Prescribed and Nonprescribed Medicines—Types and Use of Medicine." National Center for Health, Statistics Series 10, No. 29. Washington, D.C.: U. S. Dept. of Health, Education & Welfare.
Smith, Ralph Lee: *The Health Hucksters.* New York: Thomas Y. Crowell, 1960.
Cohen, Sidney: *The Drug Dilemma.* New York: McGraw-Hill Book Co., 1971.
Carroll, Charles R.: *Alcohol Use, Non-use and Abuse.* Dubuque, Iowa: Wm. C. Brown Co., 1970.

Further Suggestions

All teachers are urged to obtain a copy of the *Resource Book for Drug Abuse Education* ($1.25), available from The American Association for Health, Physical Education and Recreation, and to write for a list of publications on drug, alcohol, and smoking education from The Tane Press, 2814 Oak Lawn Ave., Dallas, Texas, 75219. The latter has many materials for both the pupil and teacher.

ALCOHOL EDUCATION

The subject of alcoholism should be treated as a disease, and not a matter of ethics, morals, or law.* This malady, which is increasing rapidly in our society, especially among teenagers, affects persons from all walks of life. Many thousands of children are the victims of neglect, battering, or physical abuse from one parent or in some cases both alcoholic parents, and many elementary school children are already well aware of the damage that can result from excessive drinking.

Found below are resource units the teacher might well use as guides in developing a preventive educational program in this area for children. It is suggested that units in this area begin at grade 3 and that all teachers in grades 3–6 develop through committee assignments teaching units for each grade which would include all of the suggested areas found below:

Objectives
1. To help students understand why people drink alcoholic beverages.
2. To make children aware of the types and uses of alcohol.
3. To present scientifically valid information to help children understand the physiological, psychological, and socio-economic effects of alcohol on people.

---

* See the splendid materials, *Teaching About Drugs, A Curriculum Guide, K–12* available from the American School Health Association.

4. To help students develop the ability to make intelligent decisions concerning the use of alcohol in everyday situations.

Areas To Be Covered
1. Types of alcohol.
   a. Ethyl (grain) alcohol—contained in alcoholic beverages.
   b. Methyl (wood) alcohol—industrial and medical applications; a poison if taken internally.
2. Uses of alcohol.
   a. Ethyl alcohol: a "stimulant" in social situations; a health measure; a psychological "crutch."
   b. Methyl alcohol: industrial uses (solvents, antifreeze, varnishes, shoe polish, etc.); medical uses (preservative for specimens, solvent for drugs, instrument sterilization, "rubbing" alcohol); extreme danger if taken internally.
3. Why *most* people drink.
   a. Adults: social drinking for physical and emotional relaxation; drinking at suggestion of medical doctor.
   b. Young people: experimentation, status seeking, rebellion against authority, "kicks."
4. Behavioral effects of alcohol on the drinker.
   a. Relaxation.
   b. Feeling of well-being.
   c. Problem drinking and alcoholism.
5. Legal controls and regulations on alcoholic beverages.

Activities
1. Have the children conduct research, then discuss the two basic types of alcohol—ethyl and methyl. Areas of research and discussion might include:
   a. What chemical elements is each composed of? What other substances include these elements?
   b. What are the differences between ethyl and methyl alcohol? What are the similarities? How can one type be safe to drink and the other be poisonous?
   c. Discuss the medical and industrial uses of methyl alcohol.
2. Divide the class into teams and have each group work on the project "How alcohol affects the body." Have each group make charts, graphs, diagrams, etc. which illustrate alcohol's effect on one of the following:
   a. Appetite and nutrition.
   b. Weight (gain and loss).
   c. Nerve depressant (sedative in small amounts; anesthetic in large amounts.)
   d. Brain activity—possible change in muscle coordination and speech.
   e. Central nervous system.
   f. Circulatory system.
   g. Body temperature.
   h. Body resistance to colds, pneumonia, and disease.
   i. Diseases related to liver, kidneys, heart, and arteries.
3. Discuss: "What are the behavioral effects of drinking?" (See booklet, "It's Best to Know about Alcohol," available from the Alcoholism and Drug Addiction Research Foundation of Ontario, 24 Harbord St., Toronto 5, Ontario, Canada. It illustrates the effects on the body and mind of various amounts of liquor. Other agencies listed in "Teaching Aids" section may have similar material.)
   a. Effect on judgment.
   b. Effect on inhibitions.
   c. Narcotic effect. (After class has gotten into unit on drugs . . . raise the question, "Is alcohol a narcotic?")

4. Have the students make tables showing physiological effects of alcohol and tobacco on the body.
   a. Discuss similarities, differences.
   b. How does advertising of tobacco and alcohol compare or contrast? (Your class already has made a scrapbook of tobacco information; have them compile a similar one about alcoholic beverages.)
5. As a followup to the comparison tables, have the youngsters research legal controls on alcohol—federal, state, and local.
   a. Legal drinking age.
   b. Prohibition: steps leading to passage of 18th Amendment; why it was unenforceable, for all practical purposes; and repeal (21st Amendment).
   c. Bootlegging.
   d. Federal and state controls on distilleries and breweries; protections against unlicensed and unregulated producers of alcohol.
   e. Traffic laws related to drunken driving.
   f. Why are there more federal and state legal controls on alcoholic beverages than on tobacco?
6. Have the children debate a topic such as "The drinking age should be lowered to 18 (or raised to 21)" or "There is nothing wrong with parents serving alcoholic beverages to their own children at home."
7. Arrange for high school students to debate or conduct a panel discussion based on questions asked by our students.
8. Have students make their own filmstrip on alcohol. Let each student select a topic to illustrate. Tape the picture together and roll your filmstrip through an opaque projector. Have each student explain his picture.

Teaching Aids
1. Single copy of pamphlet, "Thinking About Drinking," is available free from U.S. Department of Health, Education and Welfare. Welfare Administration, Children's Bureau, Publications Distribution Section, Room G024 HEW South, 330 C St. NW, Washington, D.C. 20201.
2. A teacher's kit including six pamphlets and a three-booklet teacher's guide is available for 75c from Publications Division. National Council on Alcoholism, Inc., 2 Park Ave., New York City 10016. (A student kit containing five of the same pamphlets costs 40c.)
3. Other sources of studies, pamphlets, etc.
   a. American Medical Association, 535 N. Dearborn St., Chicago, Ill. 60610.
   b. Rutgers University Center of Alcoholic Studies, New Brunswick, N.J. 08903.
   c. National Safety Council, 425 N. Michigan Ave., Chicago, Ill. 60601.
   d. Alcohol and Drug Addiction and Research Foundation of Ontario, 24 Harbord St., Toronto 5, Ontario, Canada.

SMOKING EDUCATION

Research shows that many children start experimenting in smoking tobacco and/or marijuana and trying glue sniffing in the intermediate grades and are regular users of these products by the 8th or 9th grade. In Cincinnati, Ohio, a survey showed that 22% of school children started to smoke at the age of 10 years or younger, and 60% between the ages of 11 to 13.[3] It is also known that chances for a child beginning to smoke at an early age are greater if his parents, brothers or sisters smoke and that school under achievers are more apt to develop the habit at an early age.

---

[3] Streit, William: "Students Express Views on Smoking." *Journal of School Health* 37 (March, 1967):153–154.

Although it has been estimated that one-third of all senior high schools now allow students to smoke outside the building, but on school property many schools still will not allow students to smoke while there, in spite of parent permission to do so.

One of the best sources of materials now available in the area of smoking education for children is the Berkeley Elementary School Health Curriculum Project in Smoking and Health Education. This program consists of the following:*

> *The health curriculum model* consists of three intensive units of study— one each at the fifth-, sixth-, and seventh-grade levels. Each unit is organized around a body system and all that impinges on it. They run about 8 to 10 weeks during the school year, are very comprehensive in their coverage of health education content, and involve maximal integration with other basic curriculum areas. The emphasis is on working toward the basic objectives of education, developing understanding and appreciation of the body and skills for prevention of disease, and encouraging youth to make their own sound decisions about personal and environmental factors that affect health. A wide variety of classroom education techniques and resources, materials and human, are used throughout. Great stress is placed on pupil motivation and activity of individuals and small groups dealing with real-life issues, and on involvement of school administration, parents, and community health personnel.

> *The teacher training model* involves establishment of two successful class-room examples of each unit at its grade level in one school of a district. Each participating district (each team of trainees), in addition to developing the unit in their two classrooms, is required to work with their administrators to develop and conduct similar training for other teachers at their grade level in their district within the first year. After establishment of a "success model" at the fifth-grade level involving two enthusiastic teachers, a team including administration and supervisors and groups of youngsters, succeed-ing waves of teachers are trained.

> *The teacher training* involves 2 weeks in-depth training of teams of class-room teachers and administrators. Each team typically includes: two classroom teachers, their building principal, and one or two additional cur-riculum support personnel—most generally nurses, health educators, or curriculum supervisors. Teacher trainers are frequently involved. The first year training deals with the fifth-grade level unit, the second year the sixth-grade level unit, and the third year the seventh-grade level unit. The training activities, methods, and resources parallel those employed in the classroom curriculum model. In addition to the practical training, each team utilizes approximately $2000 worth of classroom resources for conduct of the program in their two classrooms. (Primarily models, filmstrips, films, texts, charts, tapes, etc.) Carefully developed and sequentially arranged sets of materials applicable to class organization, individual pupil desk work, group projects, and parent and community involvement are included. Monitoring by training center staff is maintained on a regular basis at each area after the initial training. A communications system among all trainees is also operant. Team members are reconvened for a follow-up session about 9 months after training. During 1973 six training centers are providing training to 50 school districts in 15 states. Well over 300 elementary schools are deeply involved in the model program.

Found below is a sample resource unit which utilizes the conceptual approach to health education for use as a model by teachers when planning their own unit on smoking education for the intermediate grades:

---

* Materials reproduced by permission. Information concerning this program may be obtained from Dr. Roy Davis, Chief, Community Program Development Branch, National Clearinghouse for Smoking and Health, Department of Health, Education and Welfare, 5401 Westbard Avenue, Room 500, Bethesda, Maryland 20016.

BASIC AREA: THE USE AND ABUSE OF TOBACCO, ALCOHOL AND OTHER DRUGS

CONCEPT: The use and effects of mood and behavior modifying substances result from a complexity of factors.

Subconcept: The wide variety of mood and behavior modifiers and their effects imply certain human needs and necessary controls of these substances.

Intermediate Level

CONTENT	Code	MOTIVATING QUESTIONS Physical—A Mental-Emotional—B Sociocultural—C	LEARNING EXPERIENCES
. The use of tobacco can be harmful to the health.			As a motivator, have a teacher-made pre-test on smoking to see how much the students know.
. Forms of tobacco in use	ABC	What are the most popular forms of tobacco in use today?	Collect samples of packages and labels of each of the different forms of tobacco and create a display.
	A	How do they differ?	Conduct a demonstration with a smoking machine using cigars and cigarettes, to illustrate differences in ingredients. Let students build their own smoking machines if possible.
			Use a pipe cleaner and wipe the inside of a freshly used pipe stem. Discuss results with class.
. Tobacco in history	ABC	Where did tobacco originate? Who were some of the early originators of tobacco?	Assign a research project to the class on the history of tobacco in this country.
. The effects of the use of tobacco	ABC	What were some of the original uses of tobacco among the early users?	Show a film on the history of tobacco and discuss the film with the class.
. Smoking	AB	What are some of the effects of tobacco smoke on the body systems, including heart, lungs, circulation, nerves?	Conduct a demonstration using the smoking machine. Place a fish in the water flask of the machine and watch what happens to it when smoke begins to get into the flask. Describe the action. (Be sure to revive the fish with fresh water as soon as he acts peculiarly.)

		Questions	Suggested Activities
	AB	How does smoking affect one's appetite? His breath?	Divide the class into four groups. Have each group write to one recognized source for information about the effects of smoking. Have each group read the material and discuss the effects of smoking on the body functions. Share the results of the discussion with the rest of the class.
	B	Does smoking "calm the nerves"? How?	Show film on the effects of smoking.
	ABC	What are some of the diseases related to smoking?	Make several transparencies of graphs showing the relationship between smoking and certain diseases and smoking and life expectancy, showing age, sex, and other similar comparisons. Use the opaque projector to present information on these relationships.
	ABC	How do the effects of smoking compare in adults and young people?	
	ABC	How do the effects of steady cigarette, cigar and pipe smoking compare to the incidence of disease and other difficulties related to smoking? Why?	
	ABC	How are persons informed of the possible effects of smoking?	Have students research antismoking messages sent out through the various media. Report back to class.
		What are some of the special groups of people to whom cigarette advertising is directed, such as women, young people, and men?	Divide class into four groups. Group A should collect magazine advertisements of cigarettes and mount them. Study how the smoker is enticed by highlighting the slogan used, etc. Group B might draw a figure of the human body and locate diseases associated with smoking. Group C would collect and mount newspaper articles about smoking, and group D would compile a list of undesirable results of smoking. Invite parents and others to see the exhibit.
. Chewing . Snuff	AB	What are some of the effects of other tobacco on the human body?	Assign two students oral reports, after research, on snuff and chewing tobacco. Discuss their effects and compare them with smoking.
	ABC	Are they similar to or different from the effects of smoking? How? Why?	
. Reasons for using tobacco			

* Reproduced by permission of the Texas Education Agency, Austin, Texas.

CHAPTER 17

family life and sex education

The need exists today to help children become aware of their roles in life. The school, since it is the only institution which reaches all children over a prolonged time period, has both a challenging opportunity and obligation to contribute to their knowledge and understanding of the roles both sexes play, as well as to correct the distorted view of life they receive from television, movies, and certain magazines and books.

The principal goal of any program in family life education or human sexuality should be to affect behavior and to help children develop into effective family members (in their primary group) and in the overall family of man (in their secondary group). This program should be largely concerned with shaping values and standards of conduct and responsibilities as human beings. Good teaching in this area goes far beyond learning the names of body parts, the facts of pregnancy, or the function of the organs of reproduction.

Children are greatly affected, in many ways more than adults, by our so-called new morality, openness about sex, family mobility, and the rising divorce rate in our society. The facts that one out of every four marriages ends in a divorce, that the average family will move every four years, that both syphilis and gonorrhea are increasing at an alarming rate, as are pregnancies among early teenagers, give us enough evidence for the need of a greatly improved educational program in the area of human sexuality.

Sex education should be an integral part of the health education program on every grade level. However, since the words "sex education" usually bring quick and strong negative reaction from some parents, religious groups, or other adults, schools have increasingly been including materials in this area under the titles of "Family Life Education" or "Developing Wholesome Life Relationships." Regardless of what the material is called, it contains valuable information children should receive. The home, school, church, and community should work closely together in this area, for the education of children is not the sole responsibility of the school. The school must, however, support and provide education which is neglected or inadequate in the home.

Increasingly, educators are becoming aware that sex education possibilities abound in everyday classroom activities, and that since children are receiving some kind of information on their own from their equally uninformed peers or from older youngsters who are misinformed, it is the duty of the school to begin a graded program in the first school year that presents true information and helps young people shape desirable attitudes toward their own and the opposite sex. What children think and feel about themselves and others is far more important than knowing the answers to questions concerning human reproduction.

Young children are curious about themselves and about all aspects of life around them. They need to be given frank but brief answers to their simple questions, such as "Where do babies come from?" or "Why do babies need fathers?" They are not ready for or interested in learning the lengthy facts of reproduction, but do seek the answers to their simple questions. The films they watch, the television programs they see, the magazines their parents take, the billboard advertisements all about them play up sex and the "sexy." Consequently, an awakening appetite toward "finding out about things" is whetted to the degree that many of their questions are amazingly wise and often show surprised adults that children are far more aware of what is going on around them than they think. Above all, the teacher of elementary school children must be able to answer the many questions youngsters ask about life or to guide them to the needed information with dignity, discretion, and sincerity. Since sex is a normal human function that is the foundation of life itself, education in this area should be treated as just another part of the total school program. Facts concerning the reproductive system should be presented along with those on any of the other systems of the body. Teachers, however, must not only help children find answers to their questions but also shape desirable attitudes, values, and patterns of conduct. Classes should not be separated, although the teacher of sixth-grade girls may wish to discuss menstruation with them as a group, or there may be an occasion when she would want to talk to the boys alone. Certainly the school nurse or physician should not be brought in to speak to the class just on sex, for both should visit the classroom often to talk with the children about many aspects of good health.

In reality, sex education begins the very day of birth; it is present in one form or another when the father holds his baby daughter for the first time. Education goes on wherever there is life. It can be positive or negative, and even these contacts in the first few months of life can be of lasting importance to a child. Likewise, teaching geared toward helping pliable youngsters develop wholesome life relationships should start the first day of school. This can begin with taking the children on a tour of the building to show them where the little girls will go to the bathroom, and where the little boys will go. Throughout the primary grades "teachable moments" in this area should be capitalized upon. Oberteuffer suggests that the following teaching possibilities for sex education in the elementary grades might be used, and recommends that rather than trying to cover everything, the teacher may be wise to leave some areas untouched, while in some communities even more can be included:[1]

PRIMARY YEARS
  1. Functions of elimination as they relate to the genitalia, including protection and care.
  2. Phenomenon of birth; the coming of the baby; reproduction of plants and animals.
  3. Early social friendships, manners, and courtesies between sexes.
  4. Early conceptions of sex differences.

INTERMEDIATE YEARS
  1. Mental and physiological changes attendant upon growth; continuation of sex differences.
  2. Continuation of social and ethical relationships between the sexes, social friendships.
  3. Early lessons in hereditary influences.
  4. Basic sources of information on sex problems.

Every boy or girl is a member of a family that has representatives of those of the opposite sex. The child will need to know how to work, play, and live successfully in that closely knit group. Consequently, the school must work closely with the home to help prepare the child for his future responsibility as a parent, as well as his present role as a family member. It can do so by providing each youngster with realistic and meaningful girl-boy learning experiences in his formative years.

Guiding principles for the development of a unit or course of study in this area include the following:

  1. The home, church and school are the major and natural source for information about family life and sex development.
  2. School programs should be planned in cooperation with parents and other community organizations, such as health, welfare, church, and family-life agencies.
  3. The school should accept its responsibility for helping parents give guidance to children in problems of their growing up.
  4. The school should cooperate in community programs designed to give information about human development and should accept its responsibility for intelligent leadership and direction.
  5. Sex education should be integrated with the total health program at all grade levels and should be taught by the regular teacher with the usual class groupings.
  6. The school should provide individual guidance as well as class instruction to boys and girls in the acquisition of scientific knowledge and the development of wholesome attitudes in regard to growth and development as boys and girls.
  7. Opportunities should be provided for school personnel to acquire scientific knowledge; develop wholesome attitudes; acquire the use of a scientific vocabulary; acquaint themselves with questions (and answers) which children are likely to ask; feel secure in beginning and carrying on a program by having knowledge and the support of administrators, other teachers, and the community; understand that certain

---

[1] Oberteuffer, Delbert, *et al.*: *School Health Education.* 5th ed. New York: Harper & Row, 1972, p. 159.

personal problems of the child should be considered in private conferences.

8. Growth and development including sex education should be treated in a normal and mature manner.

9. The normal mixed groupings are usually preferable except when, in the judgment of the instructor, it is indicated that topics peculiar to one sex or age group call for separation of the sexes.

10. The teaching approach and the content of the program should give due consideration to the present understanding of the group.

Primary children can best be helped to learn about sex when the teacher answers questions as they arise, or capitalizes upon things happening around the children, such as the appearance of baby chicks at Easter or a new baby sister in the home of a pupil. As pupils advance up the academic ladder, they ask questions which require more detailed answers. Consequently, instruction in family living should become more factual, and be based upon scientific information regarding the human body. As one health education expert has suggested, there are three well-known approaches to classroom instruction: "(1) through animal and plant life (the 'birds, bees, and butterflies approach'); (2) through the anatomy and physiology involved; and (3) through human life situations."[2] Frequently, the wisest approach often is through life situations which arise naturally as boys and girls grow towards maturity.

SUGGESTED GRADED TOPICS

A graded program in family life education might well include the following topics:

Grade 1

1. The role of the father, mother, and children in a family.
2. Correct terms for the parts of the body having to do with elimination and reproduction.
3. Different toilet procedures for boys and girls.
4. The importance of sharing and being considerate of others.
5. Adult men and women who contribute to the welfare of children, such as the doctor, nurse, school janitor, policemen, etc.

Grade 2

1. Getting along with others.
2. Good sportsmanship; consideration of other classmates, parents, and family members.
3. What boys and men do at home and at work; what girls and women do.
4. How plants and animals reproduce.
5. The body, its care and function.

Grade 3

1. Steps toward independence.
2. Assuming one's own sex role in life.
3. The organs and systems of the body.
4. The beginning of life.
5. Desirable conduct patterns.
6. Personal appearance in relationship to personality and growth.
7. Family relationships which influence health.

---

[2] Oberteuffer, *op. cit.*, p. 152.

Grade 4

1. The role of the father and of the mother in the reproduction of animals and human beings.
2. How life begins.
3. Growing from an egg into a baby.
4. How we grow up.
5. Work and play with our families at home.
6. How girls and boys differ.
7. Occupations for men and women.

Grade 5

1. How animals reproduce and care for their young.
2. How the human baby grows inside the mother.
3. How mothers help babies be born.
4. The father's role in reproduction and in the family.
5. Heredity and reproduction.
6. Boy-and-girl relationships.
7. Wholesome life attitudes and values.

Grade 6

1. Body changes; how boys change, how girls change.
2. Problems of growing up.
3. Relationship between maturity and responsibility.
4. Place of the family in society; social codes and ethics.
5. Family problems and their solution for happy living.
6. Importance of wholesome sex attitudes and behavior.
7. Lives of outstanding persons of each sex.
8. Occupational choices.

CURRICULUM PLACEMENT

Education for family living can and should be correlated with all subjects included in the elementary curriculum. The following are used most often.

Social Sciences

Through study of famous historical families and personalities and their times, social studies can be an interesting and informative way of teaching family life education: George Washington and the days of early America; by tracing family customs in relationship to work and recreation; by comparing how ancient peoples reared and disciplined their children with practices of today; by showing the changing role of women throughout history; by contrasting marriage customs among primitive and civilized people, etc.

The Communicative Arts

Pupils should be provided with opportunities to write and speak about such things as why women and girls should be protected, what causes families to be unhappy or happy, how to care for babies, what to do when mother and a new baby brother or sister come home from the hospital, how we can help our mothers at mealtime, family fun, what I want to be when I grow up, and other related subjects. The possibilities of topics for use in this area are as great as a teacher's ability to utilize the right moment for doing so. She should listen carefully to what children say about the above-mentioned areas, as well as observe their behavior. Likewise, she should be on the lookout for the "sissy" or "mamma's boy" or the girl who acts and talks like a boy and wishes she were one, for these children need help. Class parties, projects, and other group activities should be initiated as a means of helping both sexes work and play cooperatively together, especially in the fourth and fifth grades, the age when both groups tend to be hypercritical of each other. Among primary children, those who are only children, excessively shy, or aggressive should be aided to contribute to group endeavors. The elementary school *is* the society of children, and each youth therein must learn to become an important, intelligent, and vital contributing member of it.

Science

Science is the foundation upon which sex education rests. It can be utilized in many ways to correlate family life education with needed scientific information about the differences between the sexes and human reproduction. Youth in the upper elementary grades are ready for detailed and more specific factual information, although many of available materials should be modified for them. Such topics as the following might well be included in the materials to be covered in instructional units on this subject:

1. The male and female reproductive organs.
2. Menstruation and nocturnal emissions.
3. Venereal diseases.
4. Pregnancy.
5. The development of the human fetus.
6. Normal and abnormal birth.
7. Heredity.
8. Infant care.
9. Reproduction of plants and animals.
10. The role of sex in mental illness.
11. Your own changing body.

It is not enough, however, merely to teach the facts about reproduction. It could be dangerous to do so, for boys and girls are naturally curious and want to see and try things out for themselves. Unless positive behavior and desirable attitudes are built into each pupil at the same time they learn the facts of life, the program can be harmful rather than beneficial.

Younger children will delight in having a class pet, feeding and caring for it, and watching it change and reproduce its own kind. Rabbits, hamsters, goldfish, chickens, or almost any other kind of small animal can be used. A new "Chick-Chick Egg Incubator" is now on the market which will enable pupils to see the entire hatching process through a plastic dome window. The correct heat and humidity can be maintained in the incubator to hatch ducks, pheasants, and quail.[3] Watching a tiny bird actually breaking out of its egg is a thrilling educational experience for any child. Each should do more than just watch, however, for all should be taught also the magic, miracle, and wonder of life.

Mathematics

Mathematics and family life education can work together in many ways. Suggested activities for doing so include:

---

[3] Write to Insta Sales Corp., Dept. M. 25, 11 E. 47th Street, New York, N.Y. 10017, for information.

1. Preparing a family budget.
2. Determining life and hospital insurance costs and learning which policies give the most benefits for the money spent on them.
3. Discovering the food costs for a baby's first year.
4. Comparing the amount of money spent on recreation from today's family budget to that spent by one's grandparents.
5. Estimating family food costs over a period of time.
6. Exploring family vacation plans in relation to family income.
7. Studying retirement insurance plans.
8. Determining the relation of take-home pay to salary.
9. Filling out income-tax forms for a married couple.
10. Finding out about loan interest rates.

Drama and Art

Dramatic and art activities are especially adaptable for correlation in this area, especially with primary children. They will learn many things by making a poster of a happy family from pictures cut out of magazines, as well as provide their teacher with new insights into what they think a happy family would be. Their feelings and emotions, many fears, hatreds, or desires can best be shown by free-hand drawings, cutouts, clay figures, or other creative endeavors. It is of paramount importance that the teacher watch these children "play house," "eat dinner with my family," or other dramatized home and family life experiences, for the children's actions can be most revealing to the trained, sensitive eye.

Suggested creative activities in this area include:

1. Act out going on a family trip.
2. Draw pictures of your family.
3. Act out a story you make up about any child in any kind of a family.
4. Show us how to play the favorite quiet game of your family.
5. Tell us about your favorite relative and why you like him.
6. Have a pet or dog show. Discuss having a pet for a friend, and how to take care of it.
7. Illustrate a story your parents or grandparents told you about any of their own experiences.
8. Give a short skit showing a typical Saturday or Sunday at your house.
9. Make a poster of what your family does on a holiday.
10. Make foreign clothes for dolls out of cloth, or clothe cardboard figures with costumes made out of colored paper. Tell us about your doll.
11. Dramatize social graces, giving each couple an assigned role to play, such as walking to school with one of the opposite sex, etc.
12. Have an art contest and choose the best painting, water color, or carving which shows human happiness. Talk about what makes people happy or sad.
13. Have each pupil make a poster of snapshots taken of happy people from all ages and walks of life. Choose the best snapshot submitted. Tell about the person shown in the photograph.
14. Conduct a class song- and motto-writing contest. Use both as a means of stressing group solidarity and good conduct.

Physical Education

It has been said that if you want to know what a child is really like, watch him play, but if you are concerned about what he might become, direct his play. Certainly the child is his real self when he is so completely engrossed in play that he forgets to be the boy his teacher wants him to be, or his mother hopes he is. Every child in every culture is culturally conditioned by adults. He is taught by adults the games of the clan, tribe, or city block, as well as those favored by his own sex, race, and religion. A boy is taught manly games, little girls are given dolls to play with, in an endeavor to teach them what boys do in contrast with what girls do. Many learn these lessons early and well, but others need extra help and patience before they do so. Even tradition enters the picture of play. Children want to be like grown-ups and thus they engage in activities once favored by adults they admire. Such games as "Run, Sheepie, Run!" or "Red Rover" are "as old as the hills," yet they remain the favorites of children throughout the ages.[4]

Other ways in which physical education can be correlated with family life education are:

1. Participating in many games and sports together, using mixed teams. Relays and other easily organized activities are especially well suited for helping boys see that girls can play skillfully, too.
2. Teaching others the favorite active team game played in your family or block.
3. Having an all-school fun night.
4. Participating in a "Share Your Adult Friends" night by having each pupil bring two admired adult friends outside his own family. Play simple active games in mixed teams with these guests, as planned and conducted by the pupils themselves.
5. Having a class cookout and have campcraft skill contests, such as wood-chopping, fire-building, or water-boiling. Evaluate the results by discussing how this experience could have been better planned and conducted so that everyone would have had a better time.
6. Learning several folk dances. Present these in costume to P.T.A. or assembly program. Learn about family groups and foreign customs through class discussions and bulletin board materials.
7. Sharing menstrual hygiene materials with girls who ask for them; answering the direct questions boys ask in the locker room or elsewhere.
8. Discussing the role exercise plays in being physically fit and attractive. Learn several basic conditioning exercises and do them regularly.
9. Playing games according to rules and good conduct; discuss the correlation between the "game of life" and the game of volleyball.
10. Learning games suitable for family backyard fun and sharing them with your own family.

The Communicative Arts

The possibilities for integrated study in this area are many. A fifth-grade class in a school in Oregon engaged in an intensive study of American Indians in their social science class. Every aspect of the life of various tribes such as the Cherokee, Blackfeet, or Iroquois was studied—their customs, family life, food, form of government, trade, problems, etc. Some pupils made a miniature Indian village, while a group of boys learned and presented the rain dance of the Cherokees, and the girls prepared and served a typical Indian meal. The group became so enthusiastic that they planned and gave an assembly program showing others what they had learned. Such experiences teach children many more things besides the differences between modern customs and ancient ones, for the children learn how to work well with

---

[4] Vannier, Maryhelen, Foster, Mildred, and Gallahue, David: *Teaching Physical Education in Elementary Schools.* 5th ed. Philadelphia: W. B. Saunders Co., 1972, p. 22.

fellow students in a cooperative venture, and how to express themselves. The same kind of an experience can be used with modification on any grade level, and people from any part of the world can be studied. Idealistic youth need to learn as much about the life of different people as possible. Our future and theirs can depend upon the experiences which boys and girls have today in our schools.

USE OF TEACHING METHODS

The following teaching methods can best be utilized in the instruction of pupils in family life education.

Problem Solving

Many aspects of sex education can be used successfully as children explore and find solutions to problems which are important to them. During this school year a group of sixth-graders studied the problem of increased juvenile delinquency in a unit on current events in their social studies class. They were amazed to learn that one cause of delinquency was inadequate and faulty home relationships among youth, irrespective of income group. Their next step was to discover what kind of family difficulties were most likely to be at the root of crime. The group spent an entire week tracking down pertinent information which helped them to learn not only much about delinquency but also a great deal about their own personal values and conduct. They were surprised to find out that sex misbehavior and faulty attitudes also played such a major role in delinquency and crime. Finally the group drew up their own code of ethics for youth and made a list of things both children and parents could do in order to become better family members.

In a fourth-grade class in a school in Minnesota, the teacher noticed that the boys usually took possession of sports equipment from the storage room, leaving the girls with only broken bats and unsewed, "beat-up" balls. She discussed this problem later in her civics class, and asked the children how it could be solved. The group spent several days discussing the rights of others, why girls should take part in sports and have the use of adequate equipment, and even studied about the lives of famous men and women athletes. Improved behavior and better understanding and respect for each other resulted.

Problem solving should not be merely limited to groups, for almost every child has his own unique set of worries about himself and relationships with others. Concern with children's problems is the duty of their teacher, who sometimes becomes so engrossed teaching subject matter that she forgets that she should also be teaching children *through* it to help them find solutions to their own personal problems. All young people need to think for themselves and control their own behavior. Abraham offers the following suggested ways in which teachers might stimulate independent thinking, and help pupils develop their own ideas and expand their horizons:

1. Let children ask and converse.
2. Ask each child often, "What do *you* think?" "How do *you* feel about this?"
3. Bring up problems of interest to children, such as "How can we figure out mileage on this map?"
4. Ask questions that dig, such as "Are you *sure?*" or "Are there any other possibilities?"

  5. Take them to as many places as your time permits.
  6. Involve them in your plans.
  7. Encourage the solution that is unusual.[5]

Class Discussions

  1. Discuss with the children their mother's and father's place and role in the family; relationships between siblings; how to function successfully in the family.
  2. Study about and see vegetables or plants grow from seeds. Discuss what causes things to grow.
  3. Read to the class the books *The Wonderful Egg* or *Bambi*. Show and discuss the pictures and story in these books.
  4. Bring a bird's nest to class. Show how the nest was built. Discuss the necessity of having a good home.
  5. Keep guppies in a bowl in the classroom. Observe them carefully every day. Draw out from the class questions they have about their observations.
  6. Discuss the proper way to use bathroom facilities at home or at school.
  7. Bring pictures to class of happy families; fathers having fun with their sons; mother-and-daughter activities. Talk about these pictures.
  8. Have each pupil tell what he wants to be when he grows up. Decide if this is a wise choice for a girl or boy to make.
  9. Have a group discussion on what fathers should do in the home, mothers' responsibilities, etc.
  10. Act out and discuss stories and poems about animal families such as "The Three Little Pigs," or "The Night before Christmas." Discuss the role and responsibility of each character.
  11. Discuss the film *Human Reproduction* in your sixth-grade class.

Special Reports

Possible topics for special reports in this field include famous men and women in various fields such as the arts or politics, family customs among certain religious groups such as the Jewish and Amish, family health problems, the changing role of the mother, family vacations, etc. Such experiences can assist children in gaining skills in speaking before a group, and also help them learn to do library research, which is necessary for the increasing numbers of students who are going on to college.

Demonstrations

Demonstrations can teach and correlate good grooming skills such as how to file fingernails correctly, cut toenails, shampoo the hair, wash the face, the kinds of clothes to wear for certain events such as church or school, etc. Since most boys will be fathers someday, they too can learn many household skills through demonstration and practice, such as cooking, washing dishes, or changing baby diapers. Girls can also learn to do many of the household tasks often done by fathers through this method of teaching, such as learning how to use a hammer, saw, and other tools, how to lay bathroom tile or kitchen linoleum, and how to paint and repair furniture. Care must be taken, however, lest too much emphasis be placed upon learning to master these skills without teaching the children why both sexes

---

[5] Abraham, Willard: "Helping Children Think." *Today's Health*, vol. 108 (June 1961).

should share and work together. The many "manly" sport skills such as throwing, batting, and catching a baseball, or kicking a football, can also be taught and shared by the boys in the group. The girls, in turn, can help them improve their dance steps. Good partners in work and play tend to become good marriage partners also.

Role Playing

Role playing can be of great value in helping the teacher gain deeper insight into individual behavior and family problems. Children do more than just act out being a father, or having a baby sister. An observant teacher can always help a child fit into a part that meets his specific needs. Role playing, coupled with music, can help children express feelings of hostility, fear, or anger, as well as make a real contribution to improved mental health. The teacher should keep in the background during these experiences and be a keen observer who focuses her attention on the child more than on what he is doing. Brief notes might be made on filing cards for each child, noting what children choose to engage in, do, and say, as well as what their reactions are. It has been said that to the skilled teacher, dramatic play is a revealing mirror of a child.

Field Trips

There are many and varied possible field trips to help children gain understanding of the role of human beings in work and play. The group will profit greatly from exploring their community and becoming acquainted with a wide variety of people in it. Trips can be taken to a zoo to observe animal families, to a dog or cat hospital to see newborn puppies and kittens, to a farm to learn how plants and animals are cared for and grow, to a local child day-care center to observe the play activities and care of young children of working mothers, to a church to see a christening or a wedding, to a pediatrician to learn what he does and how he became a baby specialist, to a flower shop to learn how seeds are planted and flowers grow, or to an airplane factory to see what work men do in contrast to that of women working in the same plant. Certainly every community resource should be used to its fullest, and can help children gain an increased understanding and appreciation of their own world.

Surveys

Suggested surveys include finding out:

1. How many in the class have brothers and sisters, and how old they are.
2. How many have both parents working, and what kind of work they do.
3. How many have only one parent.
4. How many have fathers who travel and are away from home a great deal.
5. The size of an average family in one block.
6. How many brothers and sisters each parent has.
7. What families do for home fun.
8. The average age of each parent in a family in a block.
9. How many parents are college graduates.
10. Where each member of the family was born.
11. How many times each family in the block had moved to a new house since their first child was born.
12. How many babies live in the block, including those of animals such as puppies, kittens, etc.

USE OF INSTRUCTIONAL MATERIALS

Many kinds of instructional materials can make learning about family life an exciting educational adventure. These include:

Models and Specimens

Children fortunate enough to be near the Dallas or Cleveland Health Museums can there see wonderful models showing the growth of the baby inside the mother's body month by month, and "see" how babies grow and move. Commercial models of the human body can also be used in the classroom to enable children to find answers to their frequent questions such as "Where do babies come from?" or "How does the baby get out?" Likewise, such specimens as a collection of various kinds and sizes of eggs, seeds, plants, wood, etc., can be used by the teacher to "liven up" her materials on instruction about "life."

Bulletin Boards and Posters

Boys and girls gain a better understanding of this area as well as develop creative and communicative skills with bulletin boards and posters. Suggested activities include:

1. Have each child make a poster of any aspect of family life. Help each feel secure in the group, and give each many things to do with his own hands so that he will keep them away from his own sex organs.
2. Draw pictures of a happy family spending an evening at home, at the dinner table, or going on a trip.
3. Make posters of ways each can help their families at home.
4. Have a pet show. Draw out the pupils and note their understanding of animals, how they are born, and how to care for them. Record what you learned from this experience on the class bulletin board.
5. Visit a health museum or zoo to gain information about babies or animals. Illustrate what you have seen.
6. Have a child illustrate a visit to a farm. Next, take the class to visit a dairy or other types of farm. See the young ponies, pigs, chickens, or other animals. Observe how their mother helps them.
7. Illustrate a report given on pioneers, Indians, Eskimos, primitive tribes, by making cutout feltboard figures. Compare what is learned with our own American family customs.
8. Raise a class pet. Record its weight, habits, etc., on the bulletin board.
9. Invite a local 4-H club leader to speak to the class and show illustrated materials on animal breeding.

Books

Whether used in the classroom and read aloud to the youngest children, or selected and read by older youth, books can do much to help pupils gain a clearer understanding of sex, other people, and themselves. Such books as *The Diary of Anne Frank* appeal to boys as well as girls, as do those written about famous people throughout the world. Oral or written book reports will assist the pupils in expressing themselves as well as in giving them an understanding of what they have read and its relationship to themselves. Written reports are especially valuable in helping their authors gain self-understanding, particularly if the pupils are asked to correlate any incident in the story with their own lives, or express what they feel about the actions of certain characters.

For the younger pupils, having the teacher read aloud to them can be a treat. The instructor should do more than read a story, for she should also draw out the reactions of the children to it. Recently, a young teacher in Dallas read her first-graders the book *The Wonderful Egg*. The next day she used their interest in eggs for instruction in her unit on family life education. Note how she asked leading questions in order to learn how much the pupils really knew in this area.

In our health lesson last week we learned that everyone needs to eat a good breakfast. Margaret Rose, do you remember some of the different foods we can eat to have a good breakfast?

That's right! And eggs are a very important part of a healthy breakfast. We have already learned why eggs are good for us to eat. But what else do you know about eggs? Are there any other kinds of eggs besides chicken eggs?

That's right! There are bird, fish, turtle, frog, bee, and snake eggs, just to name a few. So many different kinds of eggs!

Where can we find these different eggs? (Show poster drawings and have children see difference in places eggs are found.)

Do all these eggs look alike? (Poster again, pointing out that there are many kinds.)

Can we eat all these different kinds of eggs?

If we don't eat all of them, what else are they good for?

When we don't eat them, each different kind of egg hatches and then grows into a different kind of animal. (Show pictures.)

Where do these eggs come from?

That's right! They all are laid by their mothers. Then when they are outside their mother's body, they break their shells or coverings.

Did you know that everything else on earth that is alive started as an egg—even the plants and trees? In most plants, though, the eggs grow into seeds. Each new plant and each new animal grows to be the same kind of living thing as its parents.

Now I know that you are thinking—if everything has eggs, where are they? Trees' eggs are seeds, some animals like a bird lay their eggs and you can see those. But other animals, like my dog, have babies and you never see their eggs at all. Where are they?

You don't see them but they are there just the same. Hidden away inside the mother is a special sac—a warm, safe place where the eggs change into baby animals. They grow and grow inside their mothers until one day they come out into the world through a special tube that stretches to let them out. They are born—just as you were born one day. You grew as a tiny egg inside your mother.

At the beginning of you, you were no bigger than a dot—a tiny dot much smaller than this dot (show picture) or even a single grain of sand. So small that the dot could not be seen at all, except through a strong magnifying glass. That dot that was going to be you was like a tiny little round egg.

Something even more wonderful about this tiny egg—even though it was as tiny as a dot, it had nearly everything that it took to make you! Your eyes, hair, hands, etc. Your being able to grow from something very small and helpless into something pretty big and independent was right there in that tiny egg! Isn't that amazing?

Then the tiny egg that was you grew and grew inside your mother until you were a full-sized baby ready to be born. Then you were born with everything you needed to be a person—and it all came from the wonderful egg.[6]

---

[6] Reported in the class, Teaching Health and Physical Education in Elementary Schools, Southern Methodist University, January 8, 1961.

Radio and Television

Radio and television, like the daily newspaper and weekly magazines, have an abundance of materials which can be used by an alert teacher to help children become aware of any aspect of sex education. Cartoons seen on the television such as "Captain Kangaroo" or "Donald Duck" are especially appropriate for helping younger boys and girls learn more about families, both human and cartoon. Such radio and television programs as "Gunsmoke" or "Stagecoach West" can help children gain a better understanding of how people dressed or what they did during our pioneer days, even though these programs present fictionalized versions of the reality. Even encouraging the older pupils to listen to such serials as "All in the Family" or "Hollywood Theatre" have educational value, but only if they are fully utilized and children are helped to "see through" some of the things they see and hear. Listening to such programs for several days can even become a good introduction to such topics as family problems, the happily married couple, or problems some grown-ups face. The discriminating teacher knows just how much of what exists in the world about her is suitable for classroom use, and uses what she can, wisely and well.

Films

Almost any health film for any grade can be used for correlating such topics as posture, good grooming, growth, or nutrition with the best ways to grow up to reach maturity. *Human reproduction*, which is perhaps one of the best films available for showing the facts of life, should be used only with older pupils who are ready for such specific information. It might well be seen several times, at well-spaced intervals, in junior and senior high school, for the film contains so much well-presented information that it is impossible to absorb all of it at one time.

Sometime during this unit, the teacher should:

1. Talk individually and informally with each pupil. Discover the thoughts, fears, and attitudes toward those of the opposite sex or growing up. Gain the respect, trust, and friendship of each, however, before doing so. Evaluate the results and file summarized notes in the cumulative school record of each child.
2. Have pupils fill out the rest of several sentences similar to these given below, when the occasion best arises:
   1. I like boys because _____
   2. Girls are _____
   3. My parents think that I _____
   4. In my home, we have _____
   5. My greatest worry about growing up is that I_____
   6. I know that I am growing up because I _____
3. Read each answer carefully, keep what has been written confidential, and give assistance where needed.

DESIRABLE OUTCOMES

A well-taught and guided educational experience should produce the following desirable outcomes in terms of knowledge, attitudes, and practices:

In the primary grades, the pupils will:

1. Work and play happily together with members of their own and the opposite sex.

2. Develop interest in nature and in life.
3. Care for their own body needs and know about bodily functions.
4. Be helpful at school and at home and considerate of the rights of others.
5. Be aware of the differences between boys and girls, and know of the role each sex plays in life.
6. Understand that animals and plants as well as people reproduce themselves.
7. Know and appreciate the role each parent plays in the family.
8. Accept and be glad of their own sex.
9. Know how chickens and other animals are born.
10. Have curiosity and questions concerning sex satisfied by truthful information, and not feel ashamed or feel guilty because of their own thoughts.

In the upper elementary grades, the pupils will:

1. Understand and accept changes in their bodies.
2. Appreciate the abilities and differences between boys and girls.
3. Have many friends of both sexes; be respected by their peers and teachers.
4. Accept responsibility and be concerned about group welfare; be sensitive to situations which leave someone out or make someone feel unhappy.
5. Know how the body functions; name correctly the parts of the body.
6. Become increasingly concerned about their own personal appearance; feel secure and confident of their own ability; welcome opportunities to do new things.
7. Enjoy family life activities and share fun and happiness in their own homes.
8. Appreciate the role of the family in society; be aware of the responsibility of each parent and family member.
9. Recognize and accept their own sex role; take pride in being a girl or a boy.
10. Know how boys and girls change in adolescence.
11. Ask frank questions about sex or any aspect of family life without embarrassment or guilt feelings.
12. Belong to a closely knit circle of friends and be well liked by their classmates of both sexes.
13. Desire to have good character; belong to and take an active part in church and youth organizational activities.
14. Develop a deeper appreciation for their families, home, and school.
15. Develop social graces; desire to be popular and well respected in their school and neighborhood.
16. Have several close adult friends outside their family circle.
17. Be able to compete successfully as a member of a mixed team in class contests, physical education activities, and in games played during leisure time in the neighborhood.
18. Enjoy many outings, backyard or other home experiences with their families; take pride in being a member of their own primary group.
19. Increasingly practice good health habits and self-discipline; gain greater self-confidence and independence.
20. Possess strong, skillful bodies, take part in and enjoy a wide variety of vigorous sports, dance well; have many recreational interests.

LEARNING AIDS

There is an abundance of learning aids in this subject. The following materials are recommended:

For the Primary Grades

Films and Filmstrips
   A Story About You. Chicago, American Medical Association.

Friendship Begins at Home. (15 min.) Coronet Films.
Growing Up. (35 min.) Coronet Films.
He Acts His Age. (15 min.) McGraw-Hill.

Stories and Books for Children

Beck, C.: *How Life Is Handed On.* New York: Harcourt, Brace and Jovanovich, 1960.
Carton, L.: *Daddies; Mommies.* New York, Random House, 1969.
Earle, O.: *Squirrels In The Garden.* Morrow Press.
Hoban, Robert: *Baby Sister For Francis.* New York: Harper & Row, 1971.
Kepes, J.: *Two Little Birds and Three.* New York: Houghton Mifflin, 1969.
Lerrigo, M. O.: *Finding Yourself.* Chicago: American Medical Association, 1970.
Levine, M. L., Seligmann, J. D.: *The Wonder of Life.* New York: Simon and Schuster, 1971.
Wasson, V. P.: *The Chosen Baby.* New York: Lippincott, 1971.

For the Upper Elementary Grades

Pamphlets

Menninger, W.: "Understanding Yourself." Chicago: Science Research Associates.
"The Story of Life; Sex Education for the Ten Year Old." American Medical Association.
"From Boy to Man." Social Hygiene Association.
"Very Personally Yours." (girls) Kimberly-Clark Corp.
"Posture on Parade." (poster for girls) National Dairy Council.
"Good Grooming Chart." Bristol-Myers.
"Health for Man and Boy." American Social Hygiene Association.
"Sound Attitudes Toward Sex." American Social Hygiene Association.
"Understanding Sex." Science Research Associates.
"Its Natural." (girls) Tampax, Inc.
"Very Personally Yours." (girls) International Cellucotton Products Company.
"Your Own Story." American Social Hygiene Association.
"On Becoming a Woman." Tampax, Inc.

Films and Filmstrips

Confidence Because You Understand Menstruation. (Record and filmstrip) Personal Products Corporation.
Understanding Your Emotions (15 min.), Coronet Films.
Human Reproduction (30 min.), McGraw-Hill.
Good Grooming (30 min.), McGraw-Hill.

Posters

"Anatomical Chart on Menstruation." Tampax, Inc.
"What Happens During Menstruation," Personal Products Corp.
"Good Grooming." Bristol-Myers.
"Special Days Are Fun." National Commission on Safety Education.

Books, Magazines, and Stories for Children

Ames, Louise: *On Becoming a Woman.* New York: Dell, 1961.
Strain, Frances: *Being Born.* New York: Appleton-Century-Crofts, 1956.
Beck, Lester: *How Life Is Handed On.* New York: Harcourt, Brace and Jovanovich, 1960.
Levine, Milton, and Seligmann, Jean: *The Wonder of Life.* New York: Simon and Schuster, 1961.
Lerrigo, Marian, and Southard, Helen: *Finding Yourself; All About You; Facts Are Not Enough.* American Medical Association.
Handforth, Thomas: *Mei Li.* New York: Doubleday & Co., 1959.
Lawson, Robert: *They Were Strong and Good.* New York: Viking Press, 1960.
Burton, Virginia Lee: *Many Moons.* New York: Viking Press, 1954.
Calling All Girls. Parents Magazines, 1960.
Little Women; Blue Willow; Black Beauty; Tom Sawyer; Detective; No Children, No Pets; Just Plain Maggie; Trolley Car Family; Black Spaniel Mystery; Story

of John Paul Jones; Silver for General Washington; Horses; Mark Trail's Book of Animals; Odd Pets; Cowdog; Big Red; Gray Wolf; Yellow Eyes; First to Ride. (All of these are pocket books written especially for children. They are available for less than 50c per copy from Reader's Choice, 33 W. 42nd St., New York, N.Y. 10036, a division of Scholastic Book Services.)

Readers
Health and Personal Development Series, *You; You and Others; You're Growing Up; In the Teens.* Glenview, Ill.: Scott, Foresman and Co.
Road to Health Series, *Health Trails; Your Health and You, Keeping Healthy.* Laidlaw.
Health for Young America Series, *Health at School; Health Day by Day; Health and Fun; Health and Growth; Health and Living; Health and Happiness.* Bobbs-Merrill.
Science, Health and Safety Series, Books *III, IV, V.* Macmillan.
Safety and Health Living Series, *Helping the Body in Its Work; The Healthy Home and Community.* Ginn.
Health Action Series, *Healthy Days; Stay Healthy; Good for You; Full of Life; Here's Health.* Wilcox.
Health for Better Lving Series, *Growing Your Way; Keeping Healthy and Strong; Teamwork for Health.* Ginn.

TEACHING AIDS

The following materials are recommended teaching aids in family life education:

In the Primary Grades

Sex Education Series. Chicago: Joint Committee on Health Problems by National Education Association and American Medical Association.
Sex Education Series. Washington, D.C.: AAHPER.
Hayman, H. S.: "Basic Issues in School Sex Education," *Journal of School Health*, vol. 23, no. 1 (January, 1953), 15–17.
Kirkendall, Lester: *Sex Education as Human Relations.* New York: Ivor Publications, 1950.
Eckert, Ralph: *Sex Attitudes in the Home.* New York: Association Press, 1956.
When Children Ask about Sex. New York: Child Study Association.
How to Tell Your Child about Sex. New York: Public Affairs Committee.
Some Special Problems of Children. New York: National Association for Mental Health, 1971.
A Healthy Personality for Your Child. Washington, D.C.: Children's Bureau, Dept. of HEW, Publications no. 337, 1952, and no. 338, 1958.
Some A-to-Z's of Family Life Education. New York: Y.W.C.A. Publication Service, 600 Lexington Ave., New York, N.Y. 10022. (An outline with program suggestions, a list of resources including films, filmstrips, recordings, plays and skits, pamphlets, articles, and books.)
McHose, Elizabeth: *Family Life Education in School and Community.* New York: Teachers College, 1952.
A Guide to Teaching Health in the Elementary School. Albany: The University of the State of New York, Health Education Series Bulletin no. 2, 1959.

In the Upper Elementary Grades

Menstrual Hygiene Teaching Aid Kit. Lake Success, N.Y.: Tampax.
A Teaching Guide for Menstrual Hygiene. Miltown, N.J.: Personal Products Corporation.
Wolf, Ann: *The Parent's Manual.* New York: Simon and Schuster, 1941.
Bibby, Cyril: *Sex Education (A Guide for Parents, Teachers, and Youth Leaders).* New York: Emerson, 1946.
Jones, Marion: "At What Age Should a Girl Be Told about Menstruation?" (Pamphlet) Neenah, Wis.: Kimberly-Clark Corporation.

New Patterns in Sex Teaching. New York: Appleton-Century-Crofts, 1934.

Strain, Francis: *Sex Guidance in Family Life Education.* New York: Macmillan, 1942.

Edson, W.: "Sex in the Life of a Child. *Childcraft,* vol. 10, 1947.

Baruch, Dorothy: *New Ways in Sex Education.* New York: McGraw-Hill Book Co., 1959.

Narramore, Clyde: *How to Tell Your Child about Sex.* Grand Rapids, Mich.: Zondervan Publishing Co., 1959.

Lerrigo, Marian, and Sutherland, Helen: *A Parent's Privilege; The Story about You; Facts Are Not Enough.* Chicago: National Education Association and American Medical Association, 1955.

Hymes, James: *How to Tell Your Child about Sex.* Public Affairs Committee.

Kirkendall, Ralph: *Helping Children Understand Sex.* Chicago: Science Research Associates.

Ostrovsky, Everett: *Father to the Child.* New York: Putnam, 1960.

Some A-to-Z's of Family Life Education. New York: Y.W.C.A. Publication Service.

When Your Child Asks about Sex. New York: Child Study Association of America.

Tebbel, John: *The Magic of Balanced Living.* New York: Harper & Row, 1956.

Schweinitz, Karl D.: *Growing Up.* New York: The Macmillan Co., 1955.

The Journal of School Health; Today's Health; Journal of Health, Physical Education and Recreation.

Moser, Clarence: *Understanding Boys; Understanding Girls.* New York: Association Press, 1958.

What Every Child Needs. New York: National Association of Mental Health, 1960.

TEACHING UNITS

Found below are suggested instructional materials for teaching units in family and sex education:

Kindergarten

Objectives
1. To allow the child to express himself with his entire body and to feel comfortable in doing so.
2. To help each one to develop positive attitudes toward himself and his role in life.
3. To use correct sexual terminology without embarrassment.

Suggested Approaches
1. Terminology for anatomical differences and genital parts.
2. Personal feelings and how they relate to the privacy and the rights of others as well as one's self.
   a. Boys and girls have separate bathrooms and the reasons why.
   b. Desire for privacy is a normal desire.
   c. Acceptable bathroom behavior (alone and in groups).
3. Arrival of a new baby.
   a. Explore the role of the child in the family.
   b. Help the child develop an understanding of the new baby and his relationship to all family members.

Basic Concepts to Teach
1. All people have good and bad body feelings.
2. Every individual needs and should have privacy at certain times.
3. Sex differences between girls and boys—knowledge as well as appreciation of these differences.
4. Understand that a human baby develops inside the body of its mother in her uterus.
5. The need to feel we belong is basic to all people.
6. Every individual in the family is important.

Group Activities
1. Use correct sex terminology during ordinary conversations with the children.
2. Bathroom tour to show how facilities differ for boys and girls.
3. Male and female guinea pigs or other animals kept in classroom for the children to observe.
4. Skits and plays.

Individual Pupil Activities
1. Role playing of family situations.
2. Diagram of male and female parts on bulletin board for pupil to learn.

Pupil References
Irwin, Leslie: *Growing Every Day; You and Others.* Chicago: Lyons & Carnahan, 1965.
Zim, Herbert S.: *What's Inside of Me?* New York: William Morrow & Co., 1952.

Teacher References
Sex Education Resource Unit. Washington, D.C.: AAHPER, 1969.
Miracle of Life. Chicago: American Medical Association, 1966.
Growth Patterns and Sex Education. American School Health Association, 1967.
Baker, K. P.: *Understanding and Guiding Young Children.* Englewood Cliffs, N. J.: Prentice-Hall, 1967.
Oranstein, Irving: *Where Do Babies Come From?* New York: Pyramid Books, 1962.

Grade 1

Objectives
1. To become more familiar with the material introduced in Kindergarten.
2. To explore the makeup of many different human families as well as those of animals.

Suggested Approaches
1. Review of body parts.
   a. Anatomical differences
   b. Genital parts named accurately
2. Animal families; all animals belong to a family with a mother and father; mother and father called parents; family members are alike in many ways and different in others; babies become adults.
   a. Dog family
   b. Cat family
   c. Horse family
   d. Bear family
   e. Duck family
   f. Rabbit family
   g. Human family
3. Our family.
   a. Make-up of family: mother, father, brothers and sisters.
   b. Interactions between family members; the role each plays in the family unit.

Basic Concepts to Teach
1. Learn that some animals hatch from eggs and others develop inside body of mother until birth.
2. All animals belong to a family with a mother and father.
3. Family members are a closely knit group.
4. A family tries to live together happily with themselves and others.

Group Activities
1. Large felt board—put the animals up as you study them.

2. Field trips to zoo, farm.
3. Animal skits to help children learn how animals get food, how they live, and how they help human beings.

Individual Pupil Activities
1. Miniature felt boards.
2. Family albums showing baby pictures.

Pupil References
Boegehold, Betty: *Three To Get Ready.* New York: Harper & Row, 1965.
Hoban, Russell: *The Sorely Trying Day.* New York: Harper & Row, 1964.
Zolotow, Charlotte: *When I Have a Little Girl; When I Have a Son.* New York: Harper & Row, 1967.

Teacher References
Education for Sexuality: Concepts and Programs for Teaching. Philadelphia: W. B. Saunders Co., 1970.
The Journal of School Health. Growth Patterns and Sex Education. 1967.

Suggested references for both the children and teacher
Showers, Paul and Kay: *Before You Were a Baby.* New York: Thomas Y. Crowell Co., 1968. This is one of the finest books in the area of sex education for children. It is in this company's Let's Read and Find Out Science Series. Other highly recommended books in this series are:

The Clean Brook	*Find Out By Touching*
Ducks Don't Get Wet	*Follow Your Nose*
Look At Your Eyes	*Hear Your Heart*
My Five Senses	*My Hands*
Straight Hair — Curly Hair	*Your Skin and Mine*

Grade 2

Objectives
1. To give the children a broad look into the origin and development of the living things in their surroundings.
2. To understand the process of internal fertilization.

Suggested Approaches
1. Seed Experiment
   a. Growth of different seeds.
   b. Development; eggs grow into seeds—reproduction.
2. Living Things That Come from Eggs.
   a. Wide variety of eggs.
   b. How a baby is made: sperm, eggs, fertilization.
   c. Different ways eggs are made: fish eggs, frog eggs, hen eggs, puppies, cow, human.

Basic Concepts to Teach
1. There are many kinds of eggs.
2. Life comes from the sperm and the egg.
3. Sperm and egg join in different ways—the way they meet determines where the fertilized egg will grow into new life.

Group Activities
1. Seed chart: nature walk to find seeds, plant the seeds.
2. Make different kinds of eggs out of colored paper, clay, papier-mâché.
3. Decorate hard-boiled eggs; draw the animals which come from the eggs.
4. Demonstrate fish fertilization using a clay fish, making an opening for the eggs to drop out of.
5. Flash cards.

Individual Pupil Activities
1. Grow a flower for Mother—finger paint the flower pot.

12

2. Make a bird's nest.
3. Make a book, car, boat, etc., to see how things are put together.

Pupil References
  Darby, Gene: *What Is a Turtle?* Chicago: Benefic Press, 1960.
  Jordan, Helen: *How a Seed Grows.* New York: Thomas Y. Crowell Co., 1960.
  Schwartz, Elizabeth and Charles: *When Animals Are Babies.* New York: Holiday House, 1964.

Teacher References
  Cosgrove, Margaret: *Eggs and What Happens Inside Them.* New York: Dodd, Mead and Co., 1960.
  Julian, C. J., and Jackson, E. N.: *Modern Sex Education.* New York: Holt, Rinehart and Winston, 1967.
  Power, Jules: *How Life Begins.* New York: Simon and Schuster, 1968.
  AAHPER: *Sex Education Resource Unit.* 1969.

Audio-Visual Aids
  Kittens: Birth and Growth. (11 min.) Bailey Films. Designed to prepare children for pictures on human growth at a later grade level. Children in family are present when a mother cat gives birth to four kittens. They react in a natural manner.
  Eggs to Chickens. (10 min.) Bailey Films. Father-mother-baby relationship explained simply.
  The Day Life Begins. (23 min.) Carousel Films. Traces reproductive process from division of one-celled amoeba to the complicated workings of human birth.
  Animal Babies Grow Up. Coronet Films.
  Farmyard Babies. (11 min.) Coronet Films. What do farmyard babies look like? Sound like?
  Zoo Babies. (11 min.) Coronet Films.
  Human and Animal Beginnings. (Color, 22 min.) Henk Newenhouse. Young children express their beliefs about origin of human life in drawings.

Grade 3

Objectives
  1. To familiarize the students with types of reproduction, such as in human beings and other animals.
  2. To teach them how the family shares to protect and perfect life.

Motivational Activities
  1. Have the students build an incubator and study the growth and development of baby chicks. Have a fish or frog family with which to compare the chick development. For instructions on incubator construction refer to Burt and Brower's *Education for Sexuality.* It is also suggested that the teacher supply the class with a model of the visible woman. These can be purchased at most hobby shops or at the Health Museum at Fair Park, Dallas, Texas, or at the Cleveland, Ohio, Health Museum.

Concepts To Teach
  1. Families
     a. Birds
     b. Fish
     c. Cats and Dogs
     d. Humans: relationships and roles of family members
  2. Methods of Reproduction
     a. Eggs without parental care—fish and turtles
     b. Eggs with parental care—birds
     c. Mammals
     d. Human beings: relation and difference between human and other mammal reproduction
     e. Fertilization of each: cell division, embryo development.

3. Growth and development
   a. Physical
   b. Emotional
   c. Spiritual
   d. Intellectual
   e. Social
4. Differences between human and animal development. How family relationships play a part.

Group Activities
1. Care and observation of the chicks and the incubator.
2. Visitis to aquariums and/or health museums.

Individual Activities
1. Have each child keep an account of the growth and development of the eggs and chicks.
2. Have each child make charts of the life cycles of the animals mentioned above.

Correlation With Other Subjects
1. Arithmetic
   a. Story problems may be used dealing with time of incubation, growth of animals, pregnancy periods of the animals, etc.
2. Social Studies
   a. When studying the areas of the world, discuss the animals that could be seen in that area as well as the mating habits of those animals. (The koala bear in Australia, the seals of Alaska, etc.)
3. Language Arts
   a. Have the students write a story about their families or pets.
4. Science
   a. Discuss the anatomy of the animals and humans and the effects this has on the gestation periods of each.
5. Drama and Art
   a. Role play experiences dealing with family relationships.

Pupil References

Cosgrove, Margaret: *Eggs and What Happens Inside Them.* New York: Dodd, Mead and Company.

Darling, Louis: *Chickens and How to Raise Them.* New York: William Morrow and Co.

Gruenberg, Sidonie: *The Wonderful Story of How You Were Born.* Garden City, N. Y.: Doubleday and Co.

Kay, Helen: *A Summer to Share.* New York: Hastings House Publishers.

Levine, M. I., and Seligmann, Jean: *A Baby is Born.* New York: Golden Press. *The Wonder of Life.* New York: Golden Press.

Randall, Blossom E.: *Fun For Chris.* Chicago: Albert Whitman & Co.

Schloat, Warren G.: *The Wonderful Egg.* New York: Charles Scribner's Sons.

Selsam, Millicent: *Egg to Chick.* International Publishers Co.

Teachers References

American School Health Association: *Your Child's Questions—How to Answer Them.* New York: The Association, 1970.

Eckert, Ralph G.: *Sex Attitudes in the Home.* New York: Popular Library, 1963.

Levine, Milton I. and Seligmann, Jean: *Helping Boys and Girls Understand Their Sex Roles.* Chicago: Science Research Associates, 1952.

Power, Jules: *How Life Begins.* New York: Simon and Schuster, 1968.

Audio-Visual Aids

Your Family. (B/W or color, 11 min.) Coronet Films. Through mutual understanding, acceptance of responsibilities, cooperation, family achieves unity necessary to happy home. The role of individual in social unit of family.

How Friends Are Made. (Color, 10 min.) Independent Film Producers Co. Stresses that everybody could be friends and have friends, too. If everybody were kind, there wouldn't be an unhappy boy or girl in the world.

The Wonder of Reproduction. (B/W or color, 12 min.) Moody Institute of Science. Educational Film Division. In Uncle Bob's aquarium two boys and a girl see the beautiful fish build its bubble nest to house the eggs, the courtship of the male and female, the egg-laying and fertilization process, and the hatching of the eggs. In a second aquarium, the reproduction process of the Egyptian mouth breeder is seen.

Happy Little Hamsters. (B/W or color, 13½ min.) Henk Newenhouse. A delightful story of two hamsters, Naomi and Abdullah, and their litter of eight babies. These squirming and underdeveloped babies grow rapidly—their skin darkens, lungs develop, fur thickens, eyes and ears form, and they grow strong enough to walk. Later, children take them home for pets and the mother gets a well-earned rest. The film follows the life cycle of the hamster with narration that is both informative and entertaining.

People Are Different and Alike. Coronet Films. Shows how peope of all ages throughout the world are both alike and different in many ways.

Other Teaching Aids
Denoyer Geppert & Co., catalog of classroom materials for family life programs.

Evaluation of Results
1. Did the motivational materials stimulate questions?
2. Were the students interested in caring for the chicks, or did the teacher do all the work?
3. Did the test results show that the children really learned the basic facts included in this unit?

Grade 4

Objectives
1. To reinforce the biological aspects of sex education.
2. To teach the psychological and spiritual aspects of sexuality.

Motivational Activities
1. Place a question box in the room where any questions may be asked anonymously.
2. Continue the use of the visible woman and man or other visual aids which show the physical differences between the sexes.

Concepts To Teach
1. Heredity
   a. DNA
   b. Chromosomes and genes
   c. Fertilization and cell division
   d. Determined characteristics: pigmentation of skin, eyes, and hair; height and body build.
2. Physiological changes to take place
   a. Menstruation
   b. Seminal emissions
   c. Secondary sex characteristics
3. Psychological aspects
   a. Self-consciousness of early developers
   b. Privateness at home
   c. Need for a best friend who understands, as well as having understanding parents.
   d. Bragging by some students about their knowledge of sex.
4. Readiness for marriage
   a. Physically ready
   b. Psychologically not ready
   c. Spiritually not ready

Group Activities
1. Visitation to a hospital baby ward, if possible. If not, visit a zoo or the local dog pound to see baby animals.
2. Guest speakers—A sports hero the children admire or an adult who is skilled in talking with children, such as a physician.

Individual Activities
1. Have each child make a family tree including their immediate family's eye, hair color, etc.
2. If possible, have each child make a family tree of their pet.

Correlation With Other Subjects
1. Arithmetic
   a. Design problems may be used, dealing with heredity and the heredity formula.
2. Social Studies
   a. Study the different marriage rites of other countries.
3. Language Arts
   a. Write a paper about their grandparents, aunts, or uncles.
4. Science
   a. View various parts of the skin of people and animals; of sperm, if possible.
5. Art
   a. Have the pupils paint or draw pictures of their happy family times.

Pupil References
   Health Education Services: *The Gift of Life.* Mental Health Materials Center, 1951.
   Life Cycle Library Pamphlets. Life Cycle Library, Kotex Products. New York: Kimberly-Clark Corp., 1971.
   Menstruation booklets from Tampax, Modess, or Kotex Company. Write to the educational department of each. See appendix for addresses.
   O'Neal, Mary: *People I'd Like to Be.* Garden City, N. Y.: Doubleday & Co., 1964.
   Scheinfeld, Amram: *Why You Are You.* New York: Abelard-Schuman, 1958.

Teacher References
   Breckenridge, M. E., and Vincent, E. L.: *Child Development.* Philadelphia: W. B. Saunders Co., 1970.
   Child Study Association of America: *Sex Education and the New Morality.* New York: Columbia University Press, 1967.
   Johnson, Warren, and Belzer, E. G.: *Human Sexual Behavior and Sex Education,* 3rd ed. Philadelphia: Lea & Febiger, 1973.
   Levine, Milton I., and Seligmann, J.: *Helping Boys and Girls Understand Their Sex Roles.* Chicago: Science Research Associates, 1952.
   Sex Information and Educational Council of the United States (SIECUS): *Characteristics of Male and Female Sexual Responses.* New York, The Council, 1970.
   SIECUS: *Masturbation; Premarital Sexual-Standards; Sexuality and Sexual Learning in the Child.* New York: The Council. The Council also has a wide variety of some of the best materials in sex education available anywhere.

Audio-Visual Aids
   Human and Animal Beginnings. Henk Newenhouse. This film presents basic information about human reproduction and concepts of the family. Includes baby monkeys and mice, newborn guinea pigs and rabbits, time-lapse photographs of a hatching egg, and fish eggs in which live embryos are clearly seen. On the human side, the film includes pictures showing babies in the hospital nursery, at home with family, and animated sequences showing pre-birth growth and development and birth itself.
   Fertilization and Birth. Henk Newenhouse. As a follow-up to the subject introduced in *Human and Animal Beginnings*, this film helps the teacher answer

the primary students' questions accurately and without embarrassment, for it takes into account the reaction of children at these levels to the subject matter, an explanation of the reproductive system of fish is followed by a simple presentation of the human reproductive system and its functions, including the birth and suckling of the young in both humans and animals.

Human Growth. E. C. Brown Trust. Shows growth changes in boys and girls from ages 3 to 21. Deals especially with the changes at puberty in preparation for parenthood. The film may be used as a summary of the male and female reproductive systems and an introduction to pregnancy.

The Story of Menstruation. Walt Disney and Kimberly-Clark Corp. Although presented in cartoons, this film is good for young girls who are just starting to menstruate.

Other Teaching Aids

Denoyer Geppert & Co., catalog of classroom materials for family life programs.

Evaluation of Results

1. Were the students responsive to the films or were they embarrassed and unresponsive?
2. Did any students work on any aspect of this unit voluntarily?
3. What areas in this unit need to be retaught so that all children learn them, as was shown through testing results?

Grades 5 and 6

Objectives

1. To understand the role of the male and female in reproduction.
2. To overcome worries many students at this stage have, and guide them toward greater knowledges of changes taking place in their bodies and why these are taking place.
3. To understand the importance of hygiene and ways to achieve male and female hygiene.
4. To understand fertilization and heredity.
5. To gain knowledge of pregnancy and childbirth.
6. To recognize the value and importance of wholesome life attitudes and values.
7. To learn acceptable and unacceptable methods of showing emotions.
8. To gain the ability to talk freely, factually, and wholesomely about sexual matters.

Suggested Methods

1. Methods are numerous in this area but the teacher should use discretion, keeping in mind parental sensitivity in this area.
2. Use visual aids.
3. Class discussions are valuable in revealing what areas have not been adequately explained.
4. Allow the students to participate in planning this unit as much as possible. Find out what they want to know.

Basic Concepts

1. Reproductive cells, living vs. nonliving cells, egg cell, sperm cell.
2. Male and female reproductive system.
3. Fertilization and pregnancy.
4. Growing changes in boys.
5. Girls' preparation for motherhood.
6. Marriage and family.
7. Boy-and-girl relationships.
8. Problems of growing up.
9. Importance of healthy attitudes and behavior related to sex.
10. Reliable sources for sex education.
11. One's sexuality should be expressed as a wholesome part of his personality.

12. One should respect certain social customs, family loyalties, and life's miracles.
13. Married love.
14. Childbirth.
15. The family plan.
16. Sex roles.

Group Activities
1. Construct models of living things out of living materials such as fruits, flowers.
2. Discuss the difference between living and nonliving things.
3. Demonstrate fertilization using a plastic Easter egg and paper sperm.
4. Show the class a napkin, sanitary belt, and tampon, and explain their use.
5. Discuss growing up biologically and sociologically.
6. "Divide the class into nine groups representing each month of intra-uterine growth. Have a section of library books and materials available in your classroom. Each group will do research on the growth that takes place during their assigned month. Each group will also prepare a report to share with the class on what they have learned. Large illustrations made by the group will add more to their presentations. Later, the illustrations made by the group will be combined in one large bulletin board to show the nine-month developmental sequence." From *Education For Sexuality*. Burt & Brower, W. B. Saunders, 1970.
7. Have girls learn exercises for menstrual cramps in appropriate clothing in their physical education classes.
8. Discuss why one should use scientific terminology rather than "slang" in the study of sex education.
9. "Through a lecture-discussion, start with the basic structural unit, the cell, and 'build' a person. Include in the dialogue an analogy between the human body and a building: cells-bricks; tissues-walls; organs-rooms; systems-apartments; and organism-building." From *Sex Education Resource Unit*. AAHPER, 1967.
10. View films on human heredity, reproduction, and menstruation; discuss each.
11. Write a report including common traits of their family members and their dissimilarities.

Individual Pupil Activities
1. Have each keep a notebook of scientific terminology.
2. Have students label diagrams of the female and male reproductive systems. Have them put these in their notebooks.
3. After discussing the menstrual cycle, have each pupil summarize the cycle on paper and add this to their notebooks.
4. Have each girl construct a calendar of 12 months and record her menstrual cycle. Add this, too, to the notebook.
5. After completing the unit, each student should write a letter to an imaginary friend relating what they have learned about growing up.

Correlation With Other Subjects
1. Social Studies
   a. Discuss population problems in the different countries of the world and the effect on their society.
2. Language Arts
   a. Report on inherited family traits.
3. Drama
   a. Role play the parents' position of trying to explain sex to their children.
4. Art
   a. Living things constructed from living materials.

Pupil References

American Medical Association: *Why Girls Menstruate.* (Pamphlet) Chicago: The Association.

American Social Health Association: *Boys Want to Know and Girls Want to Know.* (Pamphlets) New York: The Association.

Archer, Elsie: *Let's Face It.* Philadelphia: J. B. Lippincott Co.

Adler, Irving and Ruth: *Evolution.* New York: The John Day Co.

Armstrong, David W.: *Questions Boys Ask.* New York: E. P. Dutton Co.

Bauer, William W.: *Moving into Manhood.* Garden City, N. Y.: Doubleday and Co.

Bauer, William W., and Varbyne, Florence: *Way to Womanhood.* Garden City, N. Y.: Doubleday and Co.

Clare, June: *The Stuff of Life.* New York: Roy Publishers.

Cornell, Betty, *All About Boys.* Englewood Cliffs, N. J.: Prentice-Hall.

Accent On You. (Pamphlet) New York: Tampax.

It's Time You Knew. (Pamphlet) New York: Tampax.

Gruenberg: *The Wonderful Story of You.* New York: Garden City Books.

Gregg, Walter H.: *A Boy and His Physique.* Chicago: National Dairy Council, 1965. (Contains growth chart for boys.)

Health Education Service: *The Gift of Life.* New York: Mental Health Association.

The Miracle of You. Neenah, Wisc.: Kimberly-Clark Corp.

Lerrigo, Marion, and Cassidy, M.: *A Doctor Talks to 9–12 Year Olds.* (Pamphlet) Chicago: Budlong Press.

Lerrigo, Marion, and Cassidy, M.: *A Story About You.* (Pamphlet) Chicago: American Medical Association.

Nilsson, Lonnart, and Rosenfeld, Albert: "Drama of Life before Birth." *Life,* July 22, 1966.

Pirkington, Roger: *Human Sex and Heredity.* New York: Franklin Watts.

All About You; Making and Keeping Friends; Understanding Sex. (Pamphlets) Chicago: Science Research Associates.

Teacher References

American Institute of Biological Sciences: *Reproduction, Growth and Development.* New York: McGraw-Hill, 1963.

Amstutz, H. Clair: *Growing Up to Love: A Guide to Sex Education for Parents.* Scottsdale, Pa.: Herald Press, 1960.

Bavin, Arthur: *Circle of Sex.* New Hyde Park, N. Y.: University Books, 1966.

Bauer, William W.: *Moving into Manhood.* Garden City, N. Y.: Doubleday & Co., 1963.

Bauer, Willaim W., and Varbyne, Florence: *Way to Womanhood.* Garden City, N. Y.: Doubleday & Co., 1965.

Breckenridge, Marian, and Vincent, E. Lee: *Child Development.* Philadelphia: W. B. Saunders Co., 1971.

Burt, John J., and Brower, Linda: *Education for Sexuality.* Philadelphia: W. B. Saunders Co., 1970.

Calderone, Mary S.: "The Development of Healthy Sexuality." *Journal of Health, Physical Education and Recreation.* Sept. 1, 1966.

A Guide For Educators on Menstrual Hygiene. Milltown, N. J.: Personal Products Co.

From Fiction to Fact. New York: Tampax.

Frias, Francis L.: *Sex Education In The Family.* Englewood Cliffs, N. J.: Prentice-Hall, 1966.

Johnson, Eric W.: *Love and Sex in Plain Language.* Philadelphia: J. B. Lippincott Co., 1965.

Josselyn, Irene M.: "The Source of Sexual Identity." *National Elementary Principal,* November, 1966.

Kilander, H.: *Sex Education In The Schools.* New York: The Macmillan Co., 1970.

Kilander, H.: *School Health Education.* 2nd ed., New York: The Macmillan Co., 1968.

Levine, Milton I., and Seligmann, Jean H.: *A Baby Is Born.* New York: Golden Press, 1966.

Kogan, Benjamin A.: *Health: Man in a Changing Environment.* New York: Harcourt, Brace & Jovanovich, 1970.

Mead, Margaret, and Wolfenstein, Martha: *Childhood in Contemporary Cultures.* Chicago: University of Chicago Press, 1963.

Read, Donald A., and Greene, Walter H.: *Creative Teaching in Health.* New York: The Macmillan Co., 1971.

Sex Education Resource Unit. Washington, D.C.: AAHPER, 1967.

Audio-Visual Aids

Girl to Woman. (Color, 18 min.) Churchill Films. Shows the physical changes that take place during adolescence in both the boy and the girl.

Growing Up. Coronet Films. Nicky and Peggy show that growing up is an uneven process that differs between boys and girls, varying with the individual's age.

CHAPTER 18

consumer education

Consumer education should begin in kindergarten. All children are consumers and must be prepared to become increasingly wise buyers of all kinds of goods. Although it is true that they have but few pennies of their own to spend, they are targets of costly advertising for toys, cereals, and other foods, as well as candy, gum, and all other products which appeal to children. As they go grocery shopping with their mothers, they pressure them to buy extra goodies for them or the family that are not needed in a well-balanced diet, such as candy or donuts.

Today's consumers of all ages are bewildered by false advertising, easy credit, and fast loans carrying hidden but costly interest rates. The teacher can help each child learn the values as well as pitfalls of buying. The Suggested Guidelines For Consumer Education, Grades K–12, published by the Office of Consumer Affairs can help each instructor, along with this chapter, devise teaching units in this area which will become alive and exciting educational experiences. The basic aim of such units should be to help students learn how and when to make their best buys and how to use their income to its greatest value. The carryover experiences of such materials should reach far into their adulthood.

SUGGESTED UNITS OF INSTRUCTIONS

Found below are suggested units of instruction in this important area for grades K to 6:

General Objectives
1. Prepare children with knowledge for making the best choice and decisions in purchasing objects and services which represent an investment in their health.
2. Develop good buying habits based upon sound criteria.

Desired Outcomes
To help the child:
1. Increase his discrimination when buying.

2. Select competent dental, medical, and other health services.
3. Know that there are governmental agencies which help by devising and holding standards in food, medicines, and services.

Kindergarten

Approach
1. Acquaint child with how money is used in buying.
2. Acquaint child with people who help him to be healthy, safe, and well fed.
3. Begin the individual's criteria for being a wise consumer.

Basic Concepts To Teach
1. There are many things from which to choose when buying something.
2. One cannot buy everything one wants, sees, or needs.
3. Choosing requires thinking as well as knowledge of what is the best.
4. Government rules help us buy things wisely.

Group Activities
1. Read, tell, and write stories about people who work for us.
   a. Farmers, dairymen
   b. Garbage collectors, policemen, firemen
   c. Salesladies, etc.
   d. Medical people
2. How food is grown, sent to market, and how supermarkets get food to sell to people.
3. Discuss and illustrate with pictures how wheat is grown, processed in bakery, and how many things are made from it. Discuss how milk is pasteurized, packaged, and delivered.
4. Learn the names and jobs done by those in the various health protective services (i.e., doctors, dentists, etc.).

Individual Activities
1. Talk with the child about things he likes to eat, play with, and where they come from in order to help him learn that they do not come ready made.
2. Let the child suggest rules for the classroom in using purchased health products, such as paper tissues, fly sprays, etc.

Correlation With Other Subjects
1. Arithmetic
   a. Practice counting with money, making and receiving change.
   b. Play grocery store with canned goods, cereal boxes, fruit, vegetables, etc., to give children practice in adding and subtracting and counting.
2. Social Studies
   a. Study people who live in different places in the country, in other countries, their customs, foods, and clothing, toys, etc.
3. Language Arts
   a. Increase vocabulary by naming professions such as doctors, nurses, and other occupations.
   b. Reading of various books which deal with such services.
4. Science
   a. Make butter.
   b. Have class make a vegetable garden, growing radishes, beans, tomatoes.
5. Drama and Art
   a. Have children draw pictures of subjects talked about, farms, bakeries, factories, doctor's office.
   b. Role playing with doctors, farmers selling food, and grocery store.
6. Physical Education
   a. Learn singing games such as "Oats and Beans and Barley Grow," "Way Down Yonder in the Paw Paw Patch," and "Old McDonald Had a Farm,"

Grade 1

Suggested Approaches
1. To acquaint the child with the process of buying and selling by using play money.
2. To further acquaint the child with people who deal in goods and service.
3. To help the child become conscious of the whole range of products available and the need to buy wisely.

Basic Concepts To Teach
1. There are many things from which to choose when buying.
2. To have a respect for the property of others so that he does not take things not belonging to him.
3. Choosing requires thinking wisely.
4. Government standards help people keep safe and healthy.

Group Activities
1. Practice buying for school parties, planning menus, etc. with play money.
2. Read aloud stories dealing with how things are made.
3. Read *The Shoemaker and the Elves*. Talk of modern shoe factory or visit one, if nearby.
4. Introduce weights and measurements such as cups, quarts, gallons, ounces. Bring scale to classroom for individual practice.
5. Visit a bakery, discuss farmers growing wheat, how it is harvested and brought to the bakery. Discuss why everything must be clean in the bakery.
6. Visit water plant and discuss the importance of good, pure water.

Individual Activities
1. Let children tell if their parents are involved in marketing and service.
2. Point out in conversations throughout the day where things in classroom came from, etc.
3. Let child tell you why he wants a certain toy for Christmas, and where and how it is made.

Correlation With Other Subjects
1. Arithmetic
    a. Continue to practice giving and receiving change, adding coins, etc.
    b. Practice adding ounces, pounds, cups, quarts, etc.
2. Social Studies
    a. Study customs of other countries and of our country.
    b. Trace the area of the country where food comes from: oranges from California and Florida, apples from Washington, etc.
3. Language
    a. Read stories such as *The First Book of Hospitals* and *The First Book of Doctors*.
4. Science
    a. Experiments in making water pure, such as bolling and purifying it with tablets.
5. Drama and Art
    a. Draw a factory, water plant, or any place the class visited.
    b. Play guessing games, such as "I'm thinking of _____ (someone who grows food)."
    c. Role play any person who deals in services, such as doctor, milkman.
6. Physical Education
    a. Singing games as listed in section for kindergarten.
    b. Play "It" using appropriate title to be it.

Films
    Fourteen Acres of Kitchen. (Color, 14 min.) Modern Talking Picture Service. History of a canning company. How foods are processed in an automated plant.

Where We Make Things. (Color, 9 min.) McGraw-Hill text film. Tony's favorite toy is an airplane. It breaks and is returned, and he is told how toys are made.

Money Experiences. Curriculum Materials. Introduces coins and provides practice in counting and making change.

Money Has Meaning. National Consumer Finance Association. Defines and illustrates barter, trading, buying, selling, earning.

Money Makes Cents. National Consumer Finance Association.

Money Needs Managing. National Consumer Finance Association.

Risa Earns Her Dime. McGraw-Hill.

The following are available from McGraw-Hill:

We Get Food From Plants and Animals.

Moving People and Goods.

Keeping The Community Informed. Carol's cat visits newspaper, T.V. offices.

Pupil References

Fairy tales such as "Jack and the Beanstalk," "Three Little Pigs," "Shoemaker and the Elves." *First Book of Hospitals; First Book of Nurses; First Book of Doctors; Being Six or So; Being Seven or So.* Glenview, Ill.: Scott, Foresman & Co.

Nursery Rhymes

"To Market, To Market," "Hot Cross Buns."

"Bread Facts for Consumer Education," AIB #142. Washington, D.C.: U.S. Dept. of Agriculture, November 1955.

Filmstrips

"Where Clothes Come From." Encyclopedia Britannica.

"From Farm To You." U.S. National Audio-Visual Center.

Teacher References

"Helping Elementary Schoolers Understand Mass Persuasion." *Social Education.* February 1967.

Packard, Vance: *Hidden Persuaders.* New York: David McKay Co., 1957.

"Consumer Champion Lays Down with the Law." *Life* 71:322 (July 16, 1971).

Krama, A.: "Basic Business for Migrant Workers' Children." *Business Education Forum* 25:16 (March 1971).

Knauer, V.: "Consumer Education and the Consumer." *Compact* 5:5 (July 1971).

Evaluation

1. During conversation with child to see if he had gained concepts.
2. Oral sample quizzes.
3. Vocabulary tests.
4. Ability to relate information and associate with other subjects as observed.

Grade 2

Suggested Approaches

1. To help each student evolve his own value system.
2. To get the student to see himself as a consumer.
3. To get the student to gain a responsibility for money.
4. To continue with change-making and buying and selling with money.
5. To explore the child's world of TV to point out consumer products.
6. To have the child develop a criteria for consuming.

Basic Concepts

1. Desirable and undesirable influences affect a person's choice of products and services.
2. Choosing requires careful thought about how to spend money wisely.
3. There are many kinds of things from which to choose.

Group Activities
1. Visit a local bank.
2. Visit a grocery store.
3. Visit a newspaper office or television station to see how advertisements are made.
4. Cite examples of television and radio advertisements for true or false advertising.
5. Find out what is in cans of food.
6. Play grocery store.
7. Have a person in public service visit the class.
8. Talk about going to the dentist.
9. Talk about going to the doctor and the school nurse.
10. Let the children talk about their sicknesses and health experiences.

Individual Activities
1. Let the students tell of their health learning experiences at home, the school, or in the community.
2. Have each child bring an ad for his favorite toy.
3. Have each child dictate a letter to the teacher about how he helps his parents when going grocery shopping with them.

Correlation
1. Arithmetic
   a. Addition and subtraction of purchases
2. Social Studies
   a. Learn of the grocery products of other countries
3. Language Arts
   a. Learn the terms of people in service positions such as a delivery man or station attendant.
4. Science
   a. Make baking soda toothpaste.
   b. Visit mints, dairies, canneries, and meat packaging plants.
5. Drama and Art
   a. Draw community helpers.
   b. Role play the duties of community helpers.
6. Physical Education
   a. Movement exploration exercises in being different consumer products—bread, furniture, etc.

Pupil References
Henry, Marguerite: *Geraldine Belinda.* New York: Platt & Munk Co., 1958.
The First Book of Hospitals; The First Book of Nurses; The First Book of Doctors; Being Seven or So. Glenview, Ill.: Scott, Foresman & Co.
"Bread Facts for Consumer Education." AIB #142. Washington, D.C.: U.S. Department of Agriculture, November 1955.

Teacher References
Consumer Reports. Published by the Consumers Union of the United States, Inc., 256 Washington St., Mt. Vernon, N. Y. 10550.
Elementary School Health Education Curriculum Guide. Texas Education Agency Publication #715.
Suggested Guidelines for Consumer Education, Grades K to 12. Washington, D.C.: Department of Health, Education and Welfare.
Knauer, Virginia: "Prepare Consumers for the Marketplace." *The Instructor.* October 1972.
Knauer, V.: "Consumer Education and the Consumer." *Compact* 5:5 (July 1971).

Audio-Visual Aids
From Farm to You. U.S. National Audiovisual Center.
Fourteen Acres of Kitchen. Modern Talking Pictures Service.
Money Experiences. Curriculum Materials.

Evaluation
1. Oral quiz.
2. Vocabulary tests.
3. Matching tests of knowledge.
4. Conversations with the class as a whole and with each child about money and how to spend it well.
5. Observations of each child as he selects food in the cafeteria.

Grade 3

Objective
1. To establish sound purchasing habits based from the beginning on sound knowledge and criteria.

Suggested Approaches
1. Field trips
2. Guest speakers
3. Bulletin boards
4. Demonstrations

Basic Concepts
1. There are many superstitions concerning health.
2. We take precautions to protect us against disease (vaccines).
3. Government has many agencies and laws protecting consumers.
4. Much propaganda and falseness in commercials.
5. Safety precautions must be taken when using medicines.
6. People are especially trained to keep us healthy.

Group Activities
1. Visit a supermarket, looking for things that help protect our foods, such as meat in the freezer, government stickers, etc.
2. Act out TV commercials pertaining to health products and discuss their effects on listener.
3. Discuss health myths, such as getting warts from handling toads, putting beefsteak on a black eye, etc.
4. Tour a milk pasteurization plant to see how milk is made pure.

Individual Activities
1. Collect advertisements from magazines and write paragraph on what each tries to make you believe.
2. Make a scrapbook showing all the people and ways in which they help us to learn about health, such as a doctor, nurse.
3. Write a report on the training of some specialist in the field of health (doctor, nurse, dentist, pharmacist).

Correlation With Other Subjects
1. Language Arts
2. Drama and Art
   a. Write a theme on some health heroes.
   a. Make collage using advertisements from magazines.
3. Science
   a. Discuss importance of pasteurization and refrigeration.
4. Physical Education
   a. Show how you can buy a good baseball glove for less money, etc.

Pupil References
Etling, Mary: *The First Book of Nurses.*
Green, Carla: *Doctors and Nurses: What Do They Do?*
Lerner, Marguerite: *Doctor's Tools.*
Thompson, Frances B.: *About Dr. John.*

Teacher References
Crowder, W. W.: "Helping Elementary School Children Understand Mass Persuasion Techniques." *Social Education Magazine.* February 1967.

Audio-Visual Aids (Materials for overhead projection)
  *How Safe Is Our Food; Additives In Our Food; The Use and Misuse of Drugs;
  Drugs and The Body.* DCA Educational Products, Inc.

Evaluation
  1. Do the students understand and appreciate the basic concepts as listed?

Grade 4

Objectives
  1. To help each student develop his own value system regarding money
     and its use.
  2. To help each student develop sound decision-making procedures based
     on his understanding of the above.
  3. To help each child understand his rights and responsibilities as a con-
     sumer in our society.
  4. To help the student to evaluate various media of advertising techniques.

Basic Concepts
  1. Desirable and undesirable influences affect a person's choice of prod-
     ucts and services.
  2. The pupils are consumers.
  3. There are sources of reliable consumer information.
  4. The consumer is protected by laws.
  5. Money and its use require understanding.

Group Activities
  1. Prepare a model medicine chest.
  2. Design labels and warnings of poison medicines, etc.
  3. Take a field trip to a dairy, baker, cannery, or the school cafeteria.
  4. Prepare a shopping list.
  5. Visit a grocery store; compare prices.
  6. Panel discussion on self-medication, including common ailments
     handled without medical aid, common remedies, and superstitions.

Individual Activities
  1. Visit the school cafeteria, cannery, dairy, and bakery to find out how
     people using food are protected.
  2. Make a collage, highlighting the emotional appeals of advertised
     products.
  3. Make your own advertisement of any product.
  4. Make a list of unsafe toys.

Correlation
  1. Arithmetic
     a. Figure the percentage of reduction in prices of sale items advertised
        in newspapers.
  2. Social Studies
     a. Learn of consumer needs in different countries such as China,
        Mexico, etc.
  3. Language Arts
     a. Individual reports or essays on people in service occupations such
        as a grocery man, etc.
  4. Science
     a. Learn the sanitary laws for food handlers.
     b. Discuss nutritional value of common foods.
  5. Drama
     a. Write and perform a play, "The Medicine Show," to show how
        people can be "taken" when buying patent medicines.
  6. Art
     a. Design advertisements for food and clothing.

7. Physical Education
   a. Discuss magazine ads for building big muscles or losing weight quickly.

Teacher References
Consumer Reports. Published by the Consumers Union of the United States, Inc., 256 Washington St., Mt. Vernon, N. Y. 10550.
Elementary School Health Education Curriculum Guide. Texas Education Agency Publication #715.
Suggested Guidelines for Consumer Education, Grades K to 12. Washington, D.C.: Department of Health, Education and Welfare.
Knauer, Virginia: "Prepare Consumers for the Marketplace." *The Instructor.* October 1972.
Knauer, Virginia: "Consumer Education and the Consumer." *Compact* 5:5 (July 1971).
Pamphlets from the Food and Drug Administration, Federal Trade Commission, and The World Health Association.
The Cancer Quacks. Washington, D. C.: Department of Health, Education and Welfare.

Pupil References
Henry, Marguerite: *Geraldine Belinda.* New York: Platt and Munk Co., 1958.
"How the FDA Works For You." The Food and Drug Administration.
Pamphlets from Department of Health, Education & Welfare, Food and Drug Administration, and the World Health Organization.

Audio-Visual Aids
Myth, Superstition, and Science.
Your Health in the Community.

Grade 5

Objectives
1. To know the individual's role as a consumer of products related to health.
2. To learn to judge value of a health product and wise purchases.
3. To understand the superstitions and misconceptions related to health goods and services.
4. To understand the value of being a knowledgeable consumer of health products and services for one's personal benefit and to benefit others by acting to keep undesirable and dangerous goods out of circulation.

Suggested Approaches
1. The approach should be factual, with emphasis placed on the students discovering facts for themselves.
2. Television, radio, magazines, etc., should be used to show how the consumer is influenced to purchase and use health products.
3. Class discussion and films will add to pupil interest.

Basic Concepts To Teach
1. The dangers of self-medication.
2. Go to competent persons for advice concerning health care.
3. There are many unqualified persons offering their services and products to the gullible public.
4. Physicians should be consulted for the diagnosis of health problems and for medication directions.
5. Advertisements are often misleading and many products on the market are harmful.

Group Activities
1. Have the students listen to TV or radio tapes of various health product advertisements; then discuss misleading words and phrases that would influence the consumer.

  2. Have the students bring a collection of labels from food and discuss them.
  3. Have students make a list of superstitions relating to health.

Individual Pupil Activities
  1. Oral or written reports on why Americans spend over 28 billion dollars for medical care each year.
  2. Have pupils define terms: fraud, quack, nostrum, quack medical device, proprietary drug, etc.
  3. Have one student make a list of health products that are advertised by television, another student do the same for radio, another for magazines and newspaper. Have a class discussion on the findings.

Correlation With Other Subjects
  1. Arithmetic
     a. Make a study of the amount of money spent annually on health products in the U. S. and for what purposes.
  2. Social Studies
     a. Study about the agencies in our society which protect the consumer.
  3. Language Arts
     a. Give a puppet show on the influence of clever advertising on the consumer.
  4. Science
     a. Study how foods are analyzed for consumer protection.
  5. Drama
     a. Role play the part of an advertiser and buyer trying to sell a health product which is really worthless.
  6. Physical Education
     a. Discuss health products that are advertised as physical "pepper-uppers" or relaxers and the dangers of using such products.

Pupil References
  Better Business Bureau.
  Current magazines, newspapers, etc.
  Kime, R. E.: *Health: A Consumer's Dilemma.* Belmont, Calif.: Wadsworth Publishing Co., 1970.

Teacher References
  Kime, R. E.: *Health: A Consumer's Dilemma.* Belmont, Calif.: Wadsworth Publishing Co., 1970.
  Consumer Reports: "The Medicine Show." Mt. Vernon, N. Y.: Consumer's Union of U. S., 1963. "Some plain truths about popular products for common ailments." A compete coverage of health products available to the consumer with reports based on actual laboratory tests.
  Community health agencies.
  Cornacchia, H. J., *et al.*: *Health in Elementary Schools.* 3rd ed., St. Louis: C. V. Mosby Co., 1970.
  Kilander, H. F.: *School Health Education.* New York: The Macmillan Co., 1968.

Audio-Visual Aids
  Tape recording of advertisements.
  Bulletin board with pamphlets from various health agencies.
  Speaker (ask a medical person to speak to the class on qualified medical care).

Checking Your Health
  All of the above films are from the United States Government Film Services, Du Art Film Laboratories.

Evaluation
  1. Can the students explain convincingly the importance of consumer education?

2. Objective and essay tests regarding observations and conversations with the students to learn how they are using the knowledge learned in this area.

Grade 6

Objectives
1. To help the student evaluate alternatives in the marketplace and how to get the best buys for his money.
2. To help the student understand his rights and responsibilities as a consumer in our society.
3. To help the student fulfill his role as a part of the free enterprise system found in America.

Basic Concepts
1. The value of having periodic health examinations and a right place to go for one.
2. Self-diagnosis and self-medication are to be avoided.
3. Quackery exists.
4. The consumer is protected to some extent by the government.
5. Scientific information should replace myths and superstitions.
6. Wise buying requires much knowledge.
7. Desirable and undesirable influences affect a person's choice of products and services.

Group Activities
1. Present a skit on quackery.
2. Design labels and warnings for products used in the home.
3. Write radio commercials and share them in class.
4. Take a field trip to an ice cream plant and discuss this experience in class.
5. Have a panel of persons from various agencies for consumer protection.
6. Have a class panel discussion on quackery.

Individual Activities
1. Give special reports on quackery.
2. Construct a list of health superstitions and food fads.
3. Visit a food store specializing in health foods and report your findings.
4. Interview your nearest druggist to find what patent medicines are most popular.

Correlation
1. Arithmetic
   a. Figure out a weekly budget for your family.
2. Social Studies
   a. Study health fads in other countries and in different parts of this country.
3. Language Arts
   a. Write a skit on the evils of false advertising.
4. Science
   a. Study illnesses caused by the use of dangerous products.
5. Drama and Art
   a. Perform the skit on medical quackery.
   b. Design labels and commercials for dishwashing products.

Pupil References
Kime, Robert E.: *Health: A Consumer's Dilemma.* Belmont, Calif.: Wadsworth Publishing Co., 1970.
Mapel, Eric: *Magic, Medicine, and Quackery.* London: Robert Hale, 1968.
Local health agencies.
Current magazines; television and radio ads.

Teacher References

Kime, Robert E.: *Health: A Consumer's Dilemma.* Belmont, Calif.: Wadsworth Publishing Co., 1970.

Kilander, H. F.: *School Health Education.* 2nd ed. New York: The Macmillan Co., 1970.

McLuhan, H. Marshall: *Understanding Media: The Extensions of Man.* New York: McGraw-Hill Book Co., 1965.

Packard, Vance O.: *The Hidden Persuaders.* New York: David McKay Co., 1957.

Audio-Visual Aids

Bulletin boards on quackery and misleading terms.

How Safe is Our Food?; Additives In Our Food. DCA Educational Products.

Myth, Superstition, and Science. Du Art Film Laboratories.

Evaluation

1. Class discussions of most important things learned in this unit.
2. Short-answer tests.
3. Analyzing the knowledge gain by students in this unit as shown in their behavior, questions, and written work.

PART FIVE

evaluating the results

The evaluation process should stimulate professional interest and arouse a desire for improving the school health program.

—Alma Nemir, M.D.

CHAPTER 19

evaluating the results

Evaluation is a method used to appraise, measure, and check progress. It is finding out where you are and carefully analyzing how you arrived there in relationship to where you want to go. It is also a process of taking stock or self-discovery so that new and better ways to gain desired goals can be found and used with renewed zest. Or, as Anderson says, it tells what is, what should be, and what should not be, and points out the following values of an evaluation program of the total health program:

1. Inventories the present status of child health and the health program.
2. Appraises the health of the individual child.
3. Appraises all aspects of the health program.
4. Measures progress.
5. Points out strengths in the program.
6. Reveals places where emphasis is needed.
7. Assists children in understanding their health condition and progress in health education.
8. Helps parents understand the health of their children and the school health program.
9. Gives the school a basis for revising both its health and general programs.
10. Provides a basis for public support and funds for school health work.[1]

PURPOSE AND SCOPE OF EVALUATION

Evaluation in health education should show that the program has had a marked and improved effect upon the health of the pupils. This is not always easy to measure, for behavior changes occur gradually and their effect may not be fully seen until the pupils reach adulthood. Evaluation should also be a process for determining to what extent the program has reached its stated objectives. The

---

[1] Anderson, C. L.: *School Health Practice*. St. Louis: C. V. Mosby Co., 1972, p. 448.

interplay between the objectives of education and health education should be continuous. The total school health program should be judged in terms of its results continuously by the school administrators, school health medical authorities, health supervisors, classroom teachers, school health council, pupils, parents, community health co-workers, and all others included or interested in the program. Such evaluation may range all the way from subjective observation to scientific measurement; it can be done by those with training in health education or methods of educational measurement or by experts in both fields. Many school administrators, pressed by taxpayers who want to get the most from their investment in public education, are including in their annual budget expenses for a scientific evaluation of their total school health program. Although this may be done by a team of experts, this type of evaluation can be an educational experience for those primarily engaged in the health program or those on the school health council. A local survey team guided by a selected health education expert might well take part in such a program. Oberteuffer suggests that any group engaged in such evaluation be first guided by the following principles:

1. Evaluation should be continuous.
2. It should embrace all the important functions of the school health program, including instruction and activities.
3. Evaluation should be cooperative. All those who are affected by the evaluation should participate in it—administrators, teachers, pupils, parents, physician, nurses, dental hygienists, nutritionists, and others.
4. It should be concerned both with end products and the means to reach these ends.
5. It should touch upon all health aspects of the school, including curriculum, administration, buildings, grounds, equipment, finances, and community relationships.
6. Evaluation should be focused upon the important values which underlie the health program of the school, and the success or failure of the program should be judged in terms of how well it meets the values held.
7. A long-range evaluation program should be so planned that no one year would involve the school in a complete study of every aspect of school health education.
8. The collection of data and keeping of records in the school have no value in themselves. Only as the data aid in evaluating the true functions of the school to educate do they attain value.[2]

There are many excellent rating scales and school health standard checklists available for evaluating the school's physical plant, health service, custodial service, health instruction programs, mental, dental, nutrition, and safety education programs.[3] Any such selected tools can assist an evaluation committee engaged in a well-planned, long-range measurement program. The results of the work done by this group should be published and made available to all school personnel and interested citizens in the community.[4] This written report might well contain the findings of the committee, what the school is actually doing in relationship to its declared objectives, and recommendations for the future betterment of the program.

[2] Oberteuffer, Delbert, et al.: *School Health Education.* 5th ed. New York: Harper & Row, 1972, pp. 322–323.
[3] See the Appendix for suggested sources.
[4] For suggestions of how the report should be written and what it might contain, see *Evaluation of Health Education and Health Services in Los Angeles Public Schools,* 1959. Available from the Los Angeles Public Schools.

EVALUATING THE PROGRAM

It must be remembered that health instruction is but one of three areas of the total health program and that it must be a part of the work done by those engaged in school health services, and all who are primarily concerned with and responsible for providing a healthful school environment. There must be a direct relationship between what is taught in the classroom and the services provided by the school and the type of school environment in which children are required by law to be 5 to 6 hours daily, 30 weeks a year for 12 or 16 years of their lives.

Evaluation of the health education program should first determine whether it is in accord with sound overall educational objectives and principles, and then measure the degree to which the health education program has reached its established objectives. Such evaluation should lead to curriculum improvement, as well as the development of better health practices and environmental conditions of the school, home, and community. It should be continuous and include the pupils. Such a study should show the weaknesses as well as the strengths of the school health program, and should be used as a guide for charting needed improvements in all three of its areas.

MEASURING INSTRUMENTS

The following instruments can be used successfully in evaluating the school program:

Records

These should include carefully kept records of the school food service department, including food choices made by the pupils, amount of milk sold, and other types of similar information; health service records, including the results of periodic weighing and measuring, physical examinations and tests, records of remedial defects corrected and as yet uncorrected, first-aid treatment given, and other pertinent information; records which show needed changes, or improvements made in the school environment, such as new, fenced-in play areas, additional fire escapes, etc.

Observations

These should include the observations made by all adults connected with the school (as well as those by each teacher of her class) of the health conditions, behavior, and attitudes of the children. The school custodian, nurse, and bus driver should report to those evaluating the school health program what they have seen children do or heard them say in relation to the opportunities provided for them by the school to learn about health.

Surveys

These should include a careful study of the health problems and needs of the school itself, then of the home, and finally of the community. The effectiveness of the school health program should be measured in terms of improvement in relationship to problems and needs in all these places.

Questionnaires and Checklists

Such records can show the interests and practices in health among parents and children. Both should be asked to answer such questions as the time children usually go to bed, what they eat for breakfast, etc., and fill out health interest forms. Careful tabulation should be made of these materials; they should be analzyed to determine the amount and degree of changes in behavior, attitudes, and interests which have taken place as a result of the health education program.

Parent Conferences

Such experiences are splendid for helping the teacher gain insight into what the child does or does not do at home for his health in relationship to what he has learned in school.

Personal Creative Work

Diaries, autobiographies, themes, poems, and other samples of personal, creative work done by each child can help adults gain needed insight concerning these pupils, as well as help them discover how effective health education experiences have been to them. Such materials are especially valuable in measuring attitudes.

Tests

Oral or written tests of knowledge, attitudes, and habits can also be used to evaluate learning results.

EVALUATING PUPIL PROGRESS

Methods of evaluating pupil progress through subjective or objective measurement of the health instruction program include:

Skill tests	Questionnaires
Written tests of knowledge, attitudes and habits	Group discussion
	Posture tests
Checklists	Attitude tests
Rating scales	Social development tests
Interviews	Health records
Case studies	Personality inventories
Diaries	Progress reports of school health
Parental opinions	service personnel
Conferences	School surveys of the use of facili-
Self-appraisal	ties, such as the lunchroom

These tests may be used for:

1. Motivation
2. Self-evaluation
3. Grading
4. Grouping
5. Diagnosing weakness
6. Guidance

SUBJECTIVE TESTS

Observation[5]

This is the most frequently used means of evaluating behavior in elementary schools. To be of value, such appraisal must be critical, precise, and skilled. Both appearance and behavior can be observed and accurate deductions made by those with trained eyes and ears.

Interviews and Conferences

Interviews and other types of counseling can reveal significant findings as the teacher talks with each child, trying to find out more about him, what he feels, thinks, knows, and does. Conferences should involve the parents, who are more informed about their own child than anyone else. Records should be kept of each conference and used to evaluate progress made by each pupil.

Self-appraisal

Check sheets, rating scales, and other such tools used by pupils can do much to stimulate interest in health and motivate the desire to improve health habits. Such methods are superior to direct questions like "What did you have for breakfast?" or "When did you brush your teeth last?", for children soon learn to give back the answers that adults desire or else tell a fib in order to gain recognition or peer status. Any type of self-appraisal record has educational value if checked by each pupil and analyzed carefully by the teacher.

Parental Opinion or Checklists

Such materials are of value only when the parents feel that they are working partners with the teacher. Those from minority or uneducated groups may use the report as a means of helping their child gain school acceptance or class status and fill out the forms dishonestly. The following type of checklist is recommended:

CHECKLIST FOR PARENTS

Does your child:	Yes	No
1. Show improved health habits?		
2. Eat a better balanced diet?		
3. Show more concern for his own safety and health?		
4. Play better with more children?		
5. Seem more concerned about caring for his own body?		
6. Use more of his leisure time in outdoor play?		
7. Go to bed earlier; get more sleep and rest?		
8. Go more willingly to the dentist?		
9. Take better care of his own teeth?		
10. Have improved health, with fewer colds or other types of illness?		

[5] See Chapter 3, "Teaching through Health Appraisal Activities," for suggestions.

HOW WELL DO I RATE?

	Credits	Possible Daily Score	Mon.	Tues.	Wed.	Thurs.	Fri.	Sat.	Sun.
Milk									
2 glasses	10	20							
4 glasses	20								
Fruit									
1 serving	5								
2 servings	10	10							
Vegetables									
2 vegetables with potatoes	10	10							
if 1 vegetable is raw	5	5							
if vegetable is yellow or leafy green									
1 serving	5								
2 servings	10	10							
if fruits and vegetables include 1 serving of tomatoes, strawberries, melons, or citrus fruits	10	10							
Cereal products whole grain enriched									
1 serving	10								
2 servings	15	15							
Eggs, cheese, meat, dried beans, or peas									
1 serving	10								
2 servings	20	20							
Total credits		100							
Deductions									
Any meal omitted		10							
Tea, coffee, soft drink		5							
Sweets between meals		5							
Total deductions		20							
Net Score For Day									

Source: A workshop report, *Techniques of Evaluation in Health Education*, George Peabody College, Nashville, Tenn., 1955, p. 15. Courtesy of George Peabody College.

Case Studies

Each case study should contain:

1. Identification of the pupil
2. Problem faced by the pupil
3. Diagnostic test data
4. Results of interviews of conferences with the pupil, parents, or other adults
5. Pupil's physical condition
6. Pupil's appearance
7. Social and emotional development
8. Mental test results

9. Special interests
10. Home conditions
11. Diagnosis of the case (beginning of the year)
12. Progress made in the case
13. Recommendations

Diaries

A daily diary can be an effective means of self-evaluation and can help the teacher gain insight into each child. In such a report, the pupil should be asked to record everything he did, thought about, or felt keenly during each day for a week. Autobiographies and constructive criticisms written by older children are also revealing and can help both the pupils and their teacher gain better understanding of each learner.

Cumulative Health Records

Such records follow the child throughout his school career and move with him as he goes from school to school. They are invaluable in helping teachers understand the physical handicaps and special needs of each pupil.

Surveys

These can be used to survey home or school hazards, check the number of glasses of milk consumed by the students, etc. Surveys may be made by observation, checklists, interviews, reading records, or any other method which will reveal people's behavior.

Skill Tests

These may include testing the ability to read a mouth thermometer correctly, use a microscope, give any aspect of first aid, use equipment safely, or any other type of technical skill.

Picture Tests

Since primary children cannot read or write well, a good way to measure their knowledge or attitude toward health is through pictures. They may either write or check an answer sheet, after seeing a picture, to tell their teacher what they "see" in it. Suggested pictures can be of such things as a toothbrush, wash cloth, microscope, nail file, traffic light showing the color red, etc. Pictures can be used with the whole class, small groups of three or four children, or pupil by pupil.

STANDARDIZED TESTS

Although there are many standardized tests available in the area of health education, there are few good ones which have been devised specifically for elementary children. The following are recommended for measuring health knowledge, habits, interests, and attitudes:

Recommended Standardized Health and Safety Tests for Elementary Schools

Tests of Health Knowledge. New York: Association Press.
Cincinnati Health Knowledge Test. Cincinnati, Ohio: Cincinnati Public Schools.
Clark, Harrison *Clark Health Habit Questionnaire.* Eugene, Ore.: University of Oregon.

Health Tests. Bloomington, Ill.: Public School Publishing.

Smith, Sara: *Evaluation of the School Health Program.* Tallahassee, Fla.: Department of Health and Physical Education, Florida State University, 1960

Health Tests. Chicago: National Achievement Tests.

A Community Bicycle Program. (3 bicycle skill tests) New York: Association of Casualty and Surety Companies, 60 John Street, New York, N.Y. 10038.

Health Education Test Forms. Washington, D. C.: American Child Health Association.

Health Information Test. New York: American Museum of Health.

Health Tests (Grades 3–8). Benjamin Sanborn, 221 East 20th Street, Chicago, Ill.

Manchester Unit Elementary Tests (Grades 5 through 8). North Manchester, Ill.: Bureau of Tests and Measurements, Manchester College.

Brewer, J. W., and Schrammel, H. E.: *Brewer-Schrammel Health Knowledge and Attitude Tests.* Emporia, Kan. : Bureau of Educational Measurement, Kansas State Teachers College.

TEACHER-DEVISED TESTS

Any of the above-mentioned standardized tests might well be studied carefully for suggested patterns by those teachers who devise their own written tests. The characteristics of any good test are that it:

1. Is easy to understand and the directions are simply stated.
2. Is easy to give, grade, and record.
3. Measures what it is supposed to measure (validity).
4. Has measurement consistency (reliability).
5. Is composed of some difficult and some easy items.
6. Challenges all who take it.
7. Is interesting and meaningful.

Written tests include objective questions which require short answers, longer essay answers to general questions, rating scales (those filled in by self or others), and problem situation questions which require short but well thought out answers.

True-and-false Tests

Educators contend that these are the poorest kind of objective test questions to use. Pupils tend to read their own meanings into each statement, it is difficult to tell the difference between a correct or incorrect statement, or the pupil may retain a false concept by not knowing wherein he made an error.

All written statements in such a test should be short and simple. Avoid using the words "never" or "always." Have the pupils use symbols (+ or 0) instead of T or F because those unsure of the answer often deliberately make the marks hard to tell apart. Other ways to score the test include encircling T if the statement is entirely true, or the F if it is only partly true, or blocking out X in the first column if the sentence is correct and encircling it if the second one is wrong. In the first grade the children might draw a face with the mouth turned down if the statement is false, or draw it with the mouth turned up if it is true.

Example: Write + if the statement is true, 0 if it is false.

0	1. Your baby teeth are not important.
+	2. Children should drink a quart of milk a day.
0	3. The red traffic light says "go."
0	4. If you are lost, sit down and cry.
0	5. Pet all dogs, even strange ones.

Multiple Choice Tests

These questions should be short, clearly written, and never copied word for word from the textbook. Care must be taken not to make all possible answers so wrong that it is obvious which one is correct, or set a pattern through which the correct answer can usually be found.

Example: Place the letter of the correct answer in the blank.
   __b__ 1. The gland that gives great strength in time of excitement or anger is the (a) pancreas, (b) adrenal, (c) thyroid, (d) pituitary.
   __d__ 2. The part of the eye that sends the message about an image to the brain is the (a) iris, (b) cornea, (c) pupil, (d) retina.
   __c__ 3. Calcium makes strong (a) muscles, (b) brain, (c) bones, (d) nerves.
   __a__ 4. A disease transmitted by a mad dog is (a) rabies, (b) pellagra, (c) anemia, (d) scurvy.
   __b__ 5. Brush the upper teeth (a) up, (b) down, (c) across, (d) around.

Matching Tests

These questions are best for measuring the mastery of "where," "when," "what," "who" types of information. They do not develop the ability to interpret or express oneself. The responses to the items to be matched should be placed alphabetically or numerically in the right-hand column. Blank spaces should be provided in the left column before each item to be matched. There should be at least two more answers in the right column than in the left.

Example: Match the items in the left column with those in the right. Some answers may be used twice.

__b__	Bone	a. Cornea
__d__	Hair	b. Marrow
__a__	Eye	c. Dentine
__f__	Blood	d. Follicle
__g__	Skin	e. Semicircular canal
		f. White corpuscle
		g. Epidermis
		h. Subconscious
		i. Crown

Fill-in Blanks

The chief drawback to this type of an examination is that pupils have difficulty filling in blanks in the exact words the teacher expects; thus, they often must be given the benefit of the doubt or cause the teacher to become irritated and more exacting as she continues to grade the paper. Also, it is time-consuming to grade such questions. One advantage to using this type of test is that the pupil is not guided to the answer.

Example: Write the correct answer in the blank provided for it below.
1. We should brush our teeth after _____ .
2. _____ has more calcium than any other food.
3. We should go to the dentist at least _____ times a year.
4. Our first teeth are called _____ teeth.
5. Every grown person should have _____ teeth.

Essay Questions

These questions are valuable in that they provide pupils with opportunities to write and read aloud complete sentences or whole paragraphs using good grammar, and to think problems through carefully. Their drawback is that they are time-consuming to read and difficult to grade objectively.

> Example: Answer the following question in not less than one hundred words. Think through your answer carefully.
>
> What seems to you to be the chief value in observing good health habits?

Rating Scales

Pupils enjoy rating and evaluating their work or habits learned in health education. The best scales for doing so are those devised by the class. Teachers can help children benefit from this type of experience by a personal follow-up conference with each child.

EXAMPLE: PUPIL'S PERSONAL EVALUATION SHEET

	Always	Frequently	Seldom	Never
1. I brush my teeth after eating.				
2. I eat fruits and vegetables every day.				
3. I drink a quart of milk daily.				
4. I usually go to bed before 9 P.M.				
5. I worry about my school work.				

Student Evaluation

Students should be given many opportunities to evaluate what progress they have made in relation to the goals set individually and by the class. The teacher should appraise their progress with them, as well as observe their reactions to what they are doing, their attitude toward her, the group, themselves, and life in general. Time should be taken frequently to discuss these reactions and problems which have arisen concerning individual or group behavior, and to formulate future goals and plans.

Deeper insight and a clearer understanding of the class as a whole, as well as the feelings of the group toward the teacher, can be gained by having each pupil write on an unsigned paper answers to the following questions at the end of a semester or a major class project.

1. Did you enjoy this experience? Why?
2. List the new things you have learned in order of importance to you.
3. What activities did you do away from school that you learned here?
4. Which person do you most admire in our class? Why?
5. How could you be like this person, if you wanted to?
6. What did you hope to do or learn that you did not?
7. What pupil do you think improved the most? In what ways?
8. Are the pupils here learning to be good citizens? In what ways?

Much information can also be gained concerning each pupil by having him complete statements which show his inner feelings, fears, or thoughts. Suggested questions include the following:

1. My greatest fear is that I _____ .
2. At night I usually dream about _____ .
3. I dislike _____ because _____ .
4. I would like to be just like _____ when I grow up
   because _____ .
5. I _____ school, because here I _____ .

There is educational value in having pupils submit sample objective test questions with their correct answers, and in their grading each other's papers in class as the teacher reads the correct answer. Such practices put children on their honor. They are less likely to be dishonest if they feel secure, if the teacher has a high degree of expectancy for each child, and if the class respects her as a leader. Every real educator will find ways to utilize any time spent in evaluating progress to its utmost. She will make good use of test findings in order to improve her skill as an effective youth leader.

EVALUATING CHANGES IN THE SCHOOL, HOME, AND COMMUNITY

A well-planned, well-conducted, and well-administered school health program should have far-reaching effects in the school, home, and community. Although these improvements are more difficult to measure, they should be included when evaluating the results of the program.

The School

An environmental school survey should give evidence of actual improvements made in the school as a result of the total school health program. A list of the things to be checked and discovered from this study should be drawn up by the principal and teachers. Such a survey might well discover the answers to the following questions.

Yes No
1. Are the seats arranged so all children can see the chalkboard, and the shades adjusted so the room is well lighted?
2. Is the room temperature checked periodically and kept around 70° in the primary grades and around 68° for the upper elementary grades?
3. Are the school grounds a safe place for the children to play?
4. Do we always have soap, towels, and warm water in the toilet rooms?
5. Is the lunchroom a relaxed, quiet place in which to eat?
6. Are our health services adequate?
7. Are our equipment and facilities checked periodically for hazards?
8. Are we supervising our stairways, corridors, halls, classrooms, and the playground enough; have fewer accidents occurred in these places?
9. Do we have enough fire and air-raid drills for the safety of all the people in our building?
10. Do our swimming pool and shower room facilities meet sanitary standards?
11. Are our toilet facilities clean, well ventilated, properly lighted, and adequate?
12. Is our curriculum well balanced and does it provide opportunities for relaxation and change of pace?

13

A survey should also be made by the cooperative efforts of the whole staff to evaluate the school health instructional program. The following questions illustrate the type of information which should be sought:[6]

Yes No

___ ___ 1. Is the program based upon an understanding of child growth and development and upon the needs inherent in this development?

___ ___ 2. Does the program deal with significant health problems as revealed through studies of the health status of individuals and health problems found in the school, home, and community?

___ ___ 3. Is the program properly related to other health education efforts within the school, home, and community?

___ ___ 4. Is health instruction a planned part of the total school health program?

___ ___ 5. Are opportunities for health education provided in the control of the school environment?

___ ___ 6. Are opportunities provided for health education in the health appraisal plan and in health counseling?

___ ___ 7. Are the health education and physical education aspects of the program interrelated?

___ ___ 8. Are sound psychological principles used in the organization and application of health teaching?

___ ___ 9. Is health teaching a definite part of teaching in other subjects?

___ ___ 10. Is there well-balanced health instruction at both elementary and secondary levels with adequate time allotment, suitable teaching materials, and well-prepared teachers?

___ ___ 11. Is there a planned program of adult health education on a community-wide basis?

___ ___ 12. Are all possible sources of help being used?

An evaluation should also be made of the school health service program in order to discover if it is fully meeting the health needs of the pupils. Records of the kinds and number of treatments given, health examination findings, and other types of recorded information should be analyzed.

A realistic measurement of the results of the total school health program should reveal if it is getting its intended job done, and if not, why. Such an evaluation can be of the greatest value when all wasteful conditions and inferior practices are eliminated, and changes made or plans modified when needed.

The Home

Although the far-reaching influences of the school health program cannot be readily seen or measured, behavior changes and new health knowledge gained by the pupils in the school should carry over into the home. Individual conferences with parents, home visits made when possible, or even telephone conversations with parents can help teachers gain needed information regarding the effectiveness of their health teaching. Obtaining such facts is well worth the effort it takes. Increasingly, public schools are conducting night classes for adults in such areas as child growth and development, nutrition, first aid and water safety, and physical fitness. These can help parents reinforce at home what is being taught at the school,

---

[6] *Health Education.* 5th ed. Washington, D.C.: National Education Association and American Medical Assocation, 1961, p. 356.

as well as give them needed information and desire to increase the health and well-being of their own families. The community-centered school is fast becoming a reality, and Americans no longer feel that only children can or should be educated at the school. In many of our larger cities, model adult education programs are being conducted which reach thousands of adults.

The Community

Surveys should be made of conditions and practices related to the well-being and safety of all who live in the community, for if the total school health program has been effective, needed improvement will result. In some cities an intensive educational program sponsored by the school has succeeded in convincing the citizens to adopt water fluoridation, take part in polio vaccination drives, or see to it that needed additional stop signals are installed near playground areas.

The schools should join hands with their local co-workers in health, such as the Red Cross, youth organizations, and the police and fire departments, and help further their efforts to make the community a cleaner, better, healthier, and safer place in which to live for all its citizens, including children.

Although community surveys will not provide teachers with the answers to educational problems, it is imperative that educators know much more than they do about the locality in which they work. The teacher who spent precious time "teaching" her class the chemical properties of water seemingly was unaware that most of her group lived in a slum area where there were no bathrooms and water had to be carried into each home from a public fountain, nor was she too concerned about the fact that many of her group were badly in need of a bath. Such examples of educational waste are unfortunately quite common.

These who engage in community surveys or capitalize upon the information gained by local community social agencies or a community health council will know more about the area in which they work and the kind of backgrounds and homes from which their pupils come. All teachers should conduct or take part in various surveys of their own school in order to gain valuable information which will enable them to become more productive, understanding, and knowledgeable teachers.

SELF-EVALUATION FOR THE TEACHER

It is not enough, however, to evaluate pupil progress, the total school health program, and changes made in the school, home, and community as a result of a well-conducted school health program. Any teacher who desires to become a productive educator should also fully evaluate her teaching results and her own health. There are many challenges that a teacher faces but perhaps none is more important than an ever-deepening desire to improve herself and her own teaching ability. Preliminary professional education is but one aspect of effective teaching. Each professional worker is obligated to herself to do her best and contribute to the growth and improvement of education and to her specialized field.

Evaluating Teaching Results

Every educator needs to know whether she is getting desired results. Such self-appraisal and evaluation should occur daily as well as periodically. The approach should be "How could I have done this better?" rather than "What did I do that was wrong?" The teacher should always be aware of whether or not her pupils were interested in the daily health lesson, motivated to improve themselves, increase their knowledge of health, or change their attitudes. Such research and "soul-searching" can go a long way toward improving teaching skill as well as the health education program itself. Such appraisal is basic if one wishes to become a skilled educator.

Some teachers are fortunate enough to work in a school system where there is a health education specialist, who serves as a consultant or supervisor. This expert should not only give every kind of assistance to the classroom teacher, but also help her evaluate her teaching results. The following evaluation checklist can be filled out by the teacher alone, or by both the teacher and supervisor and used as a basis for a helpful conference:

TEACHER'S EVALUATION SHEET

	Always	Frequently	Seldom	Never
1. Do I motivate pupil interest in learning about health?				
2. Do I talk too much and "preach" about the necessity of developing good health habits?				
3. Do I draw all pupils into class discussion?				
4. Do I use enough audio-visual aids?				
5. Do I make the fullest use of audio-visual aids?				
6. Do I use a variety of teaching methods?				
7. Do I integrate and correlate health enough with other subjects?				
8. Do the things I teach have real carry-over value and reach into the home?				
9. Are the health practices of my pupils improving?				
10. Am I observant enough of what the pupils do and say, and how they look?				
11. Do I underplan my work?				
12. Do I really try to build skill upon skill, and knowledge upon knowledge?				
13. Is every class period a positive, productive, educational one?				
14. Do I utilize community resources enough?				
15. Do I evaluate each daily lesson?				
16. Do I observe children with emotional and physical disturbances?				
17. Do I share in planning and evaluating with pupils?				
18. Do I try to understand boys and girls as individuals?				
19. Do I have a sense of humor?				
20. Do I like to teach?				
21. Do I like to teach health?				
22. Am I improving as a teacher?				

The Teacher's Health

Every teacher must be in top physical and mental condition, but there are far too many who are not. Unfortunately, these are the ones who sometimes attempt to teach children how to be healthy. The teacher's own example, however, is one of the most effective ways to change and improve the health behavior and values of children. Teaching is largely setting an example in the areas of behavior, attitudes, and character. If the teacher is healthy and respected, her pupils will want to be like her, do what she does, and follow her suggestions for their own improvement.

The following checklist will enable each teacher to see for herself if she is merely existing, or really living:

ARE YOU

LIVING?	or	EXISTING?
Score Yourself:		Rate Yourself:
5—Excellent (always)		170–136—"Living"
4—Good (most of the time)		135–110—"Acceptable"
3—Fair (half and half)		109 and below—"Existing"
2—Poor (seldom)		
1—Very Poor (never)		

HEALTH RATING SCALE[7]

DO YOU:
_____ Eat three meals every day?
_____ Include the seven basic foods in your daily diet?
_____ Drink six to eight glasses of liquid every day?
_____ Limit your "between-meal snacks" to fruit and milk?
_____ Sleep at least eight hours every night?
_____ Relax at intervals during the day?
_____ Exercise at least one hour every day (preferably out of doors)?
_____ Keep healthy—free from colds, headaches, sore throats, etc.?
_____ Keep your smoking to a minimum?
_____ See your dentist at least twice a year?
_____ Brush your teeth after every meal?
_____ Wear shoes which fit properly?
_____ Use your feet correctly when standing and walking?
_____ Carry yourself well when standing, sitting, and walking?
_____ Take mild exercise during your menstrual period?
_____ Bathe (or take a sponge bath) at least once a day while menstruating?
_____ Have a menstrual period free from pain?
_____ Have regular bowel movements?
_____ Take a daily shower or bath?
_____ Wear clean underwear and socks each day?
_____ Use a deodorant?
_____ Keep your hands and fingernails clean?
_____ Take care of your complexion?
_____ Dress appropriately for the occasion?
_____ Keep your clothes neat and clean?
_____ Keep yourself well groomed?

---

[7] Reproduced by permission from the *Student Handbook for Health Information, Posture, and Body Mechanics.* Austin: Department of Physical Education for Women, University of Texas, 1961, pp. 21–23.

PERSONALITY AND CHARACTER RATING SCALE

ARE YOU:

_____ Enthusiastic?
_____ Cooperative?
_____ Dependable?
_____ Loyal?
_____ Friendly?
_____ Receptive to new ideas?

_____ Total

IN-SERVICE TRAINING

There are two chief ways to grow professionally: (1) through in-service training, and (2) engaging in further professional pursuits.

In-service training is an on-the-job self-improvement program. Educators learn how to teach by capitalizing upon their own trial-and-error attempts. "Experience is the best teacher" is only true if one is wise enough to profit from the experience which brought success or failure. For some, the longer one stays in the profession, the greater the temptation becomes to teach in the same old way and stay in the same well-worn groove. Such teachers, who are scornfully called "professional barnacles" by some, should be reminded that the only difference between a groove and a rut is depth. Fortunately, most teachers have high professional goals and are keenly interested in improving their effectiveness as educators and leaders of youth.

Staff Meetings

Democratically led staff meetings with fellow teachers can be a splendid way to grow in understanding and appreciation of the unique and valuable contribution each makes to the school program. Such meetings should be well planned, and real problems which affect all who attend the school studied carefully. The old saying "two heads are better than one" is not necessarily true, for it depends upon the heads involved. Likewise, merely bringing a group of teachers together after a long school day to discuss unimportant business is a waste of time and effort. In order that staff meetings be beneficial, each participant must feel she has a real contribution to make to the group as well as be aware that her time is being well spent in a pursuit which will help her become a better teacher, a member of an important and successful educational team.

Curriculum Study

Increasingly, schools are providing released time for teachers to work on curriculum improvement, and regard such work as part of their job, rather than compelling them to take part in such projects after school. All schools should evaluate their programs periodically, and be aided in this task by teachers, lay citizens, youth, administrators, and supervisors. From time to time evaluation should be assisted by a small group of experts. The total school program should be revised at frequent intervals and as needed, but nothing requiring immediate revision should be allowed to remain as it is until the time comes for a major "house cleaning" or curriculum change.

Every teacher will profit greatly from engaging in the following pursuits:

1. Continually studying the purposes of education and her objectives for each class in relationship to her classroom teaching and its results.
2. Working closely with administrators, fellow teachers, lay people, and children in order to assure that all educational pursuits have meaning and value in the daily lives of each learner.
3. Working individually as well as in small committees to prepare resource units and other teaching aids.
4. Taking part in the study and discussion of the purposes of education and the improvement of the quality of American education at her own school.

Research

Many teachers fail to realize that research and experimentation which they do on their own teaching situation and effectiveness can often be far more valuable and meaningful to them and lead to their own professional growth much more than reading about the research findings of others. Although the majority of teachers have taken courses in "Tests and Measurements" or "Methods of Research," only a few ever use the research techniques they learned in college to conduct their own learning experiments, or use the other research tools to investigate their own teaching situation or educational effort.

Although much is known about how pupils learn and how to increase the rate and effectiveness of learning, much yet remains a mystery. Educators tend to teach as they have been taught and to travel along well-trodden paths. Few are courageous enough to blaze new educational trails. Far too many are doing traditional teaching in traditional ways in spite of their dim awareness of the need for new methods and great improvements of our old ones if American education is ever to improve. Great teachers are those who have found their own teaching methods, and have dared to be different and creative.

Workshops

Teacher workshops are rich sources of self-improvement. These often provide opportunities to obtain new teaching methods and materials, and help instructors gain a renewed interest in and enthusiasm for their work. Such workshops should be carefully planned by a steering committee who should select problem areas from teachers' responses to questionnaires. Health education specialists will add much to the value of a workshop. The use of films, educational displays of free and inexpensive literature and recommended books, and mimeographed materials will increase interest as well as give teachers something to take away with them.

Although it takes precious free time to attend these weekend meetings, and extra money and energy to travel long distances, teachers can find such trips valuable for gaining new ideas, materials, and friendships. Most educators do want to do a good job. The majority of them welcome opportunities to gain as well as give assistance in the raising of standards in order to obtain excellence in education.

Home Study

Correspondence extension courses are now available in many communities. Although there may be merit in securing materials via the correspondence course method, most teachers will profit more from attending an extension course and gaining inspiration, along with other things, from working with an educational authority and exchanging ideas with other teachers from other schools. Even if only one teacher from each school in the system attends such a course, her fellow instructors can profit from her experience by reading suggested new materials, her class notes, or by having her share with them the new ideas and concepts she has learned in staff meetings and workshops.

Some school systems provide scholarships to selected teachers so that they may gain further training and new materials and ideas to share with other instructors.

Professional Organizations

All teachers should be members of and contribute to professional organizations. Likewise, each should read the official publications of these groups, as well as contribute articles periodically, either individually or as a member of a committee, to them. All should attend as many local, state, regional, and national meetings of their professional organizations as possible. Increasingly, students majoring in education are taking out student memberships and attending the conventions of their professional group. The chief value for such students is that they gain a deeper respect for their chosen field and earlier become more professionally minded. Many of them become active participants on both the local and regional levels early in their careers. Certainly all who attend educational conventions, whether they are experienced teachers or beginners, return to their jobs or school from these meetings as more enthusiastic members of their profession.

Organizations which teachers of health or other classroom subjects can join with profit are the American Association for School Health, the American Association for Health, Physical Education and Recreation, American Public Health Association, and the National Education Association.

Hobbies which include reading, photography, collecting things from other places including foreign countries, and many other kinds of similar activities are especially recreational and refreshing for teachers. They can also supply them with new materials to bring into their classrooms to stimulate increased pupil interest, knowledge and understanding. Travel can also help any instructor gain new interests, perspective, and enthusiasm which will, in turn, carry over into the classroom and increase her effectiveness as an educator. There are many ways to motivate learners, but none is as powerful as a skilled, interesting, and enthusiastic teacher.

FURTHER PROFESSIONAL PURSUITS

Many large school systems require teachers to take a refresher course in a field of their choice every three years. Although doing so takes time, effort and money, these teachers usually have a rich educational experience, and return to school with renewed interest in their work. Increasingly those with a bachelor's degree are going on for graduate work to receive a master's degree. This usually takes one year, or 30 hours, of advanced work obtained in summer school or night courses. Some institutions require a written thesis, others require the student to take additional courses and write at least one long research paper.

Those who wish to advance themselves professionally, to teach on the college level, or to become national leaders in their field should seek further study beyond the master's degree. Supervisory and administrative positions increasingly require broad professional experience and a doctorate. If candidates qualify for admission and pass preliminary examinations, they then work toward the Doctor of Philosophy or Doctor of Education degree. Both degrees are similar in admission standards, matriculation procedures, residence and other time requirements. The Ed.D. tends to be more appropriate for those who wish to become education specialists while the Ph.D. comprehends more general, noneducational study. Graduate teaching fellowships, assistantships, scholarships, and loans are available for those qualified to receive them.

Each teacher, regardless of the educational level he works on, must be well selected, highly trained, and deeply desirous of becoming a professional leader who continues to grow in productive skill as an educator. Through the united efforts of every such skilled, capable, and inspired person, a happier, healthier, safer, and better world *can* become a reality. This is the time of our greatest opportunity as educators. It is also the time of our greatest challenge.

Suggested Readings

Educational Testing Service: *Making the Classroom Test: A Guide for Teachers.* Princeton, N. J.: Educational Testing Service, 1961.

Grout, Ruth: *Health Teaching In Schools.* 5th ed. Philadelphia: W. B. Saunders Co., 1968.

Read, Donald, and Greene, Walter: *Creative Teaching In Health.* New York: The Macmillan Co., 1971.

Silberman, Charles E.: *Crisis In The Classroom.* New York: Random House, 1970.

Veenker, Harold: "Evaluating Health Practice and Understanding." *Journal of Health, Physical Education and Recreation,* 37:(May 1966):39–41.

Willgoose, Carl: *Evaluation in Health Education and Physical Education.* New York: McGraw-Hill Book Co., 1961.

Willgoose, Carl: *Health Education in the Elementary School.* Philadelphia: W. B. Saunders, 1974.

appendix

PUBLISHERS OF SCHOOL HEALTH EDUCATION MATERIALS FOR THE TEACHER AND CLASS

American Association for Health, Physical Education and Recreation, 1201 16th St., N.W., Washington, D.C. 20036

American Book Company, 450 West 33rd St., New York, N.Y. 10001

Appleton-Century-Crofts, 440 Park Avenue South, New York, N.Y. 10016

Bobbs-Merrill Company, Inc., 4300 West 62nd Street, Indianapolis, Ind. 46268

W. C. Brown Company, 135 South Locust St., Dubuque, Iowa 52001

Burgess Publishing Company, 426 South 6th St., Minneapolis, Minn. 55415

The John Day Company, Inc., 257 Park Avenue South, New York, N.Y. 10010

Doubleday & Company, Inc., Garden City, New York, N.Y. 11530

Ginn and Company, 191 Spring St., Lexington, Mass. 02173

Glencoe Press, 8701 Wilshire Blvd., Beverly Hills, Calif. 90211

Harcourt, Brace & Jovanovich, Inc., 757 Third Ave., New York, N.Y. 10017

Harper & Row, 49 East 33rd St., New York, N.Y. 10016

D. C. Heath and Company, 125 Spring St., Lexington, Mass. 02173

Holbrook Press, Inc., 470 Atlantic Ave., Boston, Mass, 02210

Holt, Rinehart and Winston, Inc., 383 Madison Ave., New York, N.Y. 10017

Houghton, Mifflin Company, 2 Park St., Boston, Mass. 02107

Joint Committee on Health Problems in Education of the National Education Association and the American Medical Association, 1201 16th St., Washington, D.C. 20036

Laidlaw Brothers, Thatcher and Madison Sts., River Forest, Ill. 60305

Lea & Febiger, 600 Washington Square, Philadelphia, Pa. 19106

J. B. Lippincott Company, East Washington Square, Philadelphia, Pa. 19105

Lyons and Carnahan, 407 East 25th St., Chicago, Ill. 60616

McGraw-Hill Book Company, 1221 Avenue of the Americas, New York, N.Y. 10020

The Macmillan Company, 866 Third Ave., New York, N.Y. 10022

Charles E. Merrill Publishing Company, 1300 Alum Creek Drive, Columbus, Ohio 43216

The C. V. Mosby Company, 11830 Westline Industrial Drive, St. Louis, Mo. 63141

Prentice-Hall, Inc., Englewood Cliffs, N.J. 07632

The Ronald Press Company, 79 Madison Ave., New York, N.Y. 10016

W. B. Saunders Company, West Washington Square, Philadelphia, Pa. 19105

School Health Education Study, 3M Education Press, 3M Center, St. Paul, Minn. 55101

Scott, Foresman and Company, 1900 East Lake Ave., Glenview, Ill. 60025

Steck-Vaughn Company, P.O. Box 2028, Austin, Texas 78767

Charles C Thomas, Publisher, 301-327 East Lawrence Ave., Springfield, Ill. 62703

Van Nostrand Reinhold Company, 300 Pike St., Cincinnati, Ohio 45202

Wadsworth Publishing Company, Inc., 10 Davis Drive, Belmont, Calif. 94002

John Wiley & Sons, Inc., 605 Third Ave., New York, N.Y. 10016

SOURCES OF FREE AND INEXPENSIVE MATERIALS IN HEALTH EDUCATION

American Association for Health, Physical Education and Recreation, 1201 16th St., N.W., Washington, D.C. 20036

American Cancer Society, 219 East 52nd St., New York, N.Y. 10017

American Diabetes Association, 18 East 48th St., New York, N.Y. 10017

American Dietetic Association, 620 North Michigan Ave., Chicago, Ill. 60611

American Dental Association, Bureau of Dental Health Education, 211 East Chicago Ave., Chicago, Ill. 60611

American Dental Hygienists' Association, 211 East Chicago Ave., Chicago, Ill. 60611

American Heart Association, 44 East 23rd St., New York, N.Y. 10010

American Home Economics Association, 1600 20th St., N.W., Washington, D.C. 20036

American Institute of Baking, 400 East Ontario St., Chicago, Ill. 60611

American Medical Association, Department of Health Education, 535 North Dearborn St., Chicago, Ill. 60610

American National Red Cross, Office of Publications, 17th and D St., N.W., Washington, D.C. 20006

American Nurses' Association, 10 Columbus Circle, New York, N.Y. 10019

American Optometric Association, 7000 Chippewa, St. Louis, Mo. 63119

American Pharmaceutical Association, 2215 Constitution Ave., N.W., Washington, D.C. 20037

American Public Health Association, Inc., 1015 18th St. N.W., Washington, D.C. 20036

American School Health Association, 107 South Depeyster, Kent, Ohio 44240

American Social Health Association, 1740 Broadway, New York, N.Y. 10019

Arthritis Foundation, 1212 Avenue of the Americas, New York, N.Y. 10036

Association for Family Living, 6 North Michigan Ave., Chicago, Ill. 60602

Borden Company, Consumer's Service, 350 Madison Ave., New York, N.Y. 10017

Carnation Milk Company, Home Service Department, 5045 Wilshire Boulevard, Los Angeles, Calif. 90036

Cereal Institute, Inc., Educational Director, 135 South LaSalle St., Chicago, Ill. 60603

Consumers Union of the U.S., Inc., Mount Vernon, N.Y. 10550

Eli Lilly Company, Educational Division, 740 South Alabama St., Indianapolis, Ind. 46206

Employers Mutual of Wausau, 407 Grant St., Wausau, Wisc. 55402

Epilepsy Foundation of America, 733 15th St., N.W., Washington, D.C. 20005

Equitable Life Assurance Society of the United States, 1285 Avenue of the Americas, New York, N.Y. 10019

Evaporated Milk Association, 910 17th St., N.W., Washington, D.C. 20036

Florida Citrus Commission, Lakeland, Fla. 33802

General Mills, Inc., Education Section, 9200 Wayzata Boulevard, Minneapolis, Minn. 55426

H. J. Heinz Company, P.O. Box 57, Pittsburgh, Pa. 15230

Hogg Foundation for Mental Health, Will C. Hogg Building, The University of Texas at Austin, Austin, Texas 78712

John Hancock Mutual Life Insurance Company, Health Education Service, 200 Berkeley St., Boston, Mass. 02117

Johnson & Johnson, New Brunswick, N.J. 08903

Kellogg Company, Department of Home Economics Services, Battle Creek, Mich. 49016

Kimberly-Clark Corporation, The Life Cycle Center, Neenah, Wisc. 54956

Kraft Cheese Company, 500 Peshtigo Court, Chicago, Ill. 60690

Lederle Laboratories, Pearl River, N.Y. 10965

Lever Brothers, Educational Department, 390 Park Ave., New York, N.Y. 10022

Licensed Beverage Industries, Inc., 155 East 44th St., New York, N.Y. 10017

Maternity Center Association, 48 East 92nd St., New York, N.Y. 10028

Mental Health Materials Center, 419 Park Ave. South, New York, N.Y. 10016

Metropolitan Life Insurance Company, School Health Bureau, Health and Welfare Division, One Madison Ave., New York, N.Y. 10010

Muscular Dystrophy Associations of America, Inc., 1740 Broadway, New York, N.Y. 10019

National Association for Mental Health, Inc., 180 North Kent St., Rosslyn, Va. 22209

National Association of Hearing and Speech Agencies, 919 18th St., N.W., Washington, D.C. 20006

National Better Business Bureau, Inc., 230 Park Ave., New York, N.Y. 10017

National Board of Fire Underwriters, 85 John St., New York, N.Y. 10038

National Dairy Council, Program Service Department, 111 North Canal St., Chicago, Ill. 60606

National Easter Seal Society fo Crippled Children and Adults, 2023 West Ogden Ave., Chicago, Ill. 60612

National Education Association, 1201 16th St., N.W., Washington, D.C. 20036

National Foundation—March of Dimes, 1275 Mamaroneck Ave., White Plains, N.Y. 10605

National Health Council, 1740 Broadway, New York, N.Y. 10019

National League for Nursing, Inc., 10 Columbus Circle, New York, N.Y. 10019

National Livestock and Meat Board, 36 South Wabash Ave., Chicago, Ill. 60603

National Kidney Foundation, 315 Park Avenue South, New York, N.Y. 10010

National Multiple Sclerosis Society, 257 Park Avenue South, New York, N.Y. 10010

National Safety Council, 425 North Michigan Ave., Chicago, Ill. 60611

National Society for the *Prevention* of Blindness, Inc., 79 Madison Ave., New York, N.Y. 10016

National Tuberculosis and Respiratory Diseases Association, 1740 Broadway, New York, N.Y. 10019

Procter and Gamble Company, P.O. Box 171, Cincinnati, Ohio 45201

Public Affairs Committee, Inc., 381 Park Avenue South, New York, N.Y. 10016

School Health Education Study, 3M Education Press, 3M Center, St. Paul, Minn. 55101

Science Research Associates, Inc., 259 East Erie Street, Chicago, Ill. 60611

Scott Paper Company, Industrial Highway—Tinicum, Island Road, Philadelphia, Pa. 19153

Sex Information and Education Council of the United States (SIECUS), 1855 Broadway, New York, N.Y. 10023

Society of Public Health Educators, 81 Hillside Road, Rye, N.Y. 10580

Tampax, Inc., Educational Director, 5 Dakota Dr., Lake Success, N.Y. 11040

United Cerebral Palsy Associations, Inc., 321 West 44th St., New York, N.Y. 10036

Wheat Flour Institute, 14 East Jackson Boulevard, Chicago, Ill. 60604

HELPFUL PERIODICALS IN HEALTH EDUCATION FOR THE TEACHER

Childhood Education. Association for Childhood Education International, 3615 Wisconsin Ave., N.W., Washington, D.C. 20016

Journal of Health, Physical Education and

Recreation and *The School Health Review.* American Association for Health, Physical Education and Recreation, 1201 16th St., N.W., Washington, D.C. 20006.

Journal of the National Education Association. The National Education Association, 1201 16th St., N.W., Washington, D.C. 20006

Journal of School Health. American School Health Association, 515 East Main St., Kent, Ohio 44241

Parents' Magazine. Parents' Magazine Press, 52 Vanderbilt Ave., New York, N.Y. 10017

School Safety. National Safety Council, 425 North Michigan Ave., Chicago, Ill. 60611

Science and Children. National Science Teachers Association, 1201 16th St., N.W., Washington, D.C. 20006

Science Digest. 250 West 55th St., New York, N.Y. 10015

Science Newsletter. Science Service, 1719 N St., N.W., Washington, D.C. 20006

The Instructor Magazine. Dansville, N.Y. 14437

The Teacher. Teachers Publishing Corporation, Darien, Connecticut 06112

Today's Children. Edwards Publications, 1225 Broadway, New York, N.Y. 10001

Today's Health. American Medical Association, 535 North Dearborn St., Chicago, Ill. 60610

SUGGESTED ELEMENTARY SCHOOL HEALTH EDUCATION TEXTBOOKS:

Health For Better Living Series. Grace T. Hallock, Ross L. Allen, and Eleanor Thomas. Lexington, Mass.: Ginn and Company.

Grade 1: Health and Happy Days
Grade 2: Health in Work and Play
Grade 3: Health and Safety for You
Grade 4: Growing Your Way
Grade 5: Keeping Healthy and Strong
Grade 6: Teamwork for Health
Grade 7: Exploring the Ways of Health
Grade 8: On Your Own

Health Science Series. Herman and Nina Schneider. Boston: D. C. Heath and Company.

Kindergarten: K–1: Science Readiness Charts
                K–2: Service Around Us
Grade 1: Science for Work and Play
Grade 2: Science for Here and Now
Grade 3: Science Far and Near
Grade 4: Science in Your Life
Grade 5: Science in Our World
Grade 6: Science for Today and Tomorrow
Grade 7: Science in the Space Age
Grade 8: Science and Your Future

The New Road to Health Series. Oliver E. Byrd, M.D., Edwina Jones, Paul Landis, Edna Morgan, James S. Nicoll, Julia C. Foster, and William W. Bolton, M.D. River Forest, Ill.: Laidlaw Brothers.

Grade 1: First Steps to Health
Grade 2: Learning About Health
Grade 3: Habits for Health
Grade 4: Building for Health
Grade 5: Your Health
Grade 6: Growing in Health
Grade 7: Improving Your Health
Grade 8: Today's Health

Laidlaw Health Series. Oliver E. Byrd, M.D., Elizabeth A. Neilson, and Virginia D. Moore. River Forest, Ill.: Laidlaw Brothers. The series available in regular edition and multiethnic edition.

Grade 1: Health 1
Grade 2: Health 2
Grade 3: Health 3
Grade 4: Health 4
Grade 5: Health 5
Grade 6: Health 6
Grade 7: Health 7
Grade 8: Health 8

My Health Book Series. A Text-Workbook Series. Oliver K. Cornwell and Leslie W. Irwin. Chicago: Lyons and Carnahan.

Grade 3
Grade 4
Grade 5
Grade 6
Grade 7
Grade 8

Dimensions In Health Series. Leslie W. Irwin, Dana Farnsworth, M.D., Caroline Coonan, Sylvia Gavel, Florence Fraumeni, and Barbara Shafer. Chicago: Lyons and Carnahan.

Grade 1: All About You	Grade 5: Understanding Your Needs
Grade 2: You and Others	Grade 6: Choosing Your Goals
Grade 3: Growing Every Day	Grade 7: Foundations for Fitness
Grade 4: Finding Your Way	Grade 8: Patterns for Living

The Macmillan Science Series. J. Darrell Barnard, Celia Stendler, Benjamin Spock, and others. New York: The Macmillan Company. Also Teachers' Annotated Edition and Teachers' Manual available.

Book 1	Book 7: Science: A Search for Evidence
Book 2	Book 8: Science: A Way to Solve Problems
Book 3	Book 9: Science: A Way to the Future
Book 4	
Book 5	
Book 6	

Curriculum Foundation Series. W. W. Bauer, M.D., Dorothy Baruch, Elizabeth Montgomery, Elenore Pounds, Wallace Wesley, Helen Shacter, and Gladys Jenkins. Glenview, Ill.: Scott, Foresman and Company.

Early Grade: Just Like Me

Grade 1: Being Six	Grade 5: About Yourself
Grade 2: Seven or So	Grade 6: About All of Us
Grade 3: From Eight to Nine	Grade 7: Growing and Changing
Grade 4: Going on Ten	Grade 8: Advancing in Health

Health For All Series. William W. Bauer, M.D., Elizabeth Montgomery, Elenore Pounds, Wallace Wesley, Helen Shacter, and Gladys Jenkins. Glenview, Ill.: Scott, Foresman and Company.

Junior Primer	Book 5
Book 1	Book 6
Book 2	Book 7
Book 3	Book 8
Book 4	

*Health and Growth Series.** Julius Richmond, Orvis Harrelson, and Wallace Ann Wesley. Glenview, Ill.: Scott, Foresman and Company, 1971.

Grade 1	Grade 4
Grade 2	Grade 5
Grade 3	Grade 6

SOURCES OF AUDIO-VISUAL AIDS

Aims Instructional Media Services, Inc., P.O. Box 1010, Hollywood, Calif. 90028

Associated Films, 600 Madison Ave., New York, N.Y. 10022

Avis Films, Inc., 2408 West Olive Ave., Burbank, Calif. 91506

Bailey Films, 6509 DeLongpre Ave., Hollywood, Calif. 90028

BFA Educational Media, 2211 Michigan Ave., Santa Monica, Calif. 90404

E. C. Brown Trust, 220 Alden St., S.W., Portland, Ore. 97204

Carousel Films, 1501 Broadway, New York, N.Y. 10036

Cathedral Films, Inc., 2921 West Alameda Ave., Burbank, Calif. 91505

Cereal Learning Corp., 3 East 54th St., New York, N.Y. 10022

Churchill Films, 662 North Robertson Blvd., Los Angeles, Calif. 90069

Coronet Films, 65 East South Water St., Chicago, Ill. 60610

Creative Arts Studio, 814 H St., Washington, D.C.

---

* This series of textbooks (with the teacher's edition for each grade) is highly recommended by the author.

Curriculum Materials, 1319 Vine St., Philadelphia, Pa. 19107

Curriculum Studios, Inc., 135 Main St., Westport, Conn. 06880

Sid Davis Productions, 2429 Ocean Park Blvd., Santa Monica, Calif. 90405

DCA Educational Products, Inc., 4865 Stenton Ave., Philadelphia, Pa. 19144

Denoyer-Geppert & Co., 5235 Ravenswood Ave., Chicago, Ill. 60640

Walt Disney Educational Materials Co., 666 Busse Ave., Park Ridge, Ill. 60068

Walt Disney Productions, 800 Sonora Ave., Glendale, Calif. 91201

Walt Disney Productions, 35 South Buena Vista Ave., Burbank, Calif. 95125

DuArt Films Laboratories, Inc., 245 West 55th St., New York, N.Y. 10010

Encyclopedia Britannica Films, 425 North Michigan Ave., Chicago, Ill. 60611

Grover-Jennings Productions, P.O. Box 303, Monterey, Calif. 93940

Ideal School Supply, 1100 South Lasergne Ave., Oak Lawn, Ill. 60453

Independent Film Producers, Co., P.O. Box 501, Pasadena, Calif. 91102

International Education & Training, Inc., 1776 New Highway, Farmingdale, N.Y. 11735

The Jam Handy Corp., 2821 East Grand Blvd., Detroit, Mich. 48211

Eli Lilly & Co., Exhibits & Audiovisual Dept., Indianapolis, Ind. 46206

McGraw-Hill, Inc., 330 West 42nd St., New York, N.Y. 10036

Mass Communications Center, 1125 Amsterdam Ave., New York, N.Y. 10025

Modern Talking Pictures Services, Inc., 925 9th St., Washington, D.C.

Modern Talking Pictures Services, Inc., 1212 Avenue of the Americas, New York, N.Y. 10036

Moody Institute of Science, Educational Film Division, 12000 East Washington Blvd., Whittier, Calif. 90606

Multimedia Productions, 580 College Ave., Palo Alto, Calif. 94306

National Consumer Finance Assn., 1000 16th St., N.W., Washington, D.C. 20006

National Film Board of Canada, 680 Fifth Ave., New York, N.Y. 10019

Henk Newenhouse, 1825 Willow Road, Northfield, Ill. 60093

Henk Newenhouse, 1017 Longaker Blvd., Northbrook, Ill.

Professional Arts, Inc., P.O. Box 8484, Universal City, Calif. 91608

Society for Visual Education, 1345 Diversey Pkwy., Chicago, Ill. 60619

Turtox Products, 8200 South Hoyne Ave., Chicago, Ill. 60620

Wexler Film Productions, 801 Seward St., Los Angeles, Calif. 90038

Young America Films (See McGraw-Hill)

index

Page numbers in *italics* refer to illustrations; page numbers followed by t refer to tables.